Advances in Pain Research and Therapy
Volume 17

MYOFASCIAL PAIN AND FIBROMYALGIA

Advances in Pain Research and Therapy
Series Editor: John J. Bonica, M.D., D.Sc., F.F.A.R.C.S. (Hon.)

Titles marked with an asterisk (*) are out of print in the original edition.

Advances in Pain Research and Therapy
Volume 17

Myofascial Pain and Fibromyalgia

Editors

James R. Fricton, D.D.S., M.S.
Associate Professor
Department of Diagnostic and Surgical Sciences
University of Minnesota
School of Dentistry
Minneapolis, Minnesota

Essam A. Awad, M.D., Ph.D.
Professor and Clinical Chief
Department of Physical Medicine and Rehabilitation
University of Minnesota Health Sciences Center
Minneapolis, Minnesota

Raven Press ⬧ New York

Historically, these disorders have been described extensively but with conflicting nosology. Terms such as fibrositis, myositis, myelogelosis, interstitial myofibrositis, and muscular rheumatism have been used in past literature to reflect varying etiologies. Lately, organizations such as the American Academy of Physical Medicine and Rehabilitation, the American Rheumatological Association, the International Association for the Study of Pain, and the American Academy of Craniomandibular Disorders have made special efforts to improve understanding and consistency in terminology of muscle pain syndromes. Myofascial pain has been used most commonly for a regional muscle pain syndrome while fibromyalgia refers to a systemic muscle pain syndrome.

This volume comprises an orderly series of contributions by an outstanding group of scientists, physicians, and dentists who have a broad understanding of muscle pain. The authors represent a variety of disciplines including neuroscience, dentistry, physical medicine and rehabilitation, rheumatology, and psychiatry. They are associated with 16 universities from six different countries. This volume provides clinicians and researchers with the most current body of knowledge on both myofascial pain and fibromyalgia, with special reference to the patient care implications of recent clinical and basic science research.

James R. Fricton, D.D.S., M.S.
Essam A. Awad, M.D., Ph.D.

Acknowledgments

Much of this research was presented at the First International Symposium on Myofascial Pain and Fibromyalgia, held in May of 1989 at the University of Minnesota in Minneapolis. The goal of this symposium was to establish a high level of dialogue among clinicians and researchers interested in the subject from around the world. The success of this symposium was phenomenal and indicative of the intense interest in these disorders and the desire for further research in this area. As a result, the Second International Symposium is scheduled for 1992 in Copenhagen, Denmark.

As editors, we wish to extend our appreciation to our colleagues from Denmark, Sweden, West Germany, Czechoslovakia, Canada, and the U.S.A. who because of their special knowledge, experience, and research have contributed to this volume. We wish to specifically recognize the late Dr. Rasmus Bach-Andersen of Hvidore, Denmark whose early death a few days prior to the international conference deprived us of his own personal presence and contribution. Dr. Bach-Andersen dedicated his career to diseases of the locomotion system and especially to improve understanding of those disorders which are the subject of this book.

Our sincere thanks are also extended to Dr. Bart Galle, Darla Eckroth, and staff of the University of Minnesota Department of Continuing Education who have been instrumental in gathering this group of scientists together and to Gail Rosenbaum, Nan Stevenson and Linda Thuftedal for their secretarial and administrative support in making this book a reality. Lastly, we are grateful to Kathey Alexander, the staff of Raven Press, and Berta Steiner of Bermedica Production for their efficient collaboration, support, and encouragement in completion of this book.

James R. Fricton, D.D.S., M.S.
Essam A. Awad, M.D., Ph.D.

Contents

Contributors

Peter Arlien-Søborg, M.D. *Department of Neurology, Hvidovre Hospital University of Copenhagen, 2000 Copenhagen, Denmark*

Essam A. Awad, M.D., Ph.D. *Professor and Clinical Chief, Department of Physical Medicine and Rehabilitation, University of Minnesota Health Sciences Center, Minneapolis, Minnesota 55455*

Rasmus Bach-Andersen, M.D. *Department of Rheumatology, Hvidovre Hospital, University of Copenhagen, 2000 Copenhagen, Denmark*

Else Bartels, M.D. *Biophysics Group, Open University, Oxford, U.K.*

Ann Bengtsson, M.D., Ph.D. *Division of Rheumatology, Department of Internal Medicine, University Hospital, S-581 85 Linköping, Sweden*

Robert M. Bennett, M.D., F.R.C.P., F.A.C.P. *Professor of Medicine, Director, Division of Arthritis and Rheumatic Diseases, Oregon Health Sciences University, Portland, Oregon 97201*

Ralph L. Bowman, M.D. *Department of Medicine, Division of Rheumatology, Cedars-Sinai Medical Center, UCLA School of Medicine, Los Angeles, California and Specialty Laboratories, Inc., Santa Monica, California 90904*

Glenn T. Clark, D.D.S., M.S. *Professor and Acting Director, Dental Research Institute, University of California-Los Angeles, School of Dentistry, Los Angeles, California 90024*

Bente Danneskiold-Samsøe, M.D. *Department of Rheumatology, Frederiksberg Hospital, 2000 Copenhagen, Denmark*

Johannes Fossgreen, M.D. *Chairman, Department of Rheumatology, Physical Medicine and Rehabilitation, Aarhus Amtssygehus University Hospital, DK 8000 Aarhus C, Denmark*

James R. Fricton, D.D.S., M.S. *Associate Professor, Department of Diagnostic and Surgical Sciences, University of Minnesota, School of Dentistry, Minneapolis, Minnesota 55455*

Don L. Goldenberg, M.D. *Professor of Medicine, Tufts University School of Medicine, Chief of Rheumatology, Director of Arthritis/ Fibrositis Center, Newton-Wellesley Hospital, Newton, Massachusetts 02158*

Ole Henriksen, M.D. *Department of Magnetic Resonance, Hvidovre Hospital, University of Copenhagen, 2000 Copenhagen, Denmark*

Karl G. Henriksson, M.D. *Associate Professor of Neurology, Chief, Neuromuscular Unit, University Hospital, S-581 85 Linköping, Sweden*

Søren Jacobsen, M.D. *Department of Rheumatology, Frederiksberg Hospital, 2000 Copenhagen, Denmark*

Kai Jensen, M.D. *Department of Neurology, Gentofte Hospital, University of Copenhagen, Copenhagen, Denmark*

Karl Erik Jensen, M.D. *Department of Magnetic Resonance, Hvidovre Hospital, University of Copenhagen, 2000 Copenhagen, Denmark*

Karel Lewit, M.D. *Assistant Professor, Central Railway Health Institute, Prague, Czechoslovakia*

Glenn A. McCain, M.D., F.R.C.P. *Associate Professor of Medicine, University Hospital, University of Western Ontario, London, Ontario, Canada N6A 5A5*

Siegfried Mense, M.D. *Professor, Institut fur Anatomie un Zellbiologie, Universitat Heidelberg, D-6900 Heidelberg, Federal Republic of Germany*

H. Merskey, D.M. *Professor of Psychiatry, University of Western Ontario, Director of Research, London Psychiatric Hospital, London, Ontario, Canada N6A 4H1*

Harvey Moldofsky, M.D. *Professor of Psychiatry and Medicine, University of Toronto, Toronto, Ontario, Canada M5G 1G6*

Matthew Monsein, M.D. *Medical Director, Chronic Pain Rehabilitation Program, Sister Kenny Institute, Abbott Northwestern Hospital, Minneapolis, Minnesota 55455*

James B. Peter, M.D., Ph.D. *Department of Medicine, Division of Rheumatology, Cedars-Sinai Medical Center, UCLA School of Medicine, Los Angeles, California and Specialty Laboratories, Inc., Santa Monica, California 90904*

I. Jon Russell, M.D., Ph.D. *Associate Professor of Medicine, Director, Brady-Green Clinical Research Center, The University of Texas Health Science Center, San Antonio, Texas 78284*

Shiro Sakai, D.D.S., M.S. *Research Associate Dental Research Institute, University of California-Los Angeles, School of Dentistry, Los Angeles, California 90024*

Barry J. Sessle, Ph.D., M.D.S. *University of Toronto, School of Dentistry, Toronto, Ontario, Canada M5G 1G6*

Stuart Silverman, M.D. *Department of Medicine, Division of Rheumatology, Cedars-Sinai Medical Center, UCLA School of Medicine, Los Angeles, California 90024*

David Simons, M.D. *Clinical Professor, Department of Physical Medicine and Rehabilitation, University of California, Irvine, California 92717*

Carsten Thomsen, M.D. *Department of Magnetic Resonance, Frederiksberg Hospital, 2000 Copenhagen, Denmark*

Janet G. Travell, M.D. *Emeritus Clinical Professor of Medicine, The George Washington University School of Medicine and Health Sciences, Washington, D.C. 20037*

Daniel J. Wallace, M.D. *Department of Medicine, Division of Rheumatology, Cedars-Sinai Medical Center, UCLA School of Medicine, Los Angeles, California 90024*

Frederick Wolfe, M.D. *Clinical Professor, Department of Medicine, University of Kansas School of Medicine, Wichita, Kansas 67214*

Susan B. Wormsley, B.S. *Department of Medicine, Division of Rheumatology, Cedars-Sinai Medical Center, UCLA School of Medicine, Los Angeles, California and Specialty Laboratories, Inc., Santa Monica, California 90904*

Advances in Pain Research and Therapy
Volume 17

MYOFASCIAL PAIN AND FIBROMYALGIA

Advances in Pain Research and Therapy, Vol. 17,
edited by James R. Fricton and Essam Awad.
Raven Press, Ltd., New York © 1990.

1

Muscular Pain Syndromes

David Simons

*Department of Physical Medicine and Rehabilitation, University of California,
Irvine, California 92717*

BACKGROUND

This overview is presented from the perspective of the literature of this century that deals with muscular pain of unknown etiology. It primarily concerns questions that should help us sort out the mélange of muscle pain syndromes.

Our understanding and management of patients with musculoskeletal pain is a great void in modern medicine. Recently, the Social Security Administration of the United States government asked the Institute of Medicine of the National Science Foundation to form a committee to help them with the problem of patients who ask for disability payments for disabling chronic pain. These patients were regularly denied benefits because no disease could be found on *routine* medical examination that would account for their pain. Over half of the cases submitted to adjudication were eventually found deserving of payments. The Social Security Administration was asking for guidance on how to tell if the applicant really did have disabling pain when there was no acceptable medical diagnosis for its cause. The closest the committee could come to an answer was to recommend further study of the subject (1).

What is missing in conventional medical understanding? This committee report (1) paid no attention to fibromyalgia syndrome (FS) (fibrositis), barely mentioned somatic (articular) dysfunctions, and reluctantly included myofascial pain syndrome (MPS) as a diagnosis to be seriously considered. In this overview each of these will be considered and some of their interactions will be examined.

The problem is not a dearth of literature on the subject. In fact, the wealth of literature has been a major impediment because it has been, and the evidence strongly indicates it still is, a frustrating Babel. The confusion arises because, to date, the diagnosis of these patients with musculoskeletal pain has been totally dependent on the history and physical examination. None of the modern laboratory or imaging methods has been successful in establishing a diagnostic "gold standard" for any of the many points of view from which these patients are examined.

The failure to find simple solutions suggests that musculoskeletal pain syndromes are often complex, manifold, or both. This line of thinking raises three questions. If the problem is complex, how can we best identify the components and their relationships? If it is manifold, how can we best distinguish the different conditions that are now confusingly intertwined? Third, what research strategies will optimize our chance of locating "gold standard" diagnostic tests for individual pieces of the problem? One of the most exciting features of the First International Symposium on Myofascial Pain and Fibromyalgia, held in Minneapolis, Minnesota, is the remarkable recent progress toward finding useful objective tests.

Through the years, individual authors have taken a wide range of signs and symptoms and have given a name to certain ones that seemed related. Innumerable times, other authors have selected the same symptoms and have given them another name. Even more devastating, authors have frequently taken an established name and identified it with a different combination of signs and symptoms. The net result is that, over time, names have become more a source of confusion than of enlightenment. Reynolds (2) documented this elegantly for fibrositis. Table 1 (below) illustrates both kinds of confusion.

The cardinal rule for gaining an understanding of this literature is to first determine as clearly as possible what group of signs and symptoms the author is really talking about before trying to interpret what the results mean. Unfortunately, much of this literature fails to provide a thorough and clear description of the symptoms and physical findings in the patients being studied. Too often, the author assumes that the reader knows exactly which definition of the condition the author has in mind. For the reasons given above, it is hazardous to draw firm conclusions from nearly all of the past literature and much of the current literature. That does not mean that all past literature is useless, but, as Bennett and associates (3) carefully pointed out, one must proceed with caution and an open mind. A tabulation of this older literature can be instructive.

Seen from the perspective of current knowledge, one can identify increasingly clear evidence of four distinct conditions that often overlap and interact to make clinical distinctions frustratingly difficult: (a) localized MPS caused by trigger points (TrPs) in muscles, (b) what appears to be a systemic disease, Fibromyalgia, (c) a non–rapid eye movement (REM) sleep disturbance, and (d) articular dysfunction. These conditions are linked by the nervous system and fascia in ways that are at present poorly understood but are receiving increasing attention.

The critical problem has been to sort out which signs and symptoms should be grouped together as one condition, and which should be dealt with separately. Since these decisions, to date, have been based purely on clinical judgment, and generally on an incomplete picture of all pertinent related findings, they are subject to great controversy, and liable to serious error. Any reader who is not clear as to the distinctions between FS and MPS is referred to Chapter 2 (*this volume*). The present chapter builds on that foundation.

THE FIRST 75 YEARS OF THIS CENTURY

Mindful of the caveats above, Table 1 is an attempt to help the reader categorize selected muscle pain literature from the first 75 years of this century. It was selected as having some relevance to what are now identified as MPS and FS. The table is based on a 1975 review of that literature (4). Review articles were selected based on subject matter regardless of title. On the other hand, Reynolds (2) examined the literature of the same era by selecting those papers that identified their subject as fibrositis regardless of the content.

Although FS is now defined (47) as a chronic pain condition with widespread pain complaints and multiple tender points (TePs), the authors before 1975 rarely identified the pain distribution and were unaware of the concept of counting TePs. Table 1 lists the features of both conditions that were recognized at that time. Tenderness of muscles is essential for the diagnosis of both conditions. Although tenderness at nonmuscular sites can occur in MPS, it is more characteristic of FS. Neither palpable findings nor referral of pain is identified as a diagnostic characteristic of FS; both contribute to the diagnosis of MPS. Response of the tender muscle to massage, spray and/ or stretch, and injection is characteristic of MPS but not FS. The reader can decide which condition was most likely included in each article or whether both were included.

Concerning the evolution of the concept of MPS, Table 1 shows that prior to about 1940 primary emphasis was placed on palpable findings and muscle tension. Then, emphasis shifted to referral of pain from tender spots in the muscles. Not until after 1975 were both features regularly incorporated in the MPS literature.

It becomes apparent that the descriptions of clinical findings in most of the papers identified as dealing with fibrositis through this period fit the characteristics of myofascial pain better than they fit those of FS, which was first defined as such in 1981 (48). The Brendstrup (1957), Miehlke (1960), Awad (1973), and Fassbender (1975) entries are of special interest because they are the most recent histological studies in this time frame. Although three of the four identified the subject as fibrositis, in all of them it is more likely that the muscle tissues examined were taut bands of TrPs than TePs evidence less tenderness and a less vigorous local twitch response, if any. Latent TrPs cause less dysfunction than active ones. Active TrPs are identified primarily by reproduction of the patient's clinical pain complaint with digital pressure on the TrP and by the elimination of that pain complaint with inactivation of the TrP. Either active or latent TrPs could readily be identified as TePs if they were located at a designated TeP site. Latent TrPs produce dysfunction of the muscle, but not pain. As Dr. Travell emphasizes (Chapter 6, *this volume*), latent TrPs represent a third phase of refractory chronic myofascial pain in which the patient does not complain of pain, but experiences referred tenderness, stiffness, and restricted range of motion.

Two terms are commonly used that are easily confused with MPS. One, the "myofascial pain dysfunction syndrome," is employed by dentists and relates strongly to the temporomandibular joint. This term refers to pain around the face and masticatory musculature and particularly in the region of the temporomandibular joint. The pain is considered psychogenic by some and of muscular origin by others (65). The other confusing term is "myofascial release technique," employed by practitioners of manual medicine. Myofascial release combines other techniques such as soft tissue and muscle energy techniques in various ways, and it means many things to many people. The object is to release stress in fascial structures and tightness of muscles through the biomechanical and neurophysiological effects of manual stretching techniques and stretching exercises (66). Myofascial release is sometimes used to relieve myofascial TrPs.

Referred Pain or Altered Sensation

An understanding of the referred changes in sensation, the referred tenderness, and the associated autonomic phenomena is essential to an understanding of MPS. As early as 1938, Kellgren (67), in conjunction with his hypertonic saline experiments (68), emphasized the importance of the referred tenderness associated with referred pain. Unless the patient winces when pressure is applied at a given point, Kellgren found it a useful guide to consider the tenderness at that point to be referred and not the source of the pain. In 1969, Selzer and Spencer (69) postulated five neurological mechanisms to explain referred pain in man. All may be applicable to TrPs: (a) convergence-projection, (b) peripheral branching of primary afferent nociceptors, (c) convergence-facilitation, (d) activity of sympathetic nerves, and (e) convergence or image projection at the supraspinal level. The first two depend on the anatomical structure of the nervous system. The remaining three result from modulation of nervous system activity and are more difficult to study in animal experiments.

1. *Convergence-projection:* Two chapters in this volume describe in detail recent experimental verification that convergence-projection is a common

property of muscle nociceptors as they make central connections in the brainstem (Chapter 4) and in a part of the lumbosacral spine (Chapter 3). This is a likely mechanism for mediating a significant part of myofascial referred pain. When sensation is referred by the convergence-projection mechanism (70), a single nerve cell in the spinal cord receives nociceptive input both from the internal organs and from nociceptors coming from the skin and/or the muscles. The brain has no way of distinguishing whether the excitation came from the somatic structures or from the visceral organ. Apparently the brain interprets any such messages as coming from somatic structures rather than from the internal visceral organ. In the case of TrPs, the pain is initiated by the muscle nociceptors but referred to the area served by other somatic receptors that converge on the same spinothalamic tract cell. Foreman et al. (71) demonstrated that in monkeys 27 or 30 spinothalamic tract cells receiving nociceptive input from muscle also received convergent input from skin and muscle afferents.

2. *Peripheral branching of primary afferent nociceptors:* When branches of a nerve supply separate parts of the body, peripheral branching of the nerve is responsible for the referred pain. In this model, the brain misinterprets messages originating from nerve endings in one part of the body as coming from the nerve branches supplying the other part of the body. Recent animal studies (72,73) demonstrate that peripheral branching of unmyelinated sensory afferent nerves is not unusual. Twenty-seven of 44 single units isolated in the rat demonstrated branching based on conduction velocity testing (72). Branching was observed occasionally in the peripheral sensory axons (74). One neuron can serve shoulder and diaphragm (75), or pericardium and arm (76).

3. *Convergence-facilitation:* The convergence-facilitation hypothesis described by Ruch and Patton (70) suggests that somatic afferent impulses normally coming from the skin in insufficient quantities to excite the spinothalamic tract fibers are facilitated by visceral impulses. In this model, afferent fibers such as polymodal nociceptors producing background activity originate in the region of perceived pain or altered sensation and tenderness. The nerve activity that modulates this input originates elsewhere, for example, at a myofascial TrP. Although it is the most difficult to verify experimentally, this is the most attractive model for explaining the bulk of referred pain and tenderness.

4. *Sympathetic nervous system activity:* Sympathetic nerves may cause pain by releasing substances that sensitize primary afferent nerve endings in the region of perceived referred pain (77,78) or possibly by restricting the flow of blood in the vessels that nourish the sensory nerve fiber itself (79). In addition to pain, a myalgic focus induced by hypertonic saline also projected areas of decreased skin temperature (80). This phenomenon has yet to be investigated in an orderly manner using modern thermographic equipment. Galletti and Procacci (81) reported that spontaneous pain from

a myalgic spot in the deltoid muscle was associated with patterns of referred pain, referred changes in skin impedance, and cutaneous hyperalgesia. The extensiveness of all patterns was markedly diminished 30 min following a stellate ganglion block, strongly indicating significant autonomic nervous system involvement. Referred changes from such an induced algogenic focus were reversed by infiltrating the stimulus site with carbocaine (82). Since some myofascial TrPs are known to strongly modulate sympathetic nervous system activity in the reference zone (59), this is a reasonably likely mechanism of pain referral from TrPs.

5. *Convergence or image projection at the supraspinal level:* If pain pathways converge peripherally and at the spinal level, it is not unreasonable that they may also converge at the thalamic or cortical level. A major function of the cortex is the formulation and projection of images (83).

How can we tell which of these five mechanisms may be responsible for the referred pain in a given situation? Fortunately a relatively simple clinical test distinguishes the first two anatomically determined mechanisms from the last three functional mechanisms. Neither convergence-projection nor peripheral nerve branching requires any afferent input from the reference zone. However, convergence-facilitation requires afferent input from the reference zone and the autonomic dysfunction model requires sympathetic efferent input to the reference zone. Thus, experiments that test persistence of referred pain when the reference zone is effectively anesthetized indicate which of the two groups of referred pain mechanisms are likely to be mediating pain. If the pain disappears, it is likely mediated by one or more of the three functional mechanisms; if it persists, it is likely to be referred by one or more of the two anatomical mechanisms. Over the years, a number of experiments exploring this question have been reported.

Clinical studies report both kinds of responses; sometimes the referred pain and tenderness disappear and sometimes they persist when the reference zone is anesthetized. Kellgren (68) produced referred pain and a corresponding area of subcutaneous tenderness by injecting 6% saline into each of three muscles. Local anesthesia and nerve block to the painful area eliminated the referred pain and tenderness. Ten years earlier Weiss and Davis (84) conducted a series of experiments on patients with referred pain of visceral origin, acute gallbladder disease, chronic appendicitis, nephrolithiasis, and salpingitis. They reported complete temporary, and sometimes lasing, relief by infiltrating the zone of referred pain with local anesthetic subcutaneously.

Theobald (85) got mixed results with a visceral nociceptive stimulus of graded intensity. Referred pain produced by low-intensity electrical stimulation of the uterus was eliminated by infiltration of the skin and subcutaneous tissues in the abdominal reference zone. Referred pain produced by stronger stimulation could not be relieved in this manner. Other investigators

(86) were unable to prevent pain referral to the forearm produced by interspinous injection of hypertonic saline despite total motor and sensory block of the upper extremity, including a stellate ganglion block.

The location to which some pains are referred can be influenced by previous traumatic or painful experiences at that location. Reynolds and Hutchins (87) found that without exception in 14 subjects mechanical stimulation of the ipsilateral maxillary osteum caused pain to be referred to a front tooth that had recently received a painful dental procedure without anesthesia. However, no referred pain was felt in a corresponding front tooth on the other side that had a comparable procedure, but with anesthesia. Furthermore, anesthetizing the tooth nearly 2 weeks following the procedure eliminated this referral of pain immediately and for at least another week. Clearly, this pain must be referred by one of the latter three mechanisms, most likely convergence-facilitation.

Both Kellgren (68) and the Vecchiet team (82) found the referred pain and referred tenderness to be located very nearly in the same region. Steinbrocker et al. (80) found them sometimes in the same and sometimes in completely different locations in response to one injection of hypertonic saline.

Seen from a myofascial TrP point of view, individual muscles evidence a remarkable variety of referred pain and autonomic phenomena. At least six descriptions of referred sensation from TrPs are identifiable:

1. Pain referred from TrPs is usually described as a localized subcutaneous ache with slightly blurred edges; the pain projects well beyond the originating TrP.
2. Several muscles, including the deltoid, gluteus maximus, and serratus posterior inferior, refer this pain locally to the immediate vicinity of the TrP.
3. Most of the TrPs in limb muscles refer pain distally rather than proximally, but neither conforming to nor restricted to a segmental or peripheral nerve distribution pattern. The biceps brachii and adductor longus muscles are examples of exceptional limb muscles that refer proximally as well.
4. The infraspinatus and tensor fasciae latae muscles refer pain into adjacent joints, giving the impression of an arthritis. The serratus posterior superior refers pain deep into the chest, emulating lung disease.
5. Rather than aching pain, TrPs in the cutaneous platysma muscle refer a prickling sensation (59).
6. TrPs may refer hypesthesia or anesthesia instead of pain (88). This could be interpreted as downward instead of upward modulation of afferent activity from the reference zone.

Similarly, at least six referred autonomic effects are observed from TrPs, some specific to a particular muscle. First, a growing literature attributes skin temperature changes to TrPs in many muscles. Thermographic hot spots are reported over the TrP area (89–91) and reduced temperature in the reference zone (59,80). Second, TrPs in one part of the trapezius muscle refer pilomotor activity down the arm (59). The sternocleidomastoid muscle refers: third, tearing of the eyes; fourth, coryza; and fifth, scleral injection homolaterally. Finally, induction of referred pain to the face by pressure on an upper trapezius TrP consistently induced reduction of temporal artery pulsations bilaterally while the pain lasted, but only the artery on the painful side showed a rebound increase in amplitude of pulsations on termination of painful stimulation. Inactivation of a TrP with pain relief induced a prolonged increase in amplitude of temporal artery pulsation on the ipsilateral side (34).

Clearly, more than one mechanism must contribute to referred pain in man. There is no guarantee that several are not operating simultaneously in some situations. Each mechanism has its proponents. Convergence-projection is currently popular in texts dealing with pain (83,92,93). It has received the most attention in physiology experiments and therefore is the mechanism about which we know the most. Axon branching was staunchly defended by Sinclair (94) and is becoming recognized as a likely cause of patients' referred pain (83,92). Convergence-facilitation has been remarkably neglected, but is a likely candidate to be one of the most common contributors to referred pain. Sympathetic nervous system mediation has a solid base of experimental evidence. Vecchiet and coworkers (82) considered the results of their referred pain and tenderness study to be due primarily to sympathetic mediated effects. Procacci hypothesized that sympathetic control of the cutaneous pain threshold is modulated by a feedback loop: afferent somatic input → central nervous system → sympathetic output to somatic site → release of algogenic autocoids (78,95). Theobald (85) was a strong proponent of supraspinal convergence as the basis for the referred pain he observed.

We see that there is much evidence for many mechanisms that refer pain, tenderness, and autonomic phenomena. However, *unless the findings are recognized as referred*, no serious consideration will be given to locating their source. The fact that at this time we are unable to identify which mechanism(s) contribute to the clinical pain phenomena with which we are concerned does not mean that their recognition is unimportant. It does suggest that this is one of the important gaps in our knowledge that must be filled before we can hope to truly understand muscle pain syndromes.

Taut Band and Local Twitch Response

Clinically, the shortened muscles characteristic of MPS have taut bands, palpable when they are accessible, and they elicit local twitch responses (LTRs) on needle penetration of the TrP. The salient features of these bands

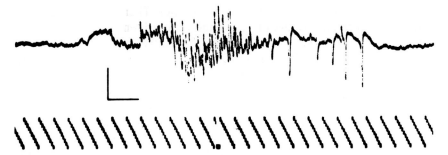

FIG. 1. Electromyographic recording of a local twitch response elicited by cross-fiber snapping palpation of a latent trigger point in the left third finger extensor muscle. A burst of complex waveforms followed by a number of more isolated action potentials is characteristic of a local twitch response. Calibrations are 500 μV and 2 msec.

have been described previously (59,96) (see also Chapter 2, *this volume*). They are considered an essential part of the pathophysiology of myofascial TrPs.

The electromyographic features of the LTR are of special interest because of their close association with the palpable taut band and TrP. This phenomenon clearly substantiates the presence of the taut band and abnormal reactivity of those muscle fibers and provides a window through which we can explore the pathophysiology of TrPs. These electromyographic features have been reported (97,98,185).

Figure 1 illustrates the electromyographic recording of a LTR that is obtained by inserting a monopolar needle electrode with its tip in the taut band 4 cm from the TrP. This twitch response was elicited by vigorous transverse snapping palpation across the TrP. One can see the quiet baseline before and after the response, with multiple action potentials and a series of relatively isolated discharges after the main burst. This prolonged complex discharge is in sharp contrast to the single biphasic action potential recorded in response to a tendon tap. Data obtained to date (99,100) indicate that the action potential is transmitted both directly from the TrP along the muscle fiber to the pickup electrode and indirectly via a reflex through the spinal cord. The LTR is valuable as a totally objective confirmatory sign that is pathognomonic of a myofascial TrP and is valuable as a research tool.

Hong's report (101) of a series of pectoralis minor MPS patients illustrates the typical overload origin of acute myofascial TrPs. It also shows how MPS can persist untreated, and that the shortening of the muscle can produce secondary nerve entrapment. When the nerve entrapment symptoms are the patient's chief complaint, they are likely to confuse the examiner. Hong reported on 17 patients who suffered whiplash injuries from automobile accidents. They all presented typical unilateral "radicular symptoms" with resting pain and tingling over the ulnar aspect of the forearm and hand.

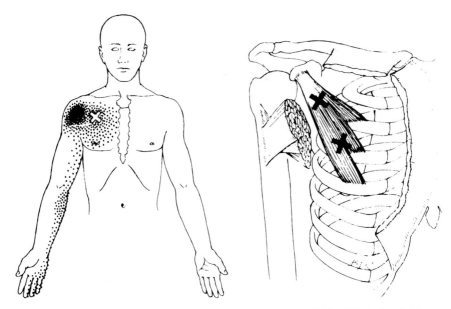

FIG. 2. Referred pain pattern (*black stipples*) and location of TrPs (*X*s) in the right pectoralis minor muscle. The muscle attaches to the coracoid process of the scapula and to the second, third, and fourth ribs deep to the pectoralis major muscle. (From Travell and Simons, ref. 59, with permission.)

Although these patients had been previously diagnosed as having cervical radiculopathy, they failed to show the typical electrodiagnostic features and failed to respond to traditional physical therapy for cervical radiculopathy. These patients had increase of pain and tingling during maximal abduction of the shoulder on the affected side and none had significant pathological findings in a cervical spine x-ray, computed tomography (CT) scan, or magnetic resonance imaging (MRI) scan, or on needle electromyography (EMG). Seven subjects had slow sensory conduction of the ulnar nerve at the thoracic outlet.

On examination, every patient had TrPs in the pectoralis minor muscle on the affected side with typical referred pain patterns (Fig. 2) and LTRs. Range of motion of the affected shoulder was reduced in all subjects. Every patient had relief of the "radicular pain" to various degrees, and five subjects became completely pain free immediately after spray-and-stretch therapy to the involved pectoralis minor muscle at the time of the initial visit. Ten patients needed TrP injection to end recurrences following treatment. At the time of the report 12 subjects considered themselves "cured."

The mechanism by which the taut band in the pectoralis minor muscle caused this brachial plexus entrapment is shown in Fig. 3. The pectoralis minor attaches to the coracoid process. The brachial plexus first hooks under

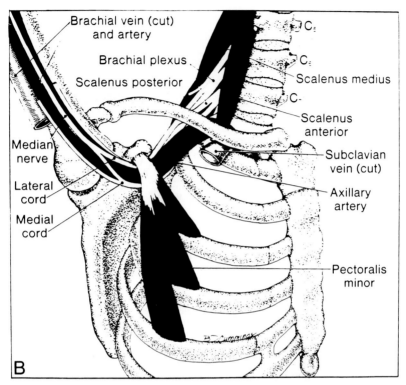

FIG. 3. Potential entrapment of the lower brachial plexus and axillary artery by the right pectoralis minor muscle during abduction of the arm. Taut bands caused by TrPs in the pectoralis minor muscle continue to exert pressure on these nerves even when the arm is in a more neutral position. (From Travell and Simons, ref. 59, with permission.)

this attachment and then passes over the first rib. The sustained compression of the nerve trunks by the shortened muscle produces a symptomatic neuropraxia. This compression was relieved, in most of the patients, by simply inactivating the TrP that caused the muscle shortening and hardening.

Involvement of Contractile Elements in the Taut Band

Danneskiold-Samsøe and coworkers (102,103) recently demonstrated the involvement of the contractile elements of muscle in the painful nodule or taut band that is characteristic of MPS. Although their first paper (102) used the term "fibrositis," it did so in the pre-1977 sense. Figure 4 illustrates the marked increase in myoglobin immediately following massage of the tender palpable firm areas in the muscle, compared with the minimal increase with similar treatment of uninvolved control muscles in 13 patients. Myoglobin

Diagnosis of Myofascial Pain Syndrome and Identification of Myofascial Trigger Points

Much of the confusion in the literature stems from the lack of tested diagnostic criteria for MPS that can determine its presence or absence and can differentiate it from other disorders. Two sets of proposed criteria are presented here. One is intended for making the clinical diagnosis of MPS and the other for use in conducting research studies. In the latter case, it is of critical importance to include only tender spots that are myofascial TrPs and not ones that are tender for other reasons. These criteria need to be studied to determine their sensitivity and specificity in diagnosing MPS. Since a gold standard does not exist to objectively confirm the diagnosis of MPS, the criteria must be tested against clinical expert opinion.

Clinical Criteria for the Diagnosis of Myofascial Pain Syndrome Caused by Active Trigger Points

To make the clinical diagnosis of MPS, the findings should include five major criteria and at least one of three minor criteria. The five MAJOR CRITERIA include:

1. Regional pain complaint.
2. Pain complaint or altered sensation in the expected distribution of referred pain from a myofascial TrP (59,96).
3. Taut band palpable in an accessible muscle (see Table 3 for examples).
4. Exquisite spot tenderness at one point along the length of the taut band.
5. Some degree of restricted range of motion, when measurable (see Table 3 for examples).

The three MINOR CRITERIA include:

1. Reproduction of clinical pain complaint, or altered sensation, by pressure on the tender spot.
2. Elicitation of a local twitch response by transverse snapping palpation at the tender spot or by needle insertion into the tender spot in the taut band.
3. Pain alleviated by elongating (stretching) the muscle or by injecting the tender spot (TrP).

NOTE: Additional symptoms such as weather sensitivity, sleep disturbance, and depression are often present but are not diagnostic because they may be attributable to chronic severe pain perpetuated by multiple mechanical and/or systemic perpetuating factors.

TABLE 3. *Likely accessibility of taut bands, local twitch response, and range of motion as criteria for trigger points in specific muscles recommended for research studies[a]*

Muscle	Taut bands palpable method	Local twitch response[b]	Range of motion applicable	Restricted movement
Adductor longus	F	+	+	Abduction of thigh
Biceps brachii (both heads)	P, F	+	±	Extension at elbow with extension of arm at glenohumeral joint
Biceps femoris	F, P	+	+	Straight leg raising (knee extension with hip flexion)
Brachioradialis	P, F	+	±	Extension of forearm
Deltoid, anterior	F	+	+	Horizontal abduction of arm
Deltoid, posterior	F	+	+	Horizontal adduction of arm
Extensor carpi radialis longus	F	+	±	Flexion and ulnar deviation of wrist
Extensor digitorum communis	F	+	+	Simultaneous flexion of fingers and wrist
Gastrocnemius	F	+	+	Dorsiflexion of foot with knee straight
Gluteus maximus	F	+	+	Flexion at hip with knee flexed
Infraspinatus	F	+	+	Reaching up behind shoulder blades (full internal rotation)
Latissimus dorsi	P	+	±	Flexion of arm with some trunk flexion to other side
Longissimus (paraspinal)	F	+	±	Spinal flexion
Masseter	F(P)	NV	+	Jaw opening
Pectoralis major	P, F	+	+	Horizontal abduction of arm
Peroneus lungus	F	+	±	Dorsiflexion and inversion of foot
Rectus femoris	F	+	+	Extension at the hip with flexion at the knee
Semimembranosus	F	+	+	Straight leg raising (knee extension with hip flexion)
Semitendinosus	F	+	+	Straight leg raising (knee extension with hip flexion)
Sternocleidomastoid	P	+	0	(Rotation of head & neck to the same side)
Teres major	F	+	±	Abduction (flexion) of arm over head with external rotation
Trapezius, upper	P, F	+	±	Lateral flexion of head to other side and rotation of head to same side
Trapezius, lower	F	+	0	(Scapular abduction with elevation)
Triceps brachii, long head	P, F	+	+	Adduction and flexion of arm with flexion of forearm

[a] *Key:* +, applicable; ±, sometimes applicable; 0, not reliably observable; P, pincer palpation preferred; F, flat palpation preferred; NV, nonvisual detection of local twitch response by palpation.

[b] A local twitch response is not considered obtainable unless a band is palpable.

Research Criteria for the Identification of Myofascial Trigger Points

For research purposes, the presence of a TrP is established if all of the following six criteria are met:

1. Identification of a taut band by palpation in an accessible muscle. (See Table 3 for expected accessibility of taut bands to palpation in the muscles recommended for research.) The accessibility to palpation of a taut band in a muscle is variable depending on thickness of adipose tissue, turgor and tension of subcutaneous tissue, thickness and tension of overlying muscles, and tension on the muscle fibers being examined.
2. Exquisitely tender spot (located at one point along a taut band if it is palpable) in the muscle belly.
3. Tender spot must cause referral of pain (or change of sensation) at a distance of at least 2 cm beyond the spot of local tenderness. Pain referral is elicited in response to needle penetration of the TrP or to pressure held for 10 sec on the tender spot before it is considered negative.
4. Restricted stretch range of motion for the primary function of that muscle, if measurable. (See Table 3 for expected applicability of range of motion measurement for specific muscles.)
5. An active TrP must have items 2 and 3 present; it must have items 1 and 4 present if they are accessible or applicable to that muscle. At least part of the clinical pain pattern (or change in sensation complaint) must be reproduced either by pressure applied transcutaneously to the tender spot or by needle penetration of the tender spot.
6. If the tender spot is penetrated with a needle as part of the experiment, it must respond with a local twitch response to be considered a TrP.

NOTE: To be considered latent, a TRP must evidence accessible items 1, 2, and 4 above. The TrP may or may not produce referred pain characteristic of that TrP; if it does refer pain, the pain should not be one that the patient has been experiencing lately. Otherwise it would be an active TrP.

For research applications, quantitative measurement of observations is of fundamental importance. Measurement of clinical TrP phenomena has been reviewed by Jaeger (105), Fischer (90,91) and Simons (96). Using the pressure algometer, two studies (106) have documented that TrPs become less sensitive with spray and stretch. A more recent double-blind, controlled pilot study (107) showed that insertion of a needle alone into a TrP is enough to reduce local TrP sensitivity, but that injection of a solution is required to reduce referred symptoms.

Attachment Tenderness

It is now becoming apparent that one of the common characteristics of the taut bands associated with myofascial TrPs is tenderness of the musculotendinous junction or tendinous attachment of that muscle. This has not been systematically studied to determine to what extent it is characteristic of all muscles, but has been noted by clinicians in many muscles of the body, and its importance emphasized by Lewit (108). What has previously been identified as a primary and a secondary TrP in some cases may be the muscle belly TrP and its attachment tenderness (59). One example is the levator scapulae muscle. The primary TrP is located at the base of the neck at TrP_1. What was identified as a secondary TrP is at the attachment of the levator scapulae over the angle of the scapula. Another example is the supraspinatus muscle, with its primary (proximal) TrP located in the belly of the muscle and the other (distal) TrP deep at the musculotendinous junction of the muscle. In both examples, the TrP in the muscle belly is of primary importance and is the one that needs to be inactivated for complete relief. The other identified TrP may be only attachment tenderness from the pull of the primary TrP's taut band. It may become necessary to modify the diagnostic criteria above to include this additional characteristic.

FIBROMYALGIA

This section briefly summarizes the variations in the number of TePs required to make the diagnosis of fibromyalgia and the impact that the variations might have on the nature of the populations selected and rejected. It concludes with a tabular review of recent FS literature to present a perspective of what the findings may mean.

Tender Point Criteria

This history of successive TeP criteria for making the diagnosis of FS is traced in Table 4. The 1977 redefinition of fibrositis by Smythe and Moldofsky (49) required a minimum of 12 TePs at 14 sites. Yunus et al. (48) in

TABLE 4. *Tender point criteria for fibromyalgia*

Minimum number of tender sites	Total number of sites examined	Term used	Source
12	14	Fibrositis	Smythe and Moldofsky, 1977 (49)
10	25	Fibrositis	Bennett, 1981 (109)
5	34	Fibromyalgia (Fibrositis)	Yunus et al., 1981 (48)
12	17	Fibrositis	Campbell et al., 1983 (110)
7	14	Fibrositis	Wolfe et al., 1985 (111)
11	18	Fibromyalgia	Wolfe et al., 1989 (47)

1981 introduced a modification of diagnostic criteria and a new name, fibromyalgia. They reduced the number of TePs required from 12 to 5 and increased the number of points examined to something in the neighborhood of 34. Yunus and associates also added major and minor criteria that affected the number of patients diagnosed with a given number of TePs. Two years later Campbell et al. (110) used an algometer and quantified the pressure applied. They required an expression of pain at less than 4 kg/1.54 cm^2. This translates to a reading of 2.6 kg on algometers that have a 1-cm^2 pressure pad. Two years after that Wolfe et al. reduced the required number of tender sites from 12 to 7 of 14 sites examined (111). In 1989, a monumental study by the Multicenter Fibromyalgia Criteria Committee (47) concluded that to diagnose FS, tenderness should be present at a minimum of 11 of 18 (9 bilateral) specified sites. This study was done with the expectation that it would become the accepted standard for the diagnosis of FS for some time to come. Dr. Fred Wolfe has been a major force in the effort to achieve this much needed standardization.

Obviously, both the number of sites to be examined and the minimum number of sites that must be tender have been difficult to resolve. In 1988, Simms et al. (112) investigated which sites should be selected for examination. They studied 75 unilateral anatomical locations in ten FS patients and ten normal control subjects. Of the previously recommended TePs, only two were included in their 19 best discriminating points. Of particular interest, they found that 15 of the 19 best discriminating points clustered in regions around the anterior shoulder, anterior chest, posterior scapula, and medial knee. Tender points within a region had similar value as discriminating points for examination.

Prevalence of Tender Points

A study done by Wolfe and Cathey (113) examined the number of TePs at 14 sites on 1,520 consecutive patients with various rheumatic diseases. The distribution of the number of TePs (Fig. 6) that resulted from this study helps to put into perspective the changes in the number of TeP sites required to diagnose FS. Most of the studies done in the name of FS to date have used the five TeP criteria initially recommended by Yunus et al. (48). Some 19.5% of this group of patients would be eligible for consideration for the diagnosis of FS according to that criterion. The 11-TeP count required by the new criteria (47) would include only about 6% of this group of patients. Not all of the 13.5% difference would be included with the reduced TeP count of Yunus et al. because they added major and minor criteria that would have eliminated some of them. However, it is clear that there is a considerable number of patients in whom there has been great difficulty determining whether or not they should be included in the diagnosis of FS.

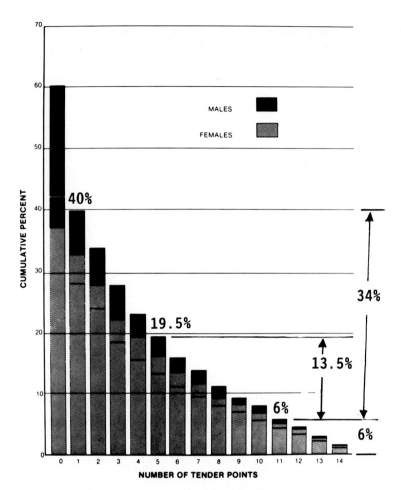

FIG. 6. Prevalence of tender points in 1,520 consecutive rheumatic disease patients. Nearly 40% of these patients had at least one tender point, 19.5% had five or more tender points, and only 6% had at least 11 tender points. Until recently, only 5 tender points were required to make the diagnosis of fibromyalgia; now 11 are required. This figure raises the question, what is wrong with the 34% of patients who have too few tender points to qualify as having fibromyalgia, but may have as many as ten tender points? (From Wolfe and Cathey, ref. 113, with permission and with annotations added.)

In addition, the graph shows that there is the much larger group of patients who have too few TePs to qualify as having FS by any proposed criteria, but who have rheumatic pain of unidentified origin. The critical question that comes to mind is, if these patients do not have FS, then what do they have (114)? Since this excluded group of patients has received little attention from investigators, there are few data as to their characteristics. The subjects in the study were classified as having various rheumatic diseases. One possibility is that many of them have regional chronic myofascial pain. This myofascial group may well include patients with less than four TePs since a MPS often starts with involvement of only one muscle.

Nature of Fibromyalgia

The cause of FS is unknown; it may be a composite of several disorders. Table 5 lists studies of FS that examined a measurable abnormality or therapeutic response. It identifies what percentage of the FS patients showed the abnormality, or what percentage responded to that specific treatment. A remarkable number of studies reported that approximately half of the patients showed the abnormality or responded to treatment and half did not. If FS patients studied have only one cause for their condition, then that cause affects individuals in a variety of different ways. If FS is caused by a composite of more than one condition, careful attention to the differences between those patients who do respond to treatment and those who do not should help to distinguish subgroups (114,150,151). One of the likely subgroups is chronic regional myofascial pain.

Table 5 is organized by organ system. This demonstrates that the cohort of patients now identified as having FS show serious involvement of multiple organ systems. This strongly suggests that fibromyalgia is a systemic disease.

Table 5 leaves little doubt that the muscles have serious problems. Many muscles are abnormally tender. Their energy supply appears to be compromised (152) and they fatigue easily. Biopsy studies to date have not been conclusive (122). The central nervous system is involved in several different ways, with mounting evidence that serotonin pathways are disturbed (153). It is not yet adequately established that FS patients as a group are psychologically disturbed (154). As shown in Table 5, autonomic nervous system function is disturbed. The studies showing abnormalities in the regulation of the immune system provide some of the most convincing evidence of systemic involvement, but in only approximately half of the patients tested. Russell (155) concluded that a central abnormality in the function of a neurotransmitter such as serotonin could account for nearly all of the clinical manifestations of FS. It is not caused by Epstein-Barr viral infection (156,157).

SLEEP

Moldofsky (158,159) (see also Chapter 13, *this volume*) has identified an alpha-delta sleep anomaly on electroencephalogram (EEG) that has been closely associated with fibrositis/fibromyalgia since its redefinition in 1977 (49). His work is of singular importance because not only do a majority of patients with the symptoms of FS have this anomalous non-REM sleep dis-

TABLE 5. *Fibromyalgia studies by systems, noting percentage of abnormal findings*

Finding or therapy	% Abnormal findings, or % responding[a]	Source
MUSCLE INVOLVEMENT		
TePs only/both/TrPs only (N = 55)	16/64/20	Bengtsson et al., 1986 (115)
LACK OF HIGH-ENERGY PHOSPHATES, BIOPSY:		
11 trapezius muscles	73	Bengtsson et al., 1986 (116)
11 tibialis anterior muscles	18	Bengtsson et al., 1986 (116)
^{31}P MAGNETIC RESONANCE SPECTROSCOPY:		
phosphocreatine peak unresponsive to exercise (N = 6)	100	Jensen et al., 1988 (117)
low phosphocreatine/inorganic ratio after exercise (N = 6)	33	Mathur et al., 1988 (118)
abnormal β-ATP/ phosphocreatine ratio in forearm after ischemic exercise (N = 12)	0	Csuka et al., 1989 (119)
Low or scattered abnormal muscle oxygen tension: trapezius (N = 10), brachioradialis (N = 4)	100	Lund et al., 1986 (120)
MUSCLE HISTOLOGY, MUSCLE BIOPSIES:		
ragged red fibers, trapezius (FS/controls) (N = 41/10)	44/0	Bengtsson et al., 1986 (121)
papillary projections (FS/control)	43/82	Yunus and Kalyan-Raman, 1988 (122)
subsarcolemmal glycogen (FS/control) (N = 21/11)	38/18	
bandlike constriction of fibers, 13 quadriceps	100	Bartels and Danneskiold-Samsøe, 1986 (123)
Fatigue of adductor pollicis (N = 8)	100	Bäckman et al., 1988 (124)
Lack of aerobic fitness	80	Bennett et al., 1989 (125)
Work loss and compromised work performance	NR	Mason et al., 1989 (126)
Pain and disability FS ≥ rheumatoid arthritis (N = 100)	NR	Russell et al., 1989 (127)
Quadriceps, weakness	NR	Bartels and Danneskiold-Samsøe, 1986 (123)
Increased fatigability	NR	Cathey et al., 1988 (128)
Fatigue reduced by guanethidine blockade	NR	Bäckman et al., 1988 (124)
Decreased blood flow in right peroneal muscles	NR	Bonefede et al., 1987 (129)
NERVOUS SYSTEM INVOLVEMENT		
Abnormal saccades (eye motility) (N = 36)	42	Rosenhall et al., 1987 (130)
Smooth pursuit eye movements deranged (fibromyalgia with dysesthesia, N = 36)	89	Rosenhall et al., 1987 (130)
Abnormal brainstem auditory-evoked responses (fibromyalgia with dysesthesia, N = 36)	31	Rosenhall et al., 1987 (131)
Alpha-delta sleep abnormality (N = 16)	94	Simms et al., 1988 (132)

TABLE 5. (*continued*)

Finding or therapy	% Abnormal findings, or % responding[a]	Source
Alpha intrusion in non-REM sleep ($N = 44$)	43	Hamm et al., 1989 (133)
One or more sleep abnormalities ($N = 44$)	75	Hamm et al., 1989 (133)
Alpha-delta pattern in stage 3–4 sleep ($N = 12$)	100	Hérrison et al., 1989 (134)
Elevated substance P in cerebrospinal fluid ($N = 30$)	100	Vaerøy et al., 1988 (135)
Numbness or tingling	84	Simms and Goldenberg, 1988 (136)

ABNORMAL IMMUNE REGULATION

Cutaneous immunoreactant deposition (5 studies), total $N = 161$	12–86	Caro, 1986 (137)
Absolute elevation of CD4 ($N = 16$)	56	Peter and Wallace, 1988 (138)
Increased incidence of DR4	37	Burda et al., 1986 (139)
Anticardiolipin antibodies ($N = 100$)	50	Romano and Romano, 1989 (140)
Increased CD4/CD8 ratios ($N = 16$)	50	Peter and Wallace, 1988 (138)
Elevated interleukin-2 ($N = 16$)	44	Peter and Wallace, 1988 (138)
Elevated interferon alpha ($N = 5/16$)	31	Peter and Wallace, 1988 (138)
Repeated grossly elevated CD4/CD8 ratios ($N = 16$)	38	Wallace et al., 1989 (141)
Low serum procollagen type III in FS with sleep disturbance ($N = 16$)	NR	Jensen et al., 1988 (142)

ABNORMAL AUTONOMIC CONTROL

Increased incidence of Raynaud's phenomenon in Fibromyalgia	NR	Ingram et al., 1987 (143)
Raynaud/Raynaud-like phenomenon by history ($N = 30$)	53	Ingram et al., 1987 (143)
Irritable bowel syndrome	49	Romano, 1988 (144)
Relief by regional sympathetic blockade	NR	Bäckman et al., 1988 (124)

RESPONSE TO THERAPY

Treatment effective, amitriptyline ($N = 10$)	50	Adachi et al., 1989 (145)
Improvement, cyclobenzaprine ($N = 60$)	NR	Bennett et al., 1988 (146)
≥50% improvement in morning stiffness and pain analog scores, amitriptyline ($N = 27$)	44	Carette et al., 1986 (147)
Long-lasting response to EMG biofeedback training ($N = 15$)	56	Ferraccioli et al., 1987 (148)
Polarized response to amitriptyline ($N = 36$)	36	Simms et al., 1988 (149)
Polarized response to cyclobenzaprine ($N = 22$)	14	Simms et al., 1988 (149)

[a] NR, % not reported.

turbance, but the reverse is also true. Individuals with situations that disturb their non-REM sleep are prone to develop pain and fatigue symptoms. Similar sleep disturbance was seen electroencephalographically in seven low back pain patients (160).

It is not yet clear that elimination of the sleep anomaly eliminates the symptoms of FS, because quantities of tricyclic medication sufficient to relieve the sleep anomaly produce intolerable side effects (161). Studies have shown that sleep-disturbing conditions, such as induced sleep deprivation (162), noise (163), automobile or industrial accidents that were psychologically but not physically traumatic (164), traumatic war-related events (165), chronic obstructive sleep apnea, nocturnal myoclonus (166–168), and acute flares of painful arthritis (166,169), induce complaints of pain and fatigue that are relieved when the cause of the sleep disturbance can be resolved. The reader is referred to Chapter 13 (*this volume*) and to Moldofsky's recent review (158) for a full summary of his findings. To describe this phenomenon, he introduced the term "rheumatic pain modulation disorder" (167).This term is particularly appealing because the sleep anomaly on which it depends can be confirmed by a sleep study. Many of the muscle pain syndromes may be pain modulation disorders of diverse etiology, and our task may be to sort them out.

The concept of modulation effects is receiving increasing attention. Bennett (170) proposed that an exaggerated reaction of skeletal muscle to microtrauma could account for the muscular findings and cold reactivity in fibromyalgia. The author of this chapter suggests that this exaggerated reaction may be an example of modulation by facilitation. The question then arises, what is causing the modulation?

Figure 7 illustrates one reason why the rheumatic pain modulation disorder may become an integral part of any *chronic* musculoskeletal pain syndrome sufficiently severe to disturb sleep. This pain modulation disorder may apply not only to FS but also to chronic regional MPS and to some fascial and articular dysfunctions. This promises to be a fertile field for investigation with much potential for benefit to patients.

INTERFACE: MYOFASCIAL PAIN SYNDROME AND FIBROMYALGIA

To understand the relationship between TrPs and TePs it would be helpful to identify why the TeP is tender. At least two possible causes are apparent:

1. Fibromyalgia is a systemic disease that causes a generalized increase in tenderness of susceptible sites throughout the body. These may be sites that are known to have especially potent connections to central pain-perception pathways, such as sites where myofascial TrPs are commonly found and at acupuncture sites that are associated with pain modulation.

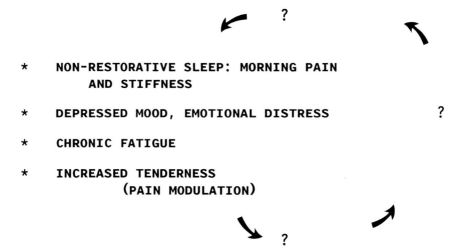

FIG. 7. The rheumatic pain modulation disorder (167) associated with non–REM sleep anomaly is characterized by morning pain and stiffness, depression, chronic fatigue, and an increased tenderness of tender points that suggests modulation of pain in the direction of increased sensitivity. One reason for the difficulty in managing the many patients with chronic pain who have a non-REM sleep anomaly may be the presence of a feedback mechanism whereby the increased sensitivity to pain contributes to disturbed sleep, which, in turn, maintains the increased sensitivity to pain.

2. The tenderness at the TeP site is caused directly or indirectly by a TrP.

This section presents examples of ways in which TrPs may be responsible for TeP tenderness. It then considers a likely relationship between chronic regional MPS and FS; it concludes with the concept of the myofascial pain modulation disorder.

Possible Trigger Point Causes of Tender Point Tenderness

Trigger point phenomena may cause tenderness at a TeP site in four ways: (a) location of a TrP precisely at the TeP site, (b) tenderness of the attachment of a muscle (harboring a TrP) at the TeP site, (c) tenderness of a taut band at the TeP site, and (d) tenderness referred to the TeP site from TrPs in a distant muscle. Table 6 identifies which of these ways are applicable to muscles that can contribute to tenderness at each of the *established* TeP sites (47). Table 6 can be very useful to those interested in distinguishing whether tenderness at TeP sites is due to TrPs or whether the TeP sites are tender for other reasons.

Table 6 demonstrates that of the nine established TeP sites all but two are located over a TrP site in a muscle. The only two non-TrP sites are the

TABLE 6. Specific trigger point phenomena that might cause tenderness at established tender point sites[a]

Tender point site	Likely site of a myofascial trigger point in	Musculotendinous junction and/or region of attachment of	Tenderness in tender taut band of a trigger point in	Likely site of tenderness referred from trigger points in
Cervical Occiput	scalenus anterior **splenius capitis**[b] obliquus capitis superior	scalenus anterior obliquus capitis superior rectus capitis posterior major	**scalenus anterior** **splenius capitis** suboccipital muscles	0 upper trapezius cervical multifidi
Second rib	internal intercostal spinalis (if present))	pectoralis major internal intercostal	**pectoralis major** internal intercostal	pectoralis major sternalis levator scapulae subscapularis serratus posterior superior
Trapezius Supraspinous	**upper trapezius** supraspinatus	0	supraspinatus **upper trapezius**	supinator triceps TrP$_1$ & TrP$_2$ Extensor carpi radialis longus
Lateral epicondyle, 2 cm distal	0	**extensor digitorum** **extensor carpi ulnaris**	extensor digitorum **extensor carpi ulnaris**	gluteus medius gluteus minimus piriformis
Buttock	gluteus medius TrP$_1$ gluteus minimus	gluteus minimus	**gluteus maximus** TrP$_2$	quadratus lumborum tensor fasciae latae gluteus maximus gluteus medius gluteus minimus vastus lateralis
Greater trochanter, site posterior to	0	superior gemellus obturator internus inferior gemellus obturator externus quadratus femoris	gluteus maximus	gracilis adductor longus vastus medialis gastrocnemius, medial head sartorius, distal TrP
Knee, medial fat pad	0	sartorius gracilis	0	

[a] TrP$_1$, trigger point number one of that muscle; TrP$_2$, trigger point number two of that muscle.
[b] Muscles appear in **bold type** if a taut band, when present, is likely to be palpable in that muscle.

greater trochanter and the medial fat pat of the knee. For example, the trapezius TeP site is a common location for TrPs in the upper trapezius muscle. This muscle has been identified as the one most likely to harbor TrPs in patients with neck and shoulder girdle pain (59,171,172).

Only two TeP sites are not over the attachment region of a muscle that is prone to develop TrPs. Those TeP sites are the trapezius and the lateral epicondyle. Even the site 2 cm distal to the lateral epicondyle is a musculotendinous junction area of the extensor digitorum and the extensor carpi ulnaris muscles. At all other TeP sites, tenderness at the musculotendinous junction or tendinous attachment of a muscle that has developed TrPs could contribute to the tenderness observed at the TeP site. This attachment tenderness is seen to develop apparently as a result of the sustained tension from a taut band associated with a TrP. Noteworthy in this regard is the cervical TeP that is directly on the points of attachment of the anterior scalene muscle, which very commonly develops TrPs.

Most of the TeP sites cover several muscles; all but one of the established TeP sites are also located over the belly of a muscle distant from where that muscle usually develops TrPs. For instance, when a tender taut band in the pectoralis major is compressed while testing the second rib TeP, the band can be readily palpated against the rib, if one examines for it. A taut band is often tender throughout its length, usually most tender at the TrP. The band can be traced laterally by palpation until one encounters the responsible TrP.

Only the cervical TeP site is in an area that is not a predictable reference zone of pain and tenderness referred from TrPs. Trigger-point reference zones characteristically develop not only pain, but also heightened sensitivity (referred tenderness). This phenomenon has been studied experimentally by injecting hypertonic saline in the muscles and eliciting both the referred pain and the referred tenderness (68,80,94). Recently Vecchiet et al. (82) examined the depth and duration of this experimentally induced referred tenderness and found that deeper tissues retained the referred tenderness for much longer periods than did skin. Clinically, referred tenderness from TrPs appears to have similar characteristics. For example, tenderness at the lateral epicondyle TeP is likely to be referred from TrPs in one of several muscles that characteristically refer pain primarily to that area: supinator TrPs, triceps brachii TrP_1 and TrP_2, and extensor carpi radialis longus TrPs.

The information for Table 6 was assembled from myofascial pain literature (35,59,173), and from an anatomy atlas (174). A taut band indicates the presence of a TrP. Therefore, those muscles in which one would expect to palpate a taut band if the tenderness at the TeP site is coming from a TrP in that muscle are presented in bold type.

Chronic Regional Myofascial Pain Syndrome

One likely interface between MPS and FS is in that group of patients who develop chronic regional MPS. Hench (175) called attention to the similarity between localized or regional FS that does not fully meet FS criteria and a regional MPS. This extension of the acute single-muscle MPS was reviewed as a separate issue (176), but the development of regional involvement was not emphasized, only incidentally mentioned. The tendency of persistent myofascial TrPs to involve additional muscles in one region (functionally related group of muscles) has been carefully noted in each muscle chapter of the text by Travell and Simons (59). This chronicity and spread of involvement leads to additional dysfunctions and therapeutically becomes a different kind of problem because of its complexity. It therefore deserves a separate term to distinguish it clearly from a simple uncomplicated single- or multiple-muscle MPS, and "chronic regional MPS" is suggested. This distinction should help to avoid statements about MPS in general that apply only to chronic regional MPS (177).

One of the most promising recent papers for opening new insights into this interface issue was that of Pellegrino et al. (104) that classified a group of patients with an autosomal dominant hereditary disorder as having fibromyalgia. However, nowhere in the paper do the authors indicate that the subjects met fibromyalgia criteria; rather, they referred to pre-1977 fibrositis reports. The findings described in their case reports sounded fully compatible with MPS. The danger is great that this important paper will be ignored because the description of the patients does not seem appropriate to the fibromyalgia literature, and the paper is not identified with the MPS literature. This issue of semantics is not trivial.

The patients likely to be most difficult to categorize are those with an insufficient number of TePs to qualify as having FS, but who have many of the other characteristics commonly associated with it. It is in these patients that careful distinction between TrPs and TePs will be most important. Sometimes, an effective way to better understand something is to clarify what it is not. As we study these interfaces in patients from both the MPS and FS point of view, we are likely to learn a lot about each condition. As Eriksson et al. (178) pointed out in the relationship between mandibular dysfunction and FS, when a considerable number of patients have two conditions, patients diagnosed as having one condition should also be examined for the other.

Myofascial Pain Modulation Disorder

The term "myofascial pain modulation disorder" is proposed to help identify a relatively small group of patients who show a remarkable distortion of their referred pain patterns. Instead of the TrPs in one region of the body each projecting pain to their usual reference zone, all TrPs in that region refer pain and tenderness to the same location. For most of the TrPs, this location is an aberrant reference zone. Commonly, this convergent focus of referred pain was the site of trauma or intense pain prior to onset of the pain modulation disorder. This fits well with the observations of Reynolds and Hutchins (87) described earlier.

The impression that the aberrant referral patterns are part of a neurological disorder is strengthened by the fact that many of these patients give a history of impact or trauma of sufficient force to have caused subtle structural damage to the sensory modulation pathways in the central nervous system.

INTERFACE: MYOFASCIAL PAIN SYNDROME AND SOMATIC DYSFUNCTION

Although somatic dysfunction was not a topic of the Symposium on Myofascial Pain and Fibromyalgia, one should not consider muscle pain syndromes without noting the important contribution of the fascial and skeletal systems. "Somatic dysfunction" is an inclusive term that includes skeletal dysfunctions that are often treated by mobilization and manipulation, fascial dysfunctions that are often treated with myofascial release techniques, and muscular dysfunctions such as myofascial TrPs that are relieved by using stretch techniques (66).

The interface between MPS and somatic dysfunction is one of the greatest voids in our knowledge. The early work of Korr et al. (179,180) on segmental facilitation described modulation of referred tenderness, motor activity, and skin conductance changes more than modulation of pain. The facilitation of motor responsiveness is especially pertinent to MPS, but remains nearly unexplored in the context of articular and fascial dysfunction. Janda, in association with others (181), is examining distortion of sequential muscular coordination associated with skeletal asymmetries and muscular imbalance. Lewit (108) has emphasized the close clinical relationship between MPS and articular dysfunctions.

One of the few clearly documented interactions between a fascial dysfunction and a MPS was recently reported in a pair of papers by Silverstolpe (182) and Skoglund (183), who reported a lesion in the thoracic erector spinae that had many characteristics of a myofascial TrP, including the electrical response to snapping palpation typical of a local twitch response (184). This can be seen by comparing the response they obtained in Figure 8A with Figure 1 and Figure 9, which is a characteristic local twitch response reported by Fricton et al. (185).

The patient was found to have a tense and tender sacrotuberous ligament that responded to massage of the attachment of the ligament on the ischial

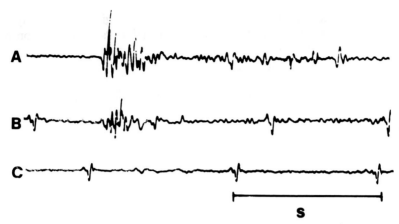

FIG. 8. Electrical activity elicited from the erector spinae muscle in response to deep palpation across the fibers in a lateral direction. The reflex response is seen to have the typical initial burst of impulses followed by afterdischarges that is characteristic of a local twitch response (see Figs. 1 and 9). (From Skoglund, ref. 183, with permission.)

tuberosity. With relief of ligamentous tension and tenderness, the tautness and tenderness of the paraspinal muscle was released and a local twitch type of response could no longer be elicited (182).

A GOLD STANDARD

The definitive solution to the quandary of how to define the component parts of the muscle pain syndromes quagmire would be a diagnostic gold standard for each component against which the clinical signs and symptoms can be tested. Three possibilities look promising.

First, research investigators of FS are valiantly striving to discern a common pathoetiology for all the abnormal findings in various organ systems. If that effort fails, at least it should lead to the identification of component syndromes that are now included in FS, effectively whittling away at the problem.

Second, little effort has been expanded in recent years on experimental investigation of the dysfunctions responsible for the referral phenomena from myofascial TrPs and on investigation of the taut band. Powerful new tools are now available. Computerized videothermography is tailor-made for investigating one autonomic component of referred pain and tenderness. The means are available for studying which sensitizing agent or agents are responsible for the hyperirritability of the TrP. The local twitch response is an unexplored window that can show us more about the nature of the taut band. Neurophysiological research has now reached the stage at which we can begin to see clearly some of the mechanisms whereby pain and altered

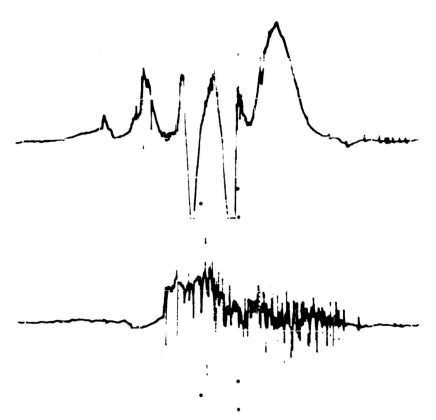

FIG. 9. Electromyographic recording of a local twitch response elicited in the upper trapezius muscle. The duration was approximately 250 msec and mean amplitude was 510 μV. (From Fricton et al., ref. 185, with permission.)

sensation are referred to distant locations. We now have a much stronger basis for clinical research that investigates these mechanisms in patients.

Third, magnetic resonance spectroscopy holds great promise for distinguishing between MPS and FS.

Magnetic Resonance Spectroscopy

Magnetic resonance spectroscopy permits measurement of the relative concentration of phosphorus-bearing compounds in tissue. The spectrogram shows discrete peaks for sugar phosphates, inorganic phosphorus, phosphocreatine, and three kinds of adenosine triphosphate (ATP) (186). These substances also represent the energy ladder that supplies muscle with the energy necessary for contraction. Equally important, they provide the energy required to maintain ion pumps such as the calcium pump for the sarcoplasmic reticulum and the sodium/potassium pump required to maintain muscle membrane excitability.

Both MPS and FS studies report evidence of an energy crisis. In the case of MPS, the energy crisis is expected to be restricted to the region of the TrP, but it apparently involves the muscles generally in FS. In addition to this difference in expected distribution, the two conditions may involve different steps in the energy ladder so that the proportions would look different. Studies to date (117,118,187) look promising, but clear answers to the above considerations are not yet available.

CONCLUDING QUESTIONS

Are MPS and FS Two Different Conditions or Are They the Ends of a Spectrum That in Reality Is Only One Condition?

The following observations indicate that MPS and FS are basically two different conditions.

1. Myofascial pain syndrome is primarily a dysfunction of one or more specific muscles. Each muscle generates characteristic patterns of referred phenomena and the severity may be modulated by mechanical and systemic factors. Evidence is rapidly mounting that FS is fundamentally a total-body systemic disease that involves multiple organ systems.
2. Patients with MPS have TrPs; patients with FS have TePs. TrPs refer pain and tenderness, on palpation they exhibit taut bands, and with adequate stimulation they evidence local twitch responses. None of these phenomena is attributed to TePs.
3. Patients with MPS are approximately equally divided between male and female. Most patients with FS are female.
4. A MPS typically begins with an acute muscle strain or chronic overuse of a specific group of muscles. FS usually begins insidiously and the patient complains of generalized pain and often of muscular fatigue.
5. Weakness in patients with MPS is limited to just the specific muscles that have TrPs. It is widespread in FS.
6. Patients with MPS characteristically have unilateral pain in one or several regions of the body. Patients with FS commonly complain of symmetrical bilateral pain.
7. The pain in MPS can be traced to myofascial TrPs in specific muscles. The pain of FS has no such identifiable origin.
8. The TrPs of MPS respond to specific therapies directed to that muscle, such as injection, spray and stretch, postisometric relaxation, and massage (59). Drugs are usually of little value. FS is treated by systemic medication and by educating the patient that FS is neither life-threat-

ening nor imaginary. Use of physical therapeutic measures is tailored to individual patients (188).

Since both MPS and FS are common conditions one would expect that a large number of patients could have a variable mixture of both afflictions. If adequate diagnostic criteria were not applied to distinguish between the two conditions in patients who had both, it would appear that there was a spectrum of patients that shifted from one condition to the other.

Clinicians who think in terms of one spectrum speak of patients evolving from having MPS to having FS as their condition becomes more severe and from having FS to having MPS as they improve (64). A mixture of the two conditions could also give this impression. With both conditions active, the patient is worse. As one condition improves, the other condition becomes more apparent. To date, I know of no discriminating experimental data that address progression from one condition to the other.

Answers to the following questions should help to clarify the interface between FS and MPS.

To What Extent and in What Way is TeP Tenderness Caused by TrP Phenomena?

Table 6 addresses this issue in some detail. Closer attention to what specific anatomical structures are responsible for TeP tenderness may help us to understand why TePs are tender.

What is the Relationship of the Systemic Perpetuating Factors of MPS to Fibromyalgia?

Do some of these systemic perpetuating factors also aggravate and perpetuate FS, or are different mechanisms, neurotransmitters, or enzyme systems involved?

What is the Role of Heredity in These Two Conditions?

Do both MPS and FS have hereditary substrates, or is the predisposition for only one of them inherited? Among those patients who do have a congenital characteristic predisposing to the condition, what is the anatomical structure or enzyme system involved?

Acknowledgments. I extend sincere thanks to Dr. Janet Travell for sharing her treasure of wisdom and knowledge of MPS with all of us and to Fred Wolfe, MD, and Lois Simons, PT, for many intense discussions on this subject but from very different points of view. The meticulous review of the manuscript by Lois was enormously valuable. The thoughtful insights of

Robert Bennett, MD, have been very helpful in making my way through this tangled web.

REFERENCES

1. Institute of Medicine. *Pain and disability: Clinical, behavioral and public policy perspectives.* Washington DC: National Academy Press, 1987.
2. Reynolds, MD. *J Hist Med Allied Sci* 1983;38:5–35.
3. Bennett, RM, Campbell S, Clark S. *Arthritis Rheum* 1985;28:1436.
4. Simons DG. *Am J Phys Med* 1975;54:289–311, and 1976;55:15–42.
5. Strauss H. *Klin Wochenschr* 1898;35:89–91, 121–123.
6. Adler I. *Med Rec* 1900;57:529–535.
7. Gowers WR. *Br Med J* 1904;1:117–121.
8. Müller A. *Z Klin Med* 1912;74:34–73.
9. Llewellyn LJ, Jones AB. *Fibrositis.* London: Heinemann, 1915.
10. Schmidt A. *Münch Med Wochenschr* 1916;63:593–595.
11. Schade H. *Z Ges Exp Med* 1919;7:275–374.
12. Port K. *Arch Orthop Unfallchir* 1920;17:465–506.
13. Stockman R. *Rheumatism and arthritis.* Edinburgh: W. Green, 1920.
14. Lange F. *Münch Med Wochenschr* 1925;72:1626–1629.
15. Lange M. *Die muskelhärten (myogelosen).* München; J.F.Lehmann's Verlag, 1931.
16. Rueff S. *Wien Arch Inn Med* 1932;23:139–154.
17. Ruhmann W. *Dtsch Arch Klin Med* 1932;173:625–645.
18. Kraus H. *Wien Klin Wochenschr* 1937;50:1356–1357.
19. Reichart A. *Dtsch Med Wochenschr* 1938;64:823–824.
20. Abel O Jr, Siebert WJ, Earp R. *J Missouri Med Assoc* 1939;36:435–437.
21. Good M. *Ann Rheum Dis* 1942;3:118–138.
22. Jordan HH. *Arch Phys Ther* 1942;23:36–54.
23. Travell J, Rinzler S, Herman J. *JAMA* 1942;120:417–422.
24. Elliott FA. *Lancet* 1944;1:47–49.
25. Gutstein RR. *Miss Valley Med J* 1944;66:114–118, 122–124.
26. Kelly M. *Ann Rheum Dis* 1946;5:69–77.
27. Bayer H. *Klin Wochenschr* 1949;27:122–126.
28. Travell J. *Miss Valley Med J* 1949;71:12-21.
29. Good MG. *Edinburgh Med J* 1949; 56:366–368.
30. Good MG. *Rheumatism* 1949;5:117–123.
31. Good MG. *Acta Med Scand* 1950;138:285–292.
32. Good MG. *Br J Phys Med* 1951;14:1–7.
33. Glogowski G, Wallraff J. *Z Orthop* 1951;80:237–268.
34. Travell J. *Arch Phys Med* 1952;33:291–298.
35. Travell J. In: Ragan C, ed. *Connective tissues; transactions of the 5th conference*, New York: Josiah Macy, Jr. Foundation, 1954;12–22.
36. Sola AE, Kuitert JH. *Northwest Med* 1955;54:980–984.
37. Long C II. *Henry Ford Hosp Med Bull* 1955;3:189–192 and 1956;4:22–28, 102–106.
38. Bonica JJ. *JAMA* 1957;164:732–738.
39. Brendstrup P, Jespersen K, Asboe-Hansen G. *Ann Rheum Dis* 1957;16:438–440.
40. Miehlke K, Schulze G, Eger W. *Z Rheumaforsch* 1960;19:310–330.
41. Cooper AL. *Arch Phys Med* 1961;42:704–709.
42. Kelly M. *J Am Geriatr Soc* 1963;11:586–596.
43. Kraft GH, Johnson EW, LaBan MM. *Arch Phys Med* 1968;49:155–162.
44. Smythe HA. In: Hollander JL, McCarty DJ, eds. *Arthritis and allied conditions*, ed 8. Philadelphia: Lea & Febiger, 1972;874–884.
45. Awad EA. *Arch Phys Med* 1973;54:449–453.
46. Fassbender HG. In: Leowi G, trans. *Pathology of Rheumatic Diseases.* New York: Springer-Verlag, 1975;303–314.

47. Wolfe F, Smythe HA, Yunus MB, Bennett RM, Bombardier C, Goldenberg DM, Tugwell P, Multicenter Fibromyalgia Criteria Committee. *Arthritis Rheum* 1989;32(4)(suppl):S47.
48. Yunus M, Masi AT, Calabro JJ, Miller KA, Feigenbaum SL. *Semin Arthritis Rheum* 1981;11:151–171.
49. Smythe HA, Moldofsky H. *Bull Rheum Dis* 1977;28:928–931.
50. Morse LH. *State Art Rev Occup Med* 1986;1:167–174.
51. Ireland DCR. *Aust Fam Physician* 1986;15:415–416, 418.
52. Sikorski JM. *Aust Fam Physician* 1988;17:81–83.
53. Fry HJH. *Lancet* 1986;2:728–731.
54. Dennett X, Fry HJH. *Lancet* 1988;1:905–908.
55. Popelianskii Ya Yu. *Revmatologikila* 1987;4:13–19.
56. Holmes GP, Kaplan JE, Gantz NM. *Ann Intern Med* 1988;108:387–389.
57. Larsson SE, Bengtsson A, Bodegård L, Henriksson KG, Larsson J. *Acta Orthop Scand* 1988;59:552–556.
58. Edwards RHT. *Eur J Appl Physiol* 1988;57:275–281.
59. Travell JG, Simons DG. *Myofascial pain and dysfunction: The trigger point manual.* Baltimore: Williams & Wilkins, 1983.
60. Littlejohn GO. *Rheum Dis Clin North Am* 1989;15:45–60.
61. Pritchard C. *Ann Intern Med* 1988;108:906 (letter).
62. Goldenberg DL, Simms RW, Geiger A, Komaroff AL. *Arthritis Rheum* 1989;32(4)(suppl):S47 (abstr).
63. Travell J. *Office hours: Day and night.* New York: The World Publishing Company, 1968;257, 274.
64. Campbell SM. *Rheum Dis Clin North Am* 1989;15:31–44.
65. Travell JG, Simons DG. *Myofascial pain and dysfunction: The trigger point manual.* Baltimore: Williams & Wilkins, 1983;168–173.
66. Greenman PE. *Principles of manual medicine.* Baltimore: Williams & Wilkins, 1989;106–112.
67. Kellgren JH. *Br Med J* 1938;1:325–327.
68. Kellgren JH. *Clin Sci* 1938;3:175–190.
69. Selzer M, Spencer WA. *Brain Res* 1969;14:331–348.
70. Ruch TC, Patton HD. *Physiology and biophysics*, ed 19. 1965;357–358. Philadelphia: WB Saunders Company.
71. Foreman RD, Schmidt RF, Willis WD. *Brain Res* 1977;124:555–560.
72. McMahon SB, Wall PD. *J Comp Neurol* 1987;261:130–136.
73. Ushiki T, Ide C. *Arch Histol Cytol* 1988;51:223–232.
74. Langford LA, Coggeshall RE. *J Comp Neurol* 1988;203:745–750.
75. Laurberg S, Sorensen KE. *Brain Res* 1985;331:160–163.
76. Alles A, Dom RM. *Brain Res* 1985;342:382–385.
77. Campbell JN, Raja SN, Meyer RA. In: Dubner R, Gebhart GF, Bond MR, eds. *Proceedings of the Vth World Congress on Pain*, Pain Research and Clinical Management Series, vol 3. Amsterdam: Elsevier, 1988;135–143.
78. Procacci P, Zoppi M. *Pain* 1981;Suppl 1:S7.
79. Roberts JT. *Am Heart J* 1948;35:369–392.
80. Steinbrocker O, Isenberg SA, Silver M, Neustadt D, Kuhn P, Schittone M. *J Clin Invest* 1953;32:1045–1051.
81. Galletti R, Procacci P. *Acta Neurovegetativa* 1966;28:495–500.
82. Vecchiet L, Galletti R, Giamberardino MA, Dragani L, Marini F. *Clin J Pain* 1988;4:55–59.
83. Fields HL. *Pain.* New York: McGraw-Hill Book Company, 1987;82–94.
84. Weiss S, Davis D. *Am J Med Sci* 1928;176:517–536.
85. Theobald GW. *Lancet* 1949;2:41–47, 94–97.
86. Feinstein B, Langton JNK, Jameson RM, Schiller F. *J Bone Joint Surg [AM]* 1954;36:981–997.
87. Reynolds OE, Hutchins HC. *Am J Physiol* 1948;152:658–662.
88. Langs HM. *Pain* 1987;Suppl. 4:S297.
89. Diakow PRP. *J Manipulative Physiol Ther* 1988;11:114–117.
90. Fischer AA. *Arch Phys Med Rehabil* 1988;69:286–291.

91. Fischer AA, Chang CH. *Thermology* 1986;1:212–215.
92. Willis WD Jr. *The Pain System* Basel: S. Karger, 1985;63–65.
93. Willis WD, Coggeshall RE. *Sensory mechanisms of the spinal cord.* New York: Plenum Press, 1978;394.
94. Sinclair DC, Weddell G, Feindel WH. *Brain* 1948;71:184–211.
95. Procacci P, Francini F, Maresca M, Zoppi M. *Pain* 1975;1:167–175.
96. Simons DG. In: Goodgold J, ed. *Rehabilitation medicine.* St. Louis: CV Mosby Co, 1988;686–723.
97. Dexter JR, Simons DG. *Arch Phys Med Rehabil* 1981;62:521.
98. Simons DG. In: Bonica JJ, Albe-Fessard D, eds. *Advances in pain research and therapy,* Vol 1. New York: Raven Press, 1976;913–918.
99. Hong C-Z, Simons DG, Statham L. *Arch Phys Med Rehabil* 1986;67:680.
100. Hong, C-Z, Simons DG, Simons L. *Arch Phys Med Rehabil* 1988;69:789.
101. Hong, C-Z. In: *First international symposium on myofascial pain and fibromyalgia,* Minneapolis, University of Minnesota, May 8–10, 1989 (abstr).
102. Danneskiold-Samsøe B, Christiansen E, Lund B, Andersen RB. *Scand J Rehab Med* 1983;15:17–20.
103. Danneskiold-Samsøe B, Christiansen E, Andersen RB. *Scand J Rheumatol* 1986;15:174–178.
104. Pellegrino MJ, Waylonis GW, Sommer A. *Arch Phys Med Rehabil* 1989;70:61–63.
105. Jaeger B. *TMJ Update* 1987;5:28–32.
106. Jaeger B, Reeves JL. *Pain* 1986;27:203–210.
107. Jaeger B, Reeves JL, Graff-Radford SB. *Proc Am Pain Soc* 1986;82 (abstr).
108. Lewit K. *Manipulative therapy in rehabilitation of the motor system* London: Butterworths, 1985.
109. Bennett RM. *West J Med* 1981;134:405–413.
110. Campbell SM, Clark S, Tindall EA, Forehand ME, Bennett RM. *Arthritis Rheum* 1983;26:817–824.
111. Wolfe F, Hawley DJ, Cathey MA, Caro X, Russell IJ. *J Rheumatol* 1985;12:1159–1163.
112. Simms RW, Goldenberg DL, Felson DT, Mason JH. *Arthritis Rheum* 1988;31:182–187.
113. Wolfe F, Cathey MA. *J Rheumatol* 1985;12:1164–1168.
114. Quimby LG, Block SR, Gratwick GM. *J Rheumatol* 1988;15:1264–1270.
115. Bengtsson A, Henriksson KG, Jorfeldt L, Kågedal B, Lennmarken C, Lindström F. *Scand J Rheumatol* 1986;15:340–347.
116. Bengtsson A, Henriksson KG, Larsson J. *Arthritis Rheum* 1986;20:817–821.
117. Jensen KE, Jacobsen S, Thomsen C, Andersen RA, Henriksen O. Paper presented to the Society of Magnetic Resonance in Medicine, San Francisco, August 22–26, 1988.
118. Mathur AK, Gatter RA, Bank WJ, Schumacher HR. *Arthritis Rheum* 1988;31(4)(suppl):S23 (abstr).
119. Csuka ME, Valen PA, Rilling W, Grist T, Wortmann RL. *Arthritis Rheum* 1989;32(1) (suppl):R33 (abstr).
120. Lund N, Bengtsson A, Thorborg P. *Scand J Rheumatol* 1986;15:165–173.
121. Bengtsson A, Henriksson KG, Larsson J. *Scand J Rheumatol* 1986;15:1–6.
122. Yunus MB, Kalyan-Raman UP. *Rheum Dis Clin North Am* 1989;15:115–134.
123. Bartels EM, Danneskiold-Samsøe B. *Lancet* 1986;1:755–757.
124. Bäckman E, Bengtsson A, Bengtsson M, Lennmarken C, Henriksson KG. *Acta Neurol Scand* 1988;77:187–191.
125. Bennett RM, Clark SR, Goldberg L, Nelson D, Bonafede RP, Porter J, Specht D. *Arthritis Rheum* 1989;32:454–460.
126. Mason JH, Simms RW, Goldenberg DL, Meenan RF. *Arthritis Rheum* 1989;32(4) (suppl.):S46 (abstr).
127. Russell IJ, Fletcher EM, Tsui J, Michalek JE. *Arthritis Rheum* 1989;32(4)(suppl):S70 (abstr).
128. Cathey MA, Kleinheksel SM, Miller S, Pitetti KH, Wolfe F. *Arthritis Rheum* 1988;31(4) (suppl):S99 (abstr).
129. Bonafede P, Nelson D, Clark S, Goldber L, Bennett R. *Arthritis Rheum* 1987;30(4) (suppl):25 (abstr).
130. Rosenhall U, Johansson G, Örndahl, G. *Scand J Rehabil Med* 1987;19:139–145.

131. Rosenhall U, Johansson G, Örndahl, G. *Scand J Rehabil Med* 1987;19:147–152.
132. Simms RW, Gunderman J, Howard G, Goldenberg DL. *Arthritis Rheum* 1988;31(4) (suppl):S100 (abstr).
133. Hamm C, Derman S, Russell IJ. *Arthritis Rheum* 1989;32(4)(suppl):S70 (abstr).
134. Hérisson C, Simon L, Touchon J, Billiard M. *Arthritis Rheum* 1989;32(4)(suppl):S70 (abstr).
135. Vaerøy H, Helle R, Førre Ø, Kåss E, Terenius L. *Pain* 1988;32:21–26.
136. Simms RW, Goldenberg DL *J Rheumatol* 1988;15:1271–1273.
137. Caro XJ. *Am J Med* 1986;81(suppl 3A):43–49.
138. Peter JB, Wallace DJ. *Arthritis Rheum* 1988;31(4)(suppl):S24 (abstr).
139. Burda CD, Cox FR, Osborne P. *Clin Exp Rheumatol* 1986;4:355–357.
140. Romano TJ, Romano I. *Arthritis Rheum* 1989;32(1)(suppl):R34 (abstr).
141. Wallace DJ, Bowman R, Wormsley SB, Peter JB. *Arthritis Rheum* 1989;32(4)(suppl):S69 (abstr).
142. Jensen LT, Jacobsen S, Hørsley-Petersen K. *Br J Rheumatol* 1988;27:496.
143. Ingram S, Nelson D, Porter J, Campbell S, Bennett R. *Arthritis Rheum* 1987;30(4) (suppl):24.
144. Romano TJ. *W Va Med J* 1988;84:16–18.
145. Adachi JD, Guyatt G, Keller J, Gordon M, Bensen WG, Tugwell PX. *Arthritis Rheum* 1989;32(1)(suppl):R9 (abstr).
146. Bennett RM, Gatter RA, Campbell SM, Andrews RP, Clark SR, Scarola JA. *Arthritis Rheum* 1988;31:1535–1542.
147. Carette S, McCain GA, Bell DA, Fam AG. *Arthritis Rheum* 1986;29:655–659.
148. Ferraccioli G, Ghirelli L, Scita F, Nolli M, Mozzani M, Fontana S, Scorsonelli M, Tridenti A, De Risio C. *J Rheumatol* 1987;14:820–825.
149. Simms RW, Felson DT, Goldenberg DL. *Arthritis Rheum* 1988;31(4)(suppl):S100 (abstr).
150. Buckelew SP. *Am J Phys Med Rehabil* 1989;68:37–41.
151. Kogstad O. *Scand J Rheumatol* 1988;17:154.
152. Henriksson KG. *Eur J Appl Physiol* 1988;57:348–352.
153. Russell IJ, Michalek JE, Vipraio GA, Fletcher EM, Wall K. *Arthritis Rheum* 1989;32(4)(suppl):S70 (abstr).
154. Goldenberg DL. *Rheum Dis Clin North Am* 1989;15:105–114.
155. Russell IJ. *Rheum Dis Clin North Am* 1989;15:149–168.
156. Buchwald D, Goldenberg DL, Sullivan JL, Komaroff AL. *Arthritis Rheum* 1987;30:1132–1136.
157. Fye KH, Whiting-O'Keefe QE, Lennette ET, Jessop C. *Arthritis Rheum* 1988;31:1455–1456.
158. Moldofsky H. *Rheum Dis Clin North Am* 1989;15:91–103.
159. Moldofsky H, Scarisbrick P, England R, Smythe H. *Psychosom Med* 1975;37:341–351.
160. Atkinson JH, Ancoli-Israel S, Slater MA, Garfin SR, Gillin JC. *Clin J Pain* 1988;4:225–232.
161. Smythe HA. *Br J Rheumatol* 1988;27:449.
162. Moldofsky H, Scarisbrick P. *Psychosom Med* 1976;38:35–44.
163. Tarnopolsky A, Watkins G, Hand DJ. *Psychol Med* 1980;10:683–698.
164. Saskin P, Moldofsky H, Lue FA. *Psychosom Med* 1986;48:319–323.
165. Lavie P, Hefez A, Halperin G, Enoch D. *Am J Psychol* 1979;136:175–178.
166. Moldofsky H, Lue FA, Saskin P. *J Rheumatol* 1987;14:124–128.
167. Moldofsky H, Tullis C, Lue FA. *J Rheumatol* 1986;13:614–617.
168. Moldofsky H, Tullis C, Quance G, Lue FA. *Can J Neurol Sci* 1986;13:52–54.
169. Moldofsky H, Lue FA, Smythe HA. *J Rheumatol* 1983;10:373–379.
170. Bennett RM. *Rheum Dis Clin North Am* 1989;15:135–147.
171. Sola AE, Rodenberger ML, Gettys BB. *Am J Phys Med* 1955;34:585–590.
172. Williams HL, Elkins EC. *Arch Phys Ther* 1942;23:14–22.
173. Travell JG, Simons DG. *Myofascial pain and dysfunction: The trigger point manual,* vol 2. Baltimore: Williams & Wilkins, (*in press*).
174. Ferner H, Staubesand J. *Sobotta atlas of human anatomy,* ed 10, vol 2. Baltimore: Urban & Schwartzenberg, 1983.
175. Hench PK. *Rheum Dis Clin North Am* 1989;15:19–29.

176. Simons DG, Simons LS. In: Tollison CD, ed. *Handbook of chronic pain management.* Baltimore: Williams & Wilkins, 1988;509–529.
177. McCain GA, Scudds RA. *Pain* 1988;33:273–287.
178. Eriksson P-O, Lindman R, Stål P, Bengtsson A. *Swed Dent J* 1988;12:141–149.
179. Korr IM. *J Am Osteopathic Assoc* 1955;54:265–282.
180. Korr IM, Wright HM, Chace JNA. *Acta Neurovegetativa* 1964;25:589–606.
181. Jull GA, Janda V. In: Twomey LT, Taylor JR, eds. *Physical therapy of the low back.* New York: Churchill Livingstone, 1987;253–278.
182. Silverstolpe L. *J Manual Med* 1989;4:28.
183. Skoglund CR. *J Manual Med* 1989;4:29–30.
184. Simons DG, Hong C-Z. *J Manual Med* 1989;4:69.
185. Fricton JR, Auvinen MD, Dykstra D, Schiffman E. *Arch Phys Med Rehabil* 1985;66:314–317.
186. Duboc D, Jehenson P, Dinh ST, Marsac C, Syrota A, Fardeau M. *Neurology* 1987;37:663–671.
187. Miller RG, Boska MD, Moussavi RS, Carson PJ, Weiner MW. *J Clin Invest* 1988;81:1190–1196.
188. Goldenberg DL. *Rheum Dis Clin North Am* 1989;15:61–71.

Advances in Pain Research and Therapy, Vol. 17,
edited by James R. Fricton and Essam Awad.
Raven Press, Ltd., New York © 1990.

2

Myofascial Pain Syndromes and the Fibromyalgia Syndrome: A Comparative Analysis

Robert M. Bennett

Department of Medicine and Division of Arthritis and Rheumatic Diseases, Oregon Health Sciences University, Portland, Oregon 97201

In the beginning there was "fibrositis," so named in 1904 by an English physician (1); in reality the concept of "muscular rheumatism" had been convincingly described by Scandinavian and German physicians in the preceding century (2–4). The term "fibrositis" encompassed a wide array of pain syndromes thought to arise from muscle and often accompanied by neurasthenia; a comprehensive description of this topic was given in the book written by Llewellyn and Jones entitled "Fibrositis (Gouty, Infective, Traumatic); So Called Chronic Rheumatism Including Villous Synovitis of Knee and Hip, and Sacroiliac Relaxation." (5). The very diversity of the problems claimed to be related to "fibrositis" coupled with a conspicuous lack of any definitive tissue pathology led many thinking physicians to consider the term "fibrositis" synonymous with a wastebasket for any poorly defined musculoskeletal pain problem. Thus it fell into disrepute with the leaders of the medical establishment and even became the subject of some derision.

In the 1950s Dr. Janet Travell started to popularize the idea of myofascial pain syndromes (MPSs). Many of her ideas were adopted by physiatrists and physical therapists, and a large body of empirical knowledge accumulated and was verified on an *ad hoc* basis, but never with the precision demanded by the current dictates of contemporary clinical science (6,7); a compendium of this knowledge appeared in the book by Travell and Simons entitled "Myofascial Pain and Dysfunction: The Trigger Point Manual" (8). On another unrelated front, a Toronto rheumatologist, Hugh Smythe, persisted in declaring that fibrositis is "alive and well" and reinforced the seminal concept that patients with a widespread musculoskeletal pain syndrome of undetermined etiology had tender areas in well-defined and reproducible

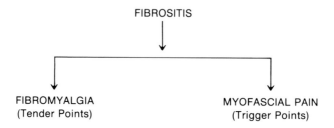

FIG. 1. The family tree of "fibrositis."

locations. His thoughts were published in the *Bulletin on the Rheumatic Diseases* (9) and, in association with the work of Harvey Moldofsky, an objective abnormality was found: a disturbance of stage 4 sleep by alpha intrusion (10). These two papers stimulated a small group of North American rheumatologists to look again at the fibrositis concept (11–16).

Fibrositis is now generally recognized to be one of the most common problems encountered by most rheumatologists in the United States and Canada (13,15–18). Chapters are devoted to it in the two major American textbooks of rheumatology, the Arthritis Foundation distributes a patient education handout on fibrositis, and it was featured in the *Disease-A-Month* series (19), a recent issue of the *Rheumatic Disease Clinics of North America* (20) and a supplement to the *American Journal of Medicine* (21). Bearing in mind the rather pejorative connotation of "fibrositis," many contemporary rheumatologists prefer the name "fibromyalgia" or the fibromyalgia syndrome (FS). Nevertheless some rheumatologists, many internists, and family physicians use the term "fibrositis" to refer to both MPS and FS, making no significant distinction between the two syndromes. Perhaps they are intuitively correct! Historically, then, fibrositis is composed of two apparently distinctive syndromes, FS and MPS (Fig. 1); whether this dichotomy is justified must now be given some scrutiny.

DEFINITIONS

A myofascial pain syndrome has been empirically defined as musculoskeletal pain arising from one or several hyperirritable spots within the belly of muscle(s) (8). The hyperirritable spot is called a trigger point (TrP) because of its propensity to cause referred pain in a distinctive distribution when stimulated; the salient features of a TrP are given in Table 1. In its simplest form MPS is due to a simple TrP. If it does not regress spontaneously, as most do, or if it is not treated effectively, other TrPs may appear in the same and adjacent muscles, giving rise to a more complex regional MPS. In turn this may be accompanied, in chronic resistant cases, by pain behavior, secondary

TABLE 1. *Definition of a myofascial pain syndrome*

1. Pain occurring in a regional distribution that can be reproduced by pressure over a trigger point.
2. A trigger point (TrP) is defined as:
   a. A tender area within the belly of a muscle.
   b. Pressure over a TrP causes pain and/or tingling in a characteristic distribution.
   c. The muscle harboring the TrP is shortened, resulting in a reduced range of motion; either stretching or contracting the muscle causes pain.
   d. The muscle harboring the TrP feels taut in the location of the TrP.
   e. Stimulating the TrP by snapping or needling often causes the muscle to contract.
   f. Injection of the TrP with a local anesthetic abolishes both the local and the referred pain.

Adapted from Travell and Simons (8).

gain considerations, and socioeconomic disruption, leading to the characteristic complex of the "chronic pain" patient.

The fibromyalgia syndrome has recently been the subject of an ambitious criteria study (22). Twenty-five investigators in 16 North American cities evaluated 263 patients with presumed FS and 250 control patients with another cause of musculoskeletal pain (e.g., neck pain, low back pain). Over 300 variables, including TrP number and intensity, were evaluated by blinded observers. The full results of this study will be published elsewhere, but in the final analysis the best criteria proved to be disarmingly simple and included widespread pain and 11 or more tender points (TePs) at 18 possible sites (Table 2). The sensitivity of these criteria was 83% and the specificity was 81%. It was of considerable interest, and somewhat unexpected, that the inclusion of symptoms such as fatigue, stiffness, modulating factors, and irritable bowel did not improve the sensitivity/specificity. Furthermore, when patients diagnosed as having primary FS were compared to those said to have secondary FS (i.e., secondary to another rheumatic disease), no

TABLE 2. *Definition of the fibromyalgia syndrome*

1. Widespread aching and pain (defined as pain in all 4 quadrants, i.e., left right/above and below the waist).
2. Eleven or more tender points out of a total of 18; defined by palpation at approximately 4 kg with the thumb pulp over the following 9 paired locations:
   a. 2 cm below lateral epicondyl of elbow
   b. Insertion of nuchal muscles into occiput
   c. Intertransverse ligaments of C5–C7
   d. Upper border of trapezius (approximately mid point)
   e. Supraspinatus, medial aspect just above scapular spine
   f. Pectoralis, over upper border of 2nd rib about 2 cm from sternum
   g. Upper gluteal area, just below iliac crest in outer quadrant
   h. Insertion of muscles into greater trochanter—about 2 cm from bone
   i. Medial condyle of femur about 2 cm above joint line on the antero-lateral aspect of the bone

From Wolfe et al., ref. 22, with permission.

significant differences were observed; thus the distinction between primary and secondary FS was abandoned. In other words, if a patient has pain all over *and* 11 or more TePs out of 18, he or she has FS irrespective of other diagnoses or test results.

AN EMERGING DILEMMA

It is evident that patients with MPS involving several separate regions will resemble patients with FS. Furthermore, it is not uncommon to see a patient who starts off with a well-defined MPS and progresses over time to a clinical picture identical to FS. Presumably patients with FS are not immune to the development of TrPs, and questions arise as to whether some TePs are in fact TrPs; this is not merely a matter of semantics, because it would have a bearing on management with specific TrP therapy, which currently is seldom employed in FS. Relevant questions in this dilemma are: (a) Are FS and MPS clinically and etiologically distinct entities? (b) Is FS a result of widespread MPS? (c) Do TePs cause pain in a referred distribution? (d) Are many of the TePs in patients with FS the same as TrPs in the same locations in MPS? (e) Are there constitutive features present in patients with a simple MPS that predispose them to develop a clinical picture identical to FS? Some of these permutations are illustrated in Fig. 2.

Before one can construct realistic hypotheses concerning the interrelationships of MPS and FS it is necessary to have a broad overview of those studies performed to date that have provided some objective or semi-objective findings and may shed light on the questions at hand—namely, what are the similarities and differences between MPS and FS and do they permit any definitive conclusions regarding pathogenesis?

MYOFASCIAL PAIN SYNDROMES

A large body of mainly empirical facts has accumulated over many years regarding the diagnosis and treatment of MPS and the relationship to TrPs; this has been amassed and set out by Travell and Simons (8). In general the basic tenets of these ideas have been substantiated by the personal observations of a large number of health professionals, but they have not been the subject of a carefully planned controlled trial. Contemporary studies of relevance to MPS are now summarized.

Myofascial Pain

Myofascial pain is generally considered to arise in muscles, although a similar pain distribution may arise from stimulation of ligaments, tendons, and

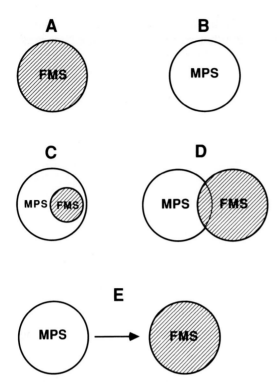

FIG. 2. Some possible associations between myofascial pain syndromes (MPS) and the fibromyalgia syndrome (FMS).

periosteum. The study by Kellgren in the late 1930s established that 6% hypertonic saline solution injected into muscle, fascia, or periosteum produced a referred pain in a broadly spinal segmental pattern (23). It was also noted that in some instances, in addition to deep referred pain, there was sometimes palpable muscle spasm and deep tenderness in the referred pain distribution. The pain was felt to be located in deeper structures rather than superficial ones, and its boundaries could be measured both by palpation of tenderness and by defining the boundaries of hyperalgesia. The pain would occur within a few seconds of the injection and last about 5 min. The areas of pain reference did not correspond to dermatomes but seemed to conform more to segmental innervation of deep somatic structures. Anesthetizing the site of the injection consistently abolished the referred effects, whereas anesthetizing the site of reference did not reduce pain.

In 1944 Elliott repeated Kellgren's experiments and basically confirmed his findings (24). In addition, Elliott performed electromyograms (EMGs) at the site of deep pain reference and found occasional but inconsistent evidence of abnormal motor discharge. He emphasized that these EMG changes were not a constant feature of referred pain and therefore the pain could not be explained as being due to muscle spasm. Travell and Bigelow in 1947 performed similar experiments and replicated Kellgren's results, except that the response between individuals as regards referred pain was quite great and did not support the idea of a fixed sclerotome distribution (6). In 1967 Hockaday and Whitty repeated Kellgren's experiments by injecting 0.1 to 0.3 ml of 6% saline into interspinous ligaments at a depth of 1 to 3 cm (25). The results were in general similar to those obtained by previous investigators, but it was noted that the referred pain was less consistent in its distribution and quality than previously described. They discussed the mechanism of deep pain referral and thought the results were most consistent with a mechanism of recruitment within the CNS at the synapse level rather than a peripheral mechanism.

Muscle Pain

Animal experiments have established that pain arising from muscle travels in the unmyelinated type C 5 (group IV fibers) after stimulation of nociceptors by 5-hydroxytryptamine, histamine, potassium, and bradykinin (26). The range of concentrations of these substances necessary to elicit pain is quite considerable (Table 3) and the result is only short lived—about 5 min. 5-Hydroxytryptamine is liberated from platelets during clotting and could be a source of pain after trauma of muscle, as would potassium release from muscle fibers. Bradykinin was the most potent stimulator of muscle nerve receptors and is responsible for a sensation of "slow" pain. In order for bradykinin to be involved in muscle pain, one would need to postulate a low-grade inflammatory reaction accompanied by the release of protein enzymes that could cause the generation of bradykinin from α_2-globulins (kininogens). Histamine can be liberated in the skin by an antidromic response as exemplified by the classical triple response of Lewis.

Epidemiology of Trigger Points

According to Travell and Simons (8), the TrP can either be active (i.e., the site of an active pain syndrome) or latent (in which case its presence is only

TABLE 3. *Activation of group IV afferent nerve fibers in the cat*

	Molar ratio
Bradykinin	1
5-Hydroxytryptamine.	30
Histamine	66
K^+ ions	4,000

From Fock and Mense, ref. 26, with permission.

apparent after elicitation of pain by palpation). There is only one study that has comprehensively looked for "hypersensitive" areas in a large number of asymptomatic adults. Sola et al. (27) palpated the shoulder girdle and neck muscles in 200 adults (100 females and 100 males) all of whom were basic airmen in the U.S. Air Force. They found one or more tender areas in 49.5% of subjects. Radiating or referred pain could only be demonstrated in 12.5%. They noted that tender areas occurred in multiples rather than as isolated phenomenan: 62.5% of subjects had more than one tender area. Of the total of 250 TePs noted, 84.7% occurred in just four muscles: the trapezius, levator scapulae, infraspinatus, and scalenes. In comparison with a previous study done by the same group on airmen with *symptomatic* myofascial shoulder pain, there was a definite correlation between asymptomatic hypersensitive areas and the areas found in the symptomatic patients.

Recently Fischer (28) used a pressure algometer to establish normal pain thresholds over muscles commonly involved with TrP syndromes; the reliability of this measuring device was established by Reeves et al. (29). This methodology lends itself to blinded control trials of myofascial TrPs and would seem to offer a convenient tool for documenting the results of therapy (30). Using the same device with a simple modification, Fischer has measured soft tissue consistency with a view to documenting the "taut band" in a quantitative fashion (31).

Thermography

Activation of the deep pain system sometimes results in a segmental activation of the autonomic nervous system as manifested by piloerection, sweating, and regional changes in blood flow. Therefore, one might expect to find characteristic changes on thermography, which measures the cutaneous temperature. The studies done to date have shown inconsistent results, with painful areas sometimes corresponding to hot spots (32) and in other instances corresponding to cold spots (8). Simons has suggested that these inconsistencies are explainable by TrPs in different locations having different effects on the sympathetic and parasympathetic nervous system, respectively (33).

Biopsies

Several investigators have biopsied "fibrositic nodules" and in some instances have attempted to compare these tissues with normal muscle, often from the same patient (34–37). The initial biopsy studies from so-called fibrositic nodules were probably performed on patients with what we now call MPS, because it is only recently that the fibromyalgia syndrome has been differentiated from MPS. In general some abnormalities have been found, such as disruption of myofibrillar structure, increased amounts of ground substance, mucopolysaccharides, multifocal loss of selected oxidated enzymes, and occasional "ragged red" fibers suggestive of mitochondrial damage. Although the consensus of these studies is that there is "something wrong with muscle," the changes are nonspecific, inconsistent, and often found in "normal" individuals. A recent study by Larsson et al. documented a decreased level of high-energy phosphates in biopsies taken from the upper part of the trapezius muscle in patients with work-related chronic myalgia with clinical findings suggestive of MPS (38). Because these findings are identical to those observed in patients with FS (39), this abnormality may represent a common denominator between FS and MPS.

Electromyographic Studies

Kellgren initially observed palpable muscle spasm after hypertonic saline injections into interspinous ligaments (23). The "taut band," previously called the "fibrositic nodule," was originally thought to represent muscle spasm, but EMG studies have shown such areas to be electrically silent (40–42). Nevertheless it is a common observation that stimulation of a TrP by needling or by snapping the involved muscle will often cause a transient twitch in more distal muscle fibers (43). Indeed, the localized twitch response has been incorporated into the definition of a TrP (8). Elliott initially reported bursts of motor activity in response to stimulation of TrPs (24). Simons identified active and latent TrPs in the quadriceps, deltoid, and peroneus longus muscles and recorded motor unit action potentials occurring in bursts of 0.2 sec at 500 μV (42). Fricton et al. used a "blinded observer" to compare the EMG response of TrPs in the upper trapezius to the uninvolved contralateral side (40). The muscles harboring TrPs showed significantly higher motor unit action potentials upon snapping than did the normal muscles.

A common problem in patients with MPS is the objective evaluation of the self-reports of limited work capacity. Hagberg and Kvarnstrom performed sophisticated EMG studies on eight men and two women who had been on extended sick leave because of a MPS involving the shoulder girdle apparently related to assembly line work (44). Myoelectric amplitude increase and mean curve frequency decrease were evaluated over time in an endurance test simulating their assembly line activity, with recordings from both the involved trapezius and the uninvolved side. All patients had a shorter duration of endurance on the more painful side. Furthermore, the endurance times was significantly reduced compared to those of healthy volunteers. No increase of motor activity was found on the painful side as compared to the pain-free side; this provided evidence against the old concept that muscle spasm was important in the etiology of these pain syndromes. The endurance time on the painful side was directly related to EMG fatigue changes, implying that the MPS had changed the work capacity of the shoulder muscles rather than invoking an explanation of lack of motivation or pain-related inhibition.

Sleep

Subjects with MPS have not been extensively studied as regards sleep abnormalities. In an analysis of 164 patients with MPSs involving the head and neck, Fricton reported that 42% self-reported poor sleep (45). Saskin et al. reported alpha intrusion into delta sleep in 21 patients with postaccident pain—some of whom probably had MPS involving the shoulder girdle on the basis of whiplash injury (46).

Psychological Studies

In general, it has not been thought that psychological factors are important in the genesis of *simple* MPSs. However, some patients with simple MPS develop more complex pain syndromes with recruitment of TrPs and the later development of pain behavior. Whether these patients represent a distinctive subpopulation that can be identified by appropriate psychometric testing has not been resolved. Fricton, in his study of 164 patients with MPS of the head and neck, noted anxiety, depression, and anger in about 20 to 25% as evaluated by a psychologist and by unspecified psychological testing (45). In a study comparing psychological distress and pain behavior in patients with MPS and low back pain, it was noted that both groups had elevations on the SCL-90R (Symptom Checklist-90, Revised), with high scores measuring somatization, obsessive/compulsive tendencies, depression, anxiety, and hostility (47). No comment was made as to whether these patients had more complex myofascial pain problems. Low back pain patients took more narcotics and sedative-hypnotic medications and showed higher levels of motor pain behavior than those with MPS.

Myoglobinemia

Liberation of myoglobin into the circulation is a characteristic feature of muscle breakdown. Danneskiold-Samsøe found that 21 out of 26 patients given massage therapy for MPS developed a significant increase in their plasma myoglobin with a maximum at 2 hr after the first treatment (48). A positive correlation was found between the amount of myoglobinemia and muscle tension and pain. The five patients who did not develop the myoglobinemia were those who did not benefit from the massage therapy [*Author's note:* These patients may have had FS.]. It was concluded that the myoglobinemia was indicative of damaged muscle fibers, thus providing a clue to a specific pathology.

Naloxone Sensitivity

A recent study described 10 patients with MPS who experienced a decrease in pain with concomitant increase in range of motion after injection of TrPs with 0.25% bupivacaine; these improvements were significantly reversed by intravenous naloxone (10 mg) compared to an intravenous placebo (49). It was suggested that this result implicated an endogenous opioid system as a mediator for the decreased pain and improved physical findings following injection of TrPs with local anesthetic.

FIBROMYALGIA SYNDROME

A generally accepted description of the fibromyalgia syndrome has only evolved over the last decade. Many patients with widespread musculo-skeletal pain and fatigue were formerly categorized as having psychogenic rheumatism or a poorly defined seronegative arthropathy. Most North American rheumatologists have embraced the term "fibrositis" or "fibromyalgia syndrome" to describe the condition of a common group of patients that accounts for about 15 to 30% of their referrals. Herein is a synopsis of the studies that have led to the recognition of an internally consistent syndrome and more recent studies that may provide some clues as to pathogenesis.

Tender Point Studies

The idea that patients with FS had tender areas on palpation that were largely unknown to the patient but were remarkably consistent from patient to patient was due to the anecdotal descriptions provided by Smythe and Moldofsky (9). In the early and mid-1980s Smythe's ideas were put to the test in double-blind controlled trials that confirmed the notion that TePs were a reproducible and internally consistent feature of patients with widespread musculoskeletal pain and fatigue (13,16,22,50–52). The first of these studies, by Yunus et al., convincingly established that FS patients were significantly different from controls as regards the number of TePs identified (16). In a study using a spring-loaded pain gauge (dolorimeter), Campbell et al. identified 22 patients from a general medical clinic who had not been previously diagnosed as having FS and compared them with 22 age- and sex-matched asymptomatic controls (13). The FS patients had a reduced pain tolerance over TeP areas compared to asymptomatic controls, but they did not differ when control points were evaluated.

Wolfe et al. quantitated TePs in all patients attending a private rheumatology clinic and noted that 60% of patients had none, those that had a few tended to have regional pain syndromes, and those that had more than seven often had widespread body pain (53). Bengtsson et al. are the only investigators to have reported on both TePs and TrPs in patients with FS (50). They found that 83.6% of their FS patients had one or more *TrPs*, and that these were more common than TePs. Scudds et al. investigated the type of painful stimuli that were discriminatory between FS patients and normal controls (51); FS patients were only differentiated from controls by a constantly changing pressure (dolorimetry), but were not different as regards the threshold for electrical stimuli or for constant pressure. Sims et al. looked at tenderness in 75 anatomical sites and noted more widespread tenderness than had previously been documented, but they also noted specific control areas where patients and controls did not differ (52).

A recent multicenter study compared patients with FS to controls with other musculoskeletal pain symptoms; this study included a TeP exam and dolorimetry by blinded observers (22). It was found that a history of widespread pain (all four quadrants) *plus* the finding of 11 or more out of 18 specified TePs was highly sensitive (88%) and specific (81%) in distinguishing patients diagnosed as having FS from patients with other musculoskeletal pain syndromes. No difference was noted between patients with primary and secondary FS, and this distinction has now been dropped. (The locations of these 18 TePs are given in Table 2.)

Sleep Disturbance

A major impetus to the scientific study of FS was the observation of Moldofsky et al. that these patients had a disturbance of stage 4 sleep characterized by a superimposition of an alpha rhythm (7.5 to 11 Hz) on the slower delta rhythm (0.5 to 2 Hz) of slow-wave sleep (10). Fibromyalgia syndrome patients have an average of 60% duration of slow-wave sleep occupied by the alpha sleep anomaly; this compares to 25% in normal subjects as well as patients with chronic insomnia or affective disorders. This sleep anomaly is not specific for FS; it has been noted in other patients with chronic pain and was originally described by Hauri and Hawkins in nine psychiatric patients with symptoms of "a general feeling of chronic somatic malaise and fatigue" (54). It is evident that the alpha sleep anomaly is not specific for fibrositis; however, Scheuler et al. found the anomaly in only 15% of healthy individuals with no specific complaints (55). Interestingly, they observed that 20 of 39 healthy individuals from six families had the anomaly and speculated that it may be genetically determined; if so, certain individuals may be constitutionally predisposed to the development of FS.

An important question is whether the sleep anomaly in FS is primary or secondary. Evidence in favor of the former was provided by Moldofsky and Scarisbrick's observation that six asymptomatic sedentary individuals subject to artificial disruption of stage 4 sleep over three consecutive nights developed diffuse aching and fatigue accompanied by increased tenderness over specific TeP areas (56). Interestingly, when the same experiment was performed on three middle-distance runners no deleterious effects were observed even though the same alpha sleep anomaly had been induced. This was the first clue that aerobic fitness may be of relevance to the development of FS (see below). It is apparent that nonrefreshing sleep may be induced by many different events, including primary sleep pathologies such as sleep apnea and nocturnal myoclonus (57,58), noise (59), rheumatoid arthritis (60), osteoarthritis (61), posttraumatic pain (46), and psychological distress (62).

Muscle Biopsies

It is evident from perusal of literature that many of the previous muscle biopsy studies said to be done in "fibrositis" patients were in fact done on patients with MPS. Three groups have reported on FS as currently defined. Kalyan-Raman et al. studied biopsies taken from the left trapezius in 12 right-handed patients with FS (63). The findings on light microscopy were not impressive, consisting of scattered hylanized fibers, occasional split fibers, and an increase in central nuclei in two biopsies. No inflammatory changes were noted. Histochemical staining with modified Gomori-trichrome, ATPase, NADH-tetrazolium reductase alcian blue with periodic acid–Schiff, and adenylate deaminase was normal apart from a "moth-eaten" appearance of some type I fibers in 42% of patients and some type II fiber atrophy in 58%. The finding of a moth-eaten appearance on NADH-tetrazolium reductase staining was also noted by Henriksson et al. in a letter to the *Lancet* (64). Electron microscopic findings in Kalyan-Raman et al.'s series were more frequent with myofibrillar lysis, subsarcolemmal accumulation of glycogen and mitochondria, and papillary projections. In a more recent follow-up study, Yunus et al. noted essentially similar findings in asymptomatic, healthy controls (65).

Bengtsson et al. studied 77 muscle biopsies from 57 patients with FS and compared them with 17 biopsies from nine healthy controls (66). Forty-one of these biopsies were taken from tender areas in the trapezius and compared to ten biopsies from trapezius in healthy controls. Twenty-two percent of the biopsies from FS patients and 10% from controls showed occasional degeneration and regeneration of muscle fibers, and in 7% there were mild inflammatory cell infiltrates. Bengtsson et al. also quantitated capillary density and found no difference between patients and controls. In 15 of the trapezius muscle biopsies from FS patients, as well as in anterior tibialis muscle biopsies, the tissues were analyzed for adenosine triphosphate

(ATP), adenosine diphosphate (ADP), adenosine monophosphate (AMP), and phosphocreatine, lactate, and pyruvate (39). The trapezii muscle of FS patients showed a significant decrease in high-energy phosphates (ATP, ADP, and phosphocreatine) compared to both the control group and the anterior tibialis biopsies of the same FS patients. It was hypothesized that these changes were due to local hypoxia and that this may be a significant feature in the pathogenesis of FS. Mathur and Gatter, using ^{31}P nuclear magnetic resonance spectroscopy, also found low levels of high-energy phosphates in flexor forearm muscles from five out of six patients with FS as compared to 22 normal controls (67). Bartels and Danneskiold-Samsøe examined the quadriceps muscle in 13 patients with "fibrositis" using a special fixation technique with examination under inverted microscope (68); the muscle fibers of patients with "fibrositis" were connected by a network of elastic fibers that were not seen in seven healthy controls. It was suggested that these fibers, by causing distortion of the microvasculature during muscle contraction, could contribute to local microvascular abnormalities in patients with FS.

Muscle Blood Flow and Oxygenation

Lund et al. used a multipoint oxygen electrode to construct histograms of oxygen pressures in the trapezius and brachioradialis muscles in patients with FS as compared with healthy controls (69). The results of this study are summarized in Table 4; it can be seen that FS patients had abnormal histograms. The oxygen electrode produces a "map" of oxygen pressures in the form of a histogram; these findings were interpreted as showing possible defects in the microcirculation in the area of fibrositis TePs. The concept that "fibrositis" symptoms, as well as those of MPS, might be due to localized muscle spasm resulting in ischemia and the accumulation of lactic acid and other waste products has often been proposed. An attempt to measure muscle blood flow in fibrositis muscles using ^{133}Xe did not show any abnormality (70). A more recent study looking at *exercising* muscle blood flow in FS, with the ^{133}Xe clearance method, did show a significantly reduced blood flow in the anterior tibialis muscle (71). Whether this finding was

TABLE 4. *Oxygen pressures using a multipoint oxygen electrode*

Tissue ( )	Number studied (FS/controls)	Number abnormal (FS/controls)
Subcutaneous tissue over trapezius	7/6	2/1
Trapezius muscle	10/8	10/0
Brachioradialis muscle	4/5	4/1

From Lund et al., ref. 69, with permission.

related to a specific tissue abnormality or was related to "detraining" is purely conjectural. The idea that FS pain is the result of muscle spasm and local hypoxia is not supported by the EMG findings or the biochemical findings of normal levels of lactate.

Electromyographic Findings

Two issues concerning FS have been addressed by electromyography: (a) Is there evidence of localized muscle spasm accounting for FS symptoms? and (b) Can the subjective weakness and apparent weakness on neuromuscular testing be objectively quantified by measuring the force generated in the adductor pollicis brevis following electrical stimulation? Kraft et al. initially reported that the resting muscles of patients with fibrositis were electrically silent (41). This was corroborated in a study by Bengtsson et al. (50). In the same paper, Bengtsson et al. documented that the force attained in the electrically stimulated adductor pollicis of FS patients was identical to that in healthy controls. In a similar vein, Stokes et al. noted similar findings of normal muscular strength on electrical stimulation of the adductor pollicis in 20 patients with "effort syndromes" compared to 20 controls—many of the patients whom they described had prominent fatigability and musculoskeletal pain and probably had FS (72). These findings suggest a normal contractility of skeletal muscle and imply that the impaired performance during voluntary activity is due to a central mechanism, possibly lack of motivation, pain, or fear of pain—or in rare cases reflex inhibition due to afferent activity in relatively asymptomatic arthropathy.

Physical Fitness

Most patients with FS exercise very little, possibly because of the perception that exertion worsens their pain or possibly because of fatigue. They perceive themselves to be weak and perform poorly on muscle testing (50,72–74). The early work of Moldofsky et al. indicated that very fit subjects seemed relatively resistant to the effect of an experimentally induced alpha sleep anomaly (56), and more recently McCain provided evidence that improving aerobic conditioning is an important adjunct in the management of FS patients (75). In a recent study, aerobic fitness was evaluated in 25 women with FS who were exercised to volitional exhaustion on an electronically braked cycle ergometer (71). They were compared to age-, sex-, and weight-matched sedentary controls. Based on their maximum oxygen uptake at exhaustion, 84% of the FS patients were below average in physical fitness. Interestingly, they did not overrate their level of physical exertion, and measurement of their respiratory quotient and ventilatory threshold based on respiratory gas exchange did not support the generation of a generalized lactic acidosis. It was concluded that FS patients are commonly aerobically unfit and that a "detraining phenomenon" may be of relevance to some of the symptomatology.

Psychometric Tests

Prior to the 1980s many patients who are now diagnosed as having FS were thought to have "psychogenic rheumatism" (76–79). Exactly what was meant by psychogenic rheumatism was never really defined: was it thought that these patients were imagining their pain, were they reacting to minimal discomfort in an inappropriate fashion, or was their psychological status predisposing them to a chronic pain syndrome? One study examined patients with fibromyalgia symptoms and TePs drawn from a general medical clinic and found no difference from matched controls on the SCL-90R, Beck Depression Inventory, and State and Trait Anxiety Score (80). In contradistinction, in another study 30 patients with FS admitted to hospital for management were compared to 30 patients with "mixed arthritis" and 30 with rheumatoid arthritis (81). On Minnesota Multiphasic Personality Inventory (MMPI) testing *all* patients had abnormalities on the hypochondriasis and hysteria scales, although the mean scale for depression did not differ in FS and rheumatoid arthritis patients. In studies drawn from patients seen in a rheumatology practice, Ahles et al. (82) and Wolfe et al. (83) found that approximately 30% of patients with FS had elevations of the hypochondriasis and hysteria scales on the MMPI. Smythe critiqued these findings and noted that many of the MMPI questions are concerned with pain and somatic symptoms and will be positive in any chronic pain condition (84).

Hudson et al. compared 31 FS patients with 14 rheumatoid arthritis patients using the Diagnostic Interview Schedule, which generates current and past diagnoses according the the *Diagnostic and Statistical Manual* (third edition) (DSM-III) criteria (85); 71% of FS patients, compared with 30% of rheumatoid patients and 12% of a normal control group, had a lifetime history of major depression. However, in only 26% of FS patients was depression present concurrently. In the same study, the Hamilton Rating Scale for depression was used to assess the degree of affective symptoms; a mean score on this study was 13.1 in FS and 7.3 in rheumatoid arthritis. These results were interpreted as indicating a psychobiological link between depression and FS, but the lack of concordance was not consistent with a causal relationship. In contradistinction, Kirmayer et al. used a similar diagnostic interview schedule and found a 20% prevalence of depressive illness in FS, compared to 8.7% in patients with rheumatoid arthritis; these figures were not statistically significant (86).

It would appear that the final answer is not yet in on the association of

22. Wolfe F, Smythe HA, Yunus MB, Bennett RM. *Arthritis Rheum* 1989;33:160–172.
23. Kellgren JH. *Clin Sci* 1938;3:175–190.
24. Elliott FA. *Lancet* 1944;1:47–49.
25. Hockaday JM, Whitty CWM. *Brain* 1967;90:481–496.
26. Fock S, Mense S. *Brain Res* 1976;105:459–469.
27. Sola AE, Rodenberger ML, Gettys BB. *Am J Phys Med* 1955;34:585–590.
28. Fischer AA. *Arch Phys Med Rehabil* 1986;67:406–409.
29. Reeves JL, Jaeger B, Graff-Radford SB. *Pain* 1986;24:313–321.
30. Fischer AA. *Clin J Pain* 1987;2:207.
31. Fischer AA. *Arch Phys Med Rehabil* 1987;68:122–125.
32. Fischer AA. *Clin Proceed Postgrad Med* 1986;99.
33. Simons DG. *Myofascial pain syndrome due to trigger points.* International Rehabilitation Medicine Association Monograph Series, no 1. Rademaker, OH: International Rehabilitation Medicine Association, 1987.
34. Awad EA. *Arch Phys Med* 1973;54:449–452.
35. Brendstrup P, Jespersen K, Asboe-Hansen G. *Ann Rheum Dis* 1957;16:438–440.
36. Glogowski G, Wallraff J. *Z Orthop* 1951;80:237–268.
37. Miehlke K, Schulze G, Eger W. *Z Rheumaforsch* 1960;19:310–330.
38. Larsson SE, Bengtsson A, Bodegard L, Henriksson KG, Larsson J. *Acta Orthop Scand* 1988;59:74–78.
39. Bengtsson A, Henriksson KG, Larsson J. *Arthritis Rheum* 1986;29:817–821.
40. Fricton JR, Auvinen MD, Dykstra D, Schiffrman E. *Arch Phys Med Rehabil* 1985;66:314–317.
41. Kraft GH, Johnson EW, LeBan MM. *Arch Phys Med Rehabil* 1968;49:155–162.
48. Simons DG. In: Bonica JJ, Albe-Fessard D, eds. *Advances in pain research and therapy,* vol 1. New York: Raven Press, 1976;913–919.
43. Dexter JR, Simons DG. *Arch Phys Med Rehabil* 1981;62:521.
44. Hagberg M, Kvarnstrom S. *Arch Phys Med Rehabil* 1984;65:522–525.
45. Fricton JR, Kroening R, Haley D, Siegart R. *Oral Surg* 1985;60:615–623.
46. Saskin P, Moldofsky H, Lue FA. *Psychosom Med* 1986;48:319–323.
47. Keefe FJ, Dolan E. *Pain* 1986;24:409.
48. Danneskiold-Samsøe B, Christiansen E, Anderson RB. *Scand J Rheum* 1986;15:154–178.
49. Fine PG, Milano R, Hard BD. *Pain* 1988;32:15–20.
50. Bengtsson A, Henriksson KG, Jorfeldt L, Kagedal B, Lennmarken C, Lindstrom F. *Scand J Rheumatol* 1986;15:340–347.
51. Scudds RA, Rollman GB, Harth M, McCain GA. *J Rheumatol* 1987;14:563–569.
52. Simms RW, Goldenberg DL, Felson DT, Mason JH. *Arthritis Rheum* 1988;31:182–187.
53. Wolfe F, Cathey MA. *J Rheumatol* 1985;12:1164–1168.
54. Hauri P, Hawkins DR. *Electroencephalogr Clin Neurophysiol* 1973;34:233–237.
55. Scheuler W, Kubicki S, Marquardt J. In: Koella WP, Obal F, Schulz H, et al. (eds). *Sleep '86.* Stuttgart: Gustav Fischer Verlag, 1988.
56. Moldofsky H, Scarisbrick P. *Psychosom Med* 1976;38:35–44.
57. Moldofsky H, Tullis C, Lue FA, Quance G, Davidson J. *Psychosom Med* 1984;46:145–151.
58. Molony RR, MacPeek DM, Schiffman PL, Frank M, Neubauer JA, Schwartzberg M, Seibold JR. *J Rheumatol* 1986;13:797–800.
59. Tarnapolsky A, Watkin G, Hand DJ. *Psychol Med* 1980;10:683–698.
60. Moldofsky H, Lue FA, Smythe HA. *J Rheumatol* 1983;10:373–379.
61. Moldofsky H, Lue FA, Saskin P. *J Rheumatol* 1987;14:124–128.
62. Lavie P, Hefez A, Halperin G. *Am J Psychiatry* 1979;136:175–178.
63. Kalyan-Raman UP, Kalyan-Raman K, Ynus MB, Masi AT. *J Rheumatol* 1984;11:808–813.
64. Henriksson KG, Bengtsson A, Larsson J, Lindstrom F, Thornell LE. *Lancet* 1982;2:1395 (letter).
65. Yunus MD, Kalyan-Raman UP, Masi AT, Aldag JC. *J Rheumatol* 1989;16:97–101.
66. Bengtsson A, Henriksson KG, Larsson J. *Scand J Rheumatol* 1986;15:1–6.
67. Mathur AK, Gatter RA. *Arthritis Rheum* 1988;31:S23.
68. Bartels EM, Danneskiold-Samsøe B. *Lancet* 1986;1:755–757.

69. Lund N, Bengtsson A, Thorborg P. *Scand J Rheumatol* 1986;15:165–173.
70. Klemp P, Nielsen HV, Korsgard J. *Scand J Rehabil Med* 1982;14:81–86.
71. Bennet RM, Clark SR, Goldberg L. *Arthritis Rheum* 1989;32:454–460.
72. Stokes MJ, Cooper RG, Edwards RHT. *Br Med J* 1988;297:1014–1016.
73. Cathey MA, Wolfe F, Kleinheksel SM. *Arthritis Care Res* 1988;1:485–498.
74. Jacobsen S, Danneskiold-Samsøe B. *Scand J Rheumatol* 1987;16:61–65.
75. McCain GA. *Am J Med* 1986;81:73–77.
76. Beetham WP Jr. *Med Clin North Am* 1979;63:433–439.
77. Boland EW. *Ann Rheum Dis* 1947;6:195–203.
78. Rotes-Querol J. *Clin Rheum Dis* 1979;5:797–805.
79. Weinberger LM. *West J Med* 1981;135:425–426 (letter).
80. Clark S, Campbell SM, Forehand ME, Tindall EA, Bennett RM. *Arthritis Rheum* 1985;28:132–137.
81. Payne TC, Leavitt F, Garron DC, Katz RS, Golden HE, Glickman PB, Vanderplate C. *Arthritis Rheum* 1982;25:213–217.
82. Ahles TA, Yunus MB, Riley SD, Bradley JM, Masi AT. *Arthritis Rheum* 1984;27:1101–1106.
83. Wolfe F, Cathey MA, Kleinheksel SM, Amos SP, Hoffman RG, Young DY, Hawley DJ. *J Rheumatol* 1984;11:500–506.
84. Smythe HA. *J Rheumatol* 1984;11:417–418.
85. Hudson JI, Hudson MS, Pliner LF, Goldenberg DL, Pope HG Jr. *Am J Psychiatry* 1985;142:441–446.
86. Kirmayer LJ, Robbins JM, Kapusta MA. *Am J Psychiatry* 1988;145:950–954.
87. McCain GA. *Rheum Dis Clin North Am* 1989;15:73–90.
88. Vaeroy H, Helle R, Forre O. *Pain* 1988;32:21–26.
89. Vaeroy H, Helle R, Frre O, Kass E, Terenius L. *J Rheumatol* 1988;15:1804–1806.
90. Yunus MB, Denko CW, Masi AT. *J Rheumatol* 1986;13:183–186.
91. Dinerman H, Goldenberg DL, Felson DT. *J Rheumatol* 1986;13:368–373.
92. Ingram S, Nelson D, Porter , Bennett RM. *Arthritis Rheum* 1987;30:513.
93. Russell IJ, Vipraio GA, Morgan WW, Bowden CL. *Am J Med* 1986;81:50–54.
94. Bengtsson A, Bengtsson M. *Pain* 1988;33:161–167.
95. Moldofsky H. *Rheum Dis Clin North Am* 1989;15:91–103.
96. Buchwald D, Goldenberg DL, Sullivan JL, Komaroff AL. *Arthritis Rheum* 1987;30:1132–1136.
97. Moldofsky H, Saskin P, Salem L. *Sleep Res* 1987;16:492.
98. Armstrong RB. *Med Sci Sports Exerc* 1984;16:529–538.
99. Hough T. *Am J Physical* 1902;7:76–92.
100. Newham DJ. *Eur J Appl Physiol* 1988;57:353–359.
100a. McCully KK, Argor Z, Boden RP, Brown RL, Rank WJ, Chance B. *Muscle Neurol* 1988;11:212–216.
101. O'Reilly KP, Warhol MJ, Fielding RA. *J Appl Physiol* 1987;63:252–256.
102. Newham DJ, Jones DA, Edwards RHT. *Muscle Nerve* 1986;9:59–63.
103. Newham DJ, Jones DA, Tolfree SEJ, Edwards RHT. *Eur J Appl Physiol* 1986;55:106–112.
104. Friden J, Seger J, Ekblom B. *Eur J Appl Physiol* 1988;57:360–368.
105. Friden J, Sjostrom M, Ekblom B. *Experientia* 1981;37:506–507.
106. Littlejohn GO. *Rheum Dis Clin North Am* 1989;15:45–60.
107. Bennett RM. *Am J Med* 1986;81:15–18.

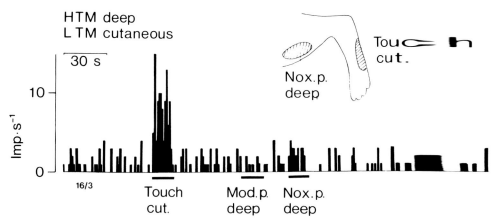

FIG. 8. Discharges of a convergent dorsal horn neuron with input from both skin and deep tissues. The cell could be activated by touching the skin (Touch cut.) of the left hindpaw and by squeezing the anterior tibial muscle (Nox. p. deep) (see *inset*). There was no response to pinching the skin overlying the anterior tibial muscle. Innocuous stimulation of the deep receptive field (Mod. p. deep) was without effect. The *bars* underneath the histogram mark the time and duration of mechanical stimulation. (Data from Hoheisel and Mense, unpublished.)

vergent input from deep tissues and skin (Fig. 8), but there were also cells that were responsive only to stimulation of skeletal muscle. (It must be kept in mind, however, that in such experiments an additional input from viscera is difficult to exclude.) A conspicuous feature of many of the neurons with deep input was the multiplicity of receptive fields, with some cells having up to four fields with LTM or HTM characteristics in deep tissues and skin (Table 1).

Dorsal horn neurons receiving input from skeletal muscle are known to be subject to a strong descending inhibition (25) and therefore can be more effectively activated by stimulation of muscle receptors after the descending pathways have been blocked by cooling of the spinal cord rostral to the recording site (Table 1). A more recent finding is that in convergent cells the deep input is more strongly inhibited by supraspinal centers than is the cutaneous input to the same cell (Fig. 9), and that the descending inhibition has a stronger effect on the HTM than on the LTM input from deep tissues. These tonic inhibitory influences are likely to suppress a great deal of the nociceptive information from skeletal muscle.

Dorsal horn neurons with deep input are modulated not only by descending pathways but also by alterations of their receptive fields. Thus it is possible to change the responsiveness of a cell to stimulation of one of its receptive fields by noxious stimulation of another field (26). An example of such a behavior is shown in Fig. 10. Initially, the neuron had three receptive fields,

TABLE 1. *Receptive field properties of cat dorsal horn neurons with deep input*[a]

| | Number of neurons | | | |
| | Spinal cord intact | | Spinal cord cooled | |
Response types (deep input/cutaneous input)	All deep tissues	Muscle	All deep tissues	Muscle
LTM	4	3	7	4
HTM	10	0	2	0
LTM, LTM	1	1	—	—
HTM, LTM	—	—	2	1
LTM /LTM	12	10	2	2
LTM /HTM	4	4	4	4
HTM /HTM	7	2	2	0
HTM /LTM	10	6	7	4
LTM /LTM, HTM	—	—	1	1
HTM /HTM, LTM	—	—	3	1
HTM /LTM, LTM	1	1	—	—
LTM, LTM/LTM	3	3	1	1
HTM, HTM/LTM	—	—	1	1
HTM, HTM/HTM	—	—	2	2
HTM, LTM/HTM	—	—	4	2
HTM, HTM/LTM, HTM	—	—	1	1
TOTAL	52	30	39	24

Data from Hoheisel and Mense (unpublished).

[a] Fifty-two cells were recorded in animals with intact neuraxes ("spinal cord intact"), and 39 cells were recorded during cooling of the spinal cord in order to block the descending inhibition ("spinal cord cooled"). The "muscle" columns are a subpopulation of the columns labeled "all deep tissues." Without spinal block, 15 of 52 cells had deep input only. The majority of these (10 cells) had HTM characteristics, but cells with exclusive HTM input from muscle were not found. The main effect of the spinal block was an increase in the proportion of neurons having multiple receptive fields in deep tissues (lower third of the table).

one in the posterior biceps muscle, another in the deep tissues of the paw, and a third in the skin of the fifth toe. All had a high mechanical threshold. Five minutes after infiltration of the receptive field in the biceps muscle with a painful dose of bradykinin, the mechanical threshold of the injected receptive field had dropped into the innocuous range and a new receptive field had appeared in the deep tissue of the fourth toe. These alterations persisted for the rest of the recording period (up to 40 min following the bradykinin injection).

These results demonstrate that the sensitivity of dorsal horn cells, which are probably involved in the mediation of deep pain, is not constant but rather subject to multifold modulatory influences. It is conceivable that under pathological conditions—which may affect the receptive fields in the periphery or the descending antinociceptive system—the excitability of the neurons is enhanced for long periods of time.

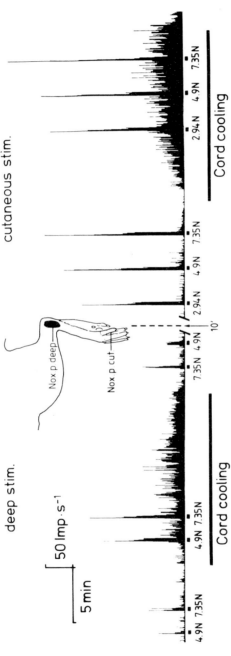

FIG. 9. Differential effect of the descending inhibition on the responses of a convergent neuron to deep and cutaneous stimulation. The cell had two receptive fields, one in the deep tissues of the ankle joint (*black*) and one in the skin of the fifth toe (*hatched*). Both had a high mechanical threshold and could be activated by noxious pressure (Nox. p.) only. Mechanical stimulation was performed with a stimulating apparatus; the applied force is given in Newtons (N). The long bars underneath the histogram of the cell's activity mark the periods of cooling of the spinal cord rostral to the recording site in order to block the descending inhibition. The cord block was followed by an increase in resting discharge and a marked enhancement of the response to stimulation of the deep receptive field (*left half* of histogram), while the reaction to cutaneous stimulation increased only slightly (*right half*) (Data from Yu and Mense, unpublished.)

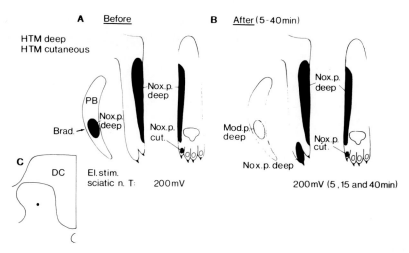

FIG. 10. Appearance of a new receptive field following noxious stimulation of skeletal muscle. Convergent dorsal horn neuron with three receptive fields in locations as indicated in **A.** All required noxious intensities of local pressure (Nox. p.) for activation. Five minutes after injection of a painful dose of bradykinin into the receptive field in the posterior biceps (PB) muscle the mechanical threshold of the injected field had dropped to innocuous levels and a new receptive field with a high threshold had appeared in the deep tissues of the fourth toe **(B).** The effect lasted for more than 40 min, at which time the recording of the cell's activity was discontinued. **C:** Location of the recording site in the dorsal horn (DC, dorsal columns). (From Hoheisel and Mense, ref. 26, with permission.)

DISCUSSION

The results of these experiments support the view that muscle pain is elicited by activation of specialized nociceptors that are connected to thin-myeli-nated and nonmyelinated afferent fibers. The nociceptors in muscle resemble those in the skin in that they have a high mechanical threshold and can be activated by chemical agents that are known to elicit pain in conscious human beings. Among these nociceptors, specialized subtypes possibly exist, such as those that respond to ischemic contractions. Although many groups III and IV muscle receptors are sensitive to a broad range of mechanical and chemical stimuli, they are probably not polymodal. The polymodality con-cept as applied to muscle receptors (14) implies that all free nerve endings belong to a single functional population that has a certain biological scatter in mechanical threshold and chemical sensitivity. According to this concept a low discharge frequency of the whole population encodes the presence of an innocuous stimulus and a high discharge rate encodes that of a noxious stimulus.

Part of the visceral receptors with slowly conducting afferent fibers appear to have such a response behavior (27), but in some areas, such as the biliary system, examples of specific nociceptors have been found (28). Therefore, it is still an open question whether visceral pain is encoded by a high discharge frequency in nonspecialized visceral afferent units or by recruitment of specific nociceptors.

The bulk of the data on receptors in skeletal muscle speaks in favor of the assumption that muscle pain is mediated by specific nociceptors. In contrast to afferent units from the viscera, where receptors with a high mechanical threshold are rare, many of the muscle receptors had a threshold in the noxious range and did not respond to physiological stimuli such as innocuous kneading or stretch. Experiments in which the reactions of groups III and IV muscle receptors to muscle contractions with and without ischemia were studied (15) have shown that there are two qualitatively different sets of receptors that are activated under these conditions. One responds to the mechanical force of the contraction irrespective of the blood supply, and the other only to ischemic contractions.

A further finding supporting the contention that the putative nociceptors are functionally distinct from the LTM receptors with slowly conducting fibers is their different termination in the spinal dorsal horn. In a study employing intraaxonal injections of a tracer into single identified fibers, the HTM (presumably nociceptive) units were found to have heavy projections to the marginal zone (lamina I), whereas the LTM afferent units lacked these terminations (29).

The excitability of the muscle nociceptors is not fixed but can be easily modulated. All patho (physio) logical alterations of the muscle tissue are likely to release endogenous sensitizing agents such as bradykinin, serotonin, and prostaglandins (PGs) of the E type. These substances are capable of lowering the mechanical threshold of nociceptors into the innocuous range. This mechanism is the most likely explanation for the tenderness of an inflamed or otherwise lesioned muscle.

It must be kept in mind that the change in the biochemical environment of the nociceptive endings can be very complex depending on the nature of the lesion. Therefore, certain combinations of chemical substances may be more effective than others. For instance, because of the potentiating action of PGE_2 on the stimulating effects of bradykinin on muscle receptors (17), a release of bradykinin together with PGE_2 will have a particularly strong sensitizing and exciting action on receptive nerve endings, whereas LTD_4 may counteract this effect. On the basis of these findings the analgesic action of acetylsalicylic acid (ASA) and other drugs that inhibit PG synthesis can be explained by the abolition of the PG-induced sensitization of nociceptors (30). An additional factor may be that the ASA-induced block of cyclooxygenase increases the substrate supply to the lipoxygenase, which may synthesize larger amounts of desensitizing LTs under these conditions. This mechanism has been considered to contribute to the analgesic action of ASA (31).

It is likely that in addition to the substances mentioned above, many more agents with as yet unknown actions may be released in pathologically altered muscle. A particularly interesting group of agents are the neuropeptides, of which calcitonin gene-related peptide (CGRP), cholecystokinin, and substance P have been shown to occur in muscle afferent fibers (32). CGRP is one of the most potent vasodilators and thus could contribute to the vascular changes during inflammation (33).

In inflamed muscle, the increase in resting activity was found to be greatest in group III receptors, while the drop in mechanical threshold was most significant in group IV endings. Thus the spontaneous inflammatory pain, which is most likely elicited by an increased activity in nociceptive afferent fibers, may be mediated predominantly by group III units, whereas the tenderness, which is probably caused by a sensitization of nociceptive receptors, may be due to activity in group IV fibers. At present, no neurophysiological explanation can be given for the sensations of weakness that are a frequent symptom of myositis (34). A speculative mechanism would be that the myositis-induced reduction in the activity of gamma motoneurons (35) leads to a decrease in afferent activity from muscle spindle primary endings, which results in a reduction of the predepolarization (or hyperpolarization) of alpha motoneurons. The hyperpolarized cells require a stronger central nervous effort to be excited, which might be felt as weakness.

At the spinal cord level, there exists a small but distinct population of dorsal horn cells that process information from muscle receptors only. However, neurons with exclusive HTM input from muscle were not found (Table 1). Apparently, muscle pain is transmitted together with other forms of deep pain by HTM neurons or together with cutaneous information by convergent neurons. The information from visceral afferents has been reported to be similarly processed by viscerosomatic (convergent) cells, but in contrast to the cells with deep input all the visceral neurons were convergent (i.e., apparently there are no dorsal horn neurons that receive visceral input exclusively) (36).

Some of the clinical characteristics of muscle pain can be explained by neurophysiological and neuroanatomical data. The diffuse nature of muscle pain may be due to the fact that the afferent fibers from a given muscle are distributed to many spinal segments (37), which makes the localization of the pain difficult. The multiplicity of the receptive fields of many dorsal horn neurons with deep input may add to this effect and could form the basis of the spread or referral of deep pain to other deep tissues. As with visceral pain, the conspicuous convergence of input from muscle and skin onto the same cell may be the neurophysiological correlate for the referral of deep pain to the skin (38,39).

The stronger descending inhibition of the deep input in convergent neurons may be an additional factor that contributes to the poor localization of muscle pain. The descending inhibition was particularly prominent in HTM (presumably nociceptive) neurons. This is a clear difference from cells processing nociceptive input from the skin, which are less influenced by the antinociceptive system than are the multireceptive (or wide dynamic range) cells (for a review, see ref. 40).

As shown in Fig. 10, the responsiveness of some of the neurons with multiple deep receptive fields could be altered for prolonged periods of time by stimulating one of these fields. The alteration usually consisted in a lowering in threshold of the nonstimulated field(s) or in the appearance of a new field. It is conceivable that the symptoms of referred deep tenderness and referral to the skin, respectively, may be related to these events (38).

These examples of an enhanced responsiveness of dorsal horn neurons probably reflect changes at the spinal cord level that lead to an increased excitability of the cells. The changes lasted for more than half an hour after a short stimulation of one receptive field, and there is evidence that strong trauma or surgical operations are highly effective in inducing such long-lasting changes in central excitability (26). Therefore, it is likely that patients with afflictions of deep tissues experience deep pain not only because of the peripheral lesion but also because the spinal neurons develop an increased excitability. The mechanisms underlying this phenomenon are unknown; a speculative explanation would be that the noxious input releases neuropeptides in the dorsal horn that influence spinal neurons (41).

CONCLUSIONS

In conclusion, the presented data demonstrate that the neurons that mediate pain from skeletal muscle and other deep tissues do not form a circuit with fixed transmission properties but are subject to strong modulatory influences. The nociceptive endings in skeletal muscle can be sensitized very easily by endogenous substances, and the excitability of dorsal horn neurons is dependent on at least two factors: activity in descending inhibitory pathways and alterations of their receptive fields.

It must be emphasized that many problems related to muscle pain are still far from being solved. One of these problems is the development of painful muscle spasms; another is the possible relevance of efferent sympathetic activity. The old concept that muscle spasms are due to a reflex activation of gamma motoneurons following a deep lesion has not been supported by the results of recent animal experiments (35), and the importance of sympathetic activity for muscle pain is not understood at all. Possibly, the "normal" animal models used are not suitable for studying these questions and must be replaced by pathological ones that show tissue alterations similar to those of patients suffering from muscle pain.

REFERENCES

1. Travell JG, Simons DG. *Myofascial pain and dysfunction: The trigger point manual.* Baltimore: Williams & Wilkins, 1983.

2. Burgess PR, Perl ER. In: Iggo A, ed. *Handbook of sensory physiology,* Vol II. Heidelberg: Springer, 1973;29–78.
3. Lloyd DPC. *J Neurophysiol* 1943;6:293–315.
4. Paintal AS. *J Physiol (Lond)* 1967;193:523–533.
5. Barker D. In: Hunt CC, ed. *Handbook of sensory physiology,* Vol III/2. Heidelberg: Springer, 1974;1–190.
6. Matthews PBC. *Mammalian muscle receptors and their central actions.* London: Arnold, 1972.
7. Mense S, Meyer H. *J Physiol (Lond)* 1985;363:403–417.
8. Mense S. *Progr Sens Physiol* 1986;6:139–219.
9. Stacey MJ. *J Anat* 1969;105:231–254.
10. Andres KH, Düring M von, Schmidt RF. *Anat Embryol* 1985;172:145–156.
11. Iggo A. *J Physiol (Lond)* 1961;155:52–53P.
12. Mense S, Schmidt RF. *Brain Res* 1974;72:305–310.
13. Paintal AS. *J Physiol (Lond)* 1960;152:250–270.
14. Kumazawa T, Mizumura K. *Brain Res* 1976;101:589–593.
15. Mense S, Stahnke M. *J Physiol (Lond)* 1983;342:383–397.
16. Mense S, Meyer H. *J Physiol (Lond)* 1988;398:49–63.
17. Mense S. *Brain Res* 1981;225:95–105.
18. Piper PJ. *Trends Pharmacol Sci* 1983;4:75–77.
19. Roberts WJ, Elardo SM. *Somatosens Res* 1985;3:33–44.
20. Di Rosa M, Giroud JP, Willoughby DA. *J Pathol* 1971;104:15–29.
21. Berberich P, Hoheisel U, Mense S. *J Neurophysiol* 1988;59:1395–1409.
22. Hoheisel U, Mense S. *Pflügers Arch* 1987;408(suppl 1):R55.
23. Schaible H-G, Schmidt RF, Willis WD. *Exp Brain Res* 1987;66:479–488.
24. Sessle BJ, Hu JW, Amano N, Zhong G. *Pain* 1986;27:219–235.
25. Hong SK, Kniffki K-D, Mense S, Schmidt RF, Wendisch M. *J Physiol (Lond)* 1979;290:129–140.
26. Hoheisel U, Mense S. *Pain* 1989;36:239–247.
27. Jänig W. *Eur J Anaesthesiol* 1985;2:319–346.
28. Cervero F. *Pain* 1982;13:137–151.
29. Hoheisel U, Lehmann-Willenbrock E, Mense S. *Neuroscience* 1989;28:495–507.
30. Ferreira SH, Moncada S, Vane JR. *Br J Pharmacol* 1973;49:86–97.
31. Schweizer A, Brom R, Glatt M, Bray MA. *Eur J Pharmacol* 1984;105:105–112.
32. Molander C, Ygge J, Dalsgaard C-J. *Neurosci Lett* 1987;74:37–42.
33. Gamse R, Posch M, Saria A, Jancsó G. *Acta Physiol Hung* 1987;69:343–354.
34. DeVere R, Bradley WG. *Brain* 1975;98:637–666.
35. Berberich P, Hoheisel U, Mense S, Skeppar P. In: Schmidt RF, ed. *Pain and afferent fibers.* Weinheim: VCH Verlagsgesellschaft 1987;165–175.
36. Tattersall JEH, Cervero F, Lumb BM. *J Neurophysiol* 1986;56:785–796.
37. Mense S, Craig AD. *Neuroscience* 1988;26:1023–1035.
38. Hockaday JM, Whitty CWM. *Brain* 1967;90:481–496.
39. Lewis T. *Pain.* (facsimile ed). London: Macmillan, 1981.
40. Iggo A, Steedman WM, Fleetwood-Walker S. *Philos Trans R Soc Lond* [B] 1985;308:235–252.
41. Hunt SP, Rossi J. *Philos Trans R Soc Lond* [B] 1985;308:283–289.

Advances in Pain Research and Therapy, Vol. 17,
edited by James R. Fricton and Essam Awad.
Raven Press, Ltd., New York © 1990.

4

Central Nervous System Mechanisms of Muscular Pain

Barry J. Sessle

Faculty of Dentistry, University of Toronto, Toronto, Ontario, Canada M5G 1G6

Most of the recent focus on central neural mechanisms underlying pain has centered on the processing of nociceptive information from superficial tissues such as skin and, in the trigeminal (Vth cranial nerve) system, the tooth pulp. Yet, except perhaps for toothache, deep pain is more commonly encountered in clinical situations than superficial pain. However, the lack of understanding of the neural mechanisms involved in pain from deep structures has led to much speculation about mechanisms related to diagnosis, therapy, and etiology and pathogenesis of pain disorders affecting deep structures. In the craniofacial region, for example, probably no dental subject generates so much controversy as the temporomandibular/temporomandibular joint/myofascial pain dysfunction syndromes, and the amount of literature on the topic each year seems to be matched only by the number of concepts and therapies advocated for the clinical management of these conditions.

Fortunately, there have been a few recent electrophysiological studies that have shed some light on the mechanisms underlying deep pain in the craniofacial region and elsewhere in the body. Some recent reviews have also appeared to which the reader is referred (1–4) to obtain an excellent background and the recent advances in knowledge of this subject. It is to be noted, however, that these reviews have focused almost exclusively on processing of deep nociceptive information in the spinal somatosensory system. Therefore, in addition to reviewing spinal mechanisms of muscle pain, a major aim of this chapter is to outline recent advances in our knowledge of primary afferent and especially central neural processes involved in pain from the craniofacial musculature. Given the frequently close clinical association of pain of the masticatory muscles with that from the temporomandibular joint (TMJ), I will also review the literature related to processing of nociceptive information from the TMJ.

PRIMARY AFFERENT MECHANISMS

Dr. Mense, in Chapter 3 (*this volume*) outlines the properties of the receptors and their associated primary afferent fibers that respond to noxious stimulation of muscle. I shall highlight some of the major features of these properties so as to put into proper perspective the properties of the central neurons receiving these afferent inputs. The early studies in this area established that some group III and IV muscle afferents could be activated by mechanical, thermal, and chemical stimuli in the noxious range (5–7). More recent studies have also established that some of these afferents show (a) progressive increase in activity with graded noxious stimuli of increasing intensity; (b) changes in activity as a result of the injection of inflammatory agents into the muscle; (c) sensitization, in that their thresholds to mechanical stimulation, for example, can be lowered by the local application of the algesic chemical bradykinin; (d) marked activation during ischemic contraction of the muscle they innervate; and (e) depression of their response to stimuli such as bradykinin by peripherally acting analgesics (e.g., acetylsalicylic acid) (2,3) (see Chapter 3, *this volume*). These response properties, thus, suggest peripheral mechanisms that may contribute to (a) the coding of the intensity of muscle pain, (b) the hyperalgesia and allodynia that may occur in an inflamed or traumatized muscle, (c) the intense pain that earmarks a contracting muscle deprived of its blood supply, and (d) the relief of muscle pain that aspirin often affords. It is also noteworthy that group III and IV primary afferents innervating limb joints also show many of these properties (e.g., sensitization and decreased threshold for activation after the injection of an inflammatory agent into the articular tissues) (2,3,8). A similar enhancement of the responsivity of joint afferents so that they become responsive to even gentle, innocuous movements has also been described in animals with an experimentally induced arthritis (2). Mense and Guilbaud and their colleagues have suggested that such sensitization of articular receptors might account for the spontaneous pain and movement-induced pain that characterize a traumatized or inflamed joint.

Groups III and IV as well as larger, faster conducting afferents supply the craniofacial musculature and the TMJ, and free nerve endings as well as more complex receptors have been found in these tissues (9,10). Only a few studies have attempted electrophysiological recordings of single afferents supplying these deep tissues, and these have focused on the larger diameter nonnociceptive afferents. There is virtually no information about the physiological properties of afferent units that are clearly nociceptive. Such afferents presumably exist in view of the pain that can be evoked from the craniofacial muscles and TMJ, the presence of free nerve endings and of afferents with diameters in the groups III and IV range that are associated with nociceptive fibers, and the occurrence of reflex effects that can be evoked by high-threshold stimulation of cranial nerve V, VII, and XII muscle afferents (9).

PRIMARY AFFERENT PROJECTIONS INTO THE CNS

While there are some conflicting data in the spinal literature on the termination sites in the spinal cord dorsal horn of muscle afferents (11–14), the general consensus now indicates that small-diameter spinal afferents from deep tissues terminate predominantly in laminae I and V of the dorsal horn as well as in the gray matter around the central canal (2,3,15).

In the craniofacial region, few studies have yet addressed the central projection sites within the trigeminal brainstem sensory nuclear complex of afferents from deep tissues, although the central projections of large-diameter jaw muscle afferents whose cell bodies are located in the trigeminal mesencephalic nucleus have been well detailed (9,16). While no study has specifically examined the projection of small-diameter afferents from craniofacial muscles and the TMJ, it does appear that deep afferents may project to each subdivision of the trigeminal brainstem complex, and terminations have been noted in regions (16–20) in which trigeminal nociceptive neurons receiving deep afferent inputs are located (see below).

ACTIVATION OF CENTRAL NEURONS

Dr. Mense also outlines some of the properties of spinal dorsal horn neurons in Chapter 3, so this section will only briefly review spinal dorsal horn mechanisms and will focus instead on trigeminal brainstem processing of deep nociceptive information.

Spinal Cord

The neural messages carried in the small-diameter nociceptive primary afferents from deep tissues are relayed onto neurons in the spinal cord dorsal horn and can then reach higher levels of the brain (e.g., thalamus, cerebral cortex) as well as spinal and brainstem regions involved in reflex and other behavioral responses to noxious inputs from muscles and joints. As mentioned above, most of the research focus on spinal nociceptive mechanisms has centered on neuronal responses to noxious stimulation of superficial structures. These studies have shown that two types of neurons are responsive to noxious cutaneous stimuli, and that these neurons are concentrated in the superficial (e.g., lamina I) and deep (e.g., laminae V/VI) layers of the spinal dorsal horn (4,21,22). The two types of cutaneous nociceptive neurons are wide dynamic range (WDR) neurons, which are excited by in-

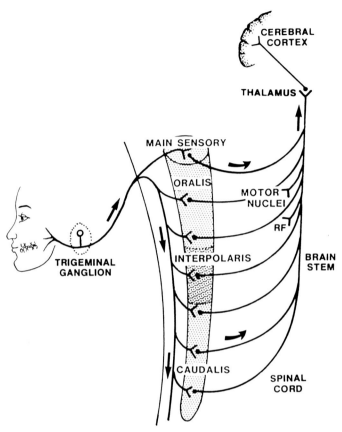

FIG. 1. The major central neural pathway transmitting sensory information from the orofacial region. The first synaptic relay of information from the face and mouth may occur on neurons at all levels of the trigeminal brainstem sensory nuclear complex, which may be subdivided, from rostral to caudal, into the main (or principal) sensory nucleus and the spinal tract nucleus; the latter consists of three subnuclei: oralis, interpolaris, and caudalis. From the brainstem complex, sensory information may then be relayed directly to the thalamus and then to the cerebral cortex, or less directly by multisynaptic pathways involving, for example, the reticular formation (RF). The sensory information relayed from a particular nucleus or subnucleus of the complex may also pass to other brainstem structures, such as the cranial nerve motor nuclei involved in reflex responses to the sensory inputs from the face and mouth. (From Sessle, ref. 32, with permission.)

the jaw-closing musculature (38,39). Similarly, neurons in adjacent regions implicated in jaw muscle reflex pathways (e.g., supratrigeminal nucleus, intertrigeminal nucleus) had also been shown to receive electrically evoked muscle afferent inputs (9,40). Given this background information, plus the finding of deep nociceptive inputs to functionally identified spinal dorsal horn neurons, and the lack of knowledge of neural mechanisms underlying

TABLE 1. *Afferent input convergence to nociceptive neurons in trigeminal subnucleus caudalis*[a]

Facial skin/oral mucosa	100%
Tooth pulp	60%
Muscle (jaw and/or tongue)	55%
TMJ	35%
Upper cervical	50%
Laryngeal mucosa (visceral)	55%

[a] Based on a population of 88 WDR and NS neurons with a mechanoreceptive field in the cat's mouth or face.

deep craniofacial pain and pathophysiological conditions such as temporo-mandibular/myofascial pain dysfunction, we have carried out several recent detailed studies of the response properties of trigeminal brainstem neurons receiving deep craniofacial afferent inputs. These studies have involved elec-trophysiological recordings of the activity of single neurons in the subnucleus caudalis or oralis of anesthetized or decerebrate (unanesthetized) cats or anesthetized rats. Each neuron was functionally identified as a LTM, WDR, or NS neuron on the basis of its *cutaneous* (or intraoral) mechanoreceptive field properties, and its responsiveness was tested to electrical, mechanical or algesic chemical stimulation of afferents supplying the jaw-closing (mas-seter or temporalis) or tongue muscles or the TMJ. Neurons not having a cutaneous mechanoreceptive field but receiving these deep afferent inputs were classified as "deep" neurons.

With respect to muscle afferent inputs, we have documented (41,42) that over 50% of the neurons classified on the basis of their *cutaneous* mechan-oreceptive field properties as cutaneous nociceptive neurons (WDR and NS) and located in laminae I/II or V/VI of the subnucleus caudalis of cats can indeed also be activated by electrical stimulation of high-threshold muscle afferents in the masseter, temporalis, or hypoglossal (XIIth cranial) nerves (Table 1). The mean latencies of these excitatory responses (between 10 and 20 msec) were two to three times longer than the responses of the neurons to cutaneous afferent inputs and are indicative of either inputs from very slowly conducting muscle primary afferents or inputs involving a multisy-naptic path. The neurons showed a graded response to stimuli of increasing intensity, suggesting that they are capable of coding the intensity of the nociceptive muscle afferent inputs. Very few neurons exclusively receiving these deep inputs were found (i.e., "deep" neurons), and less than 20% of the more than 200 LTM neurons tested received these inputs. It is also to be noted that some of the WDR and NS neurons were shown to be thalamic-projection neurons on the basis of their antidromic activation by contralateral ventrobasal thalamic stimulation. Some of these various properties are shown in Fig. 2.

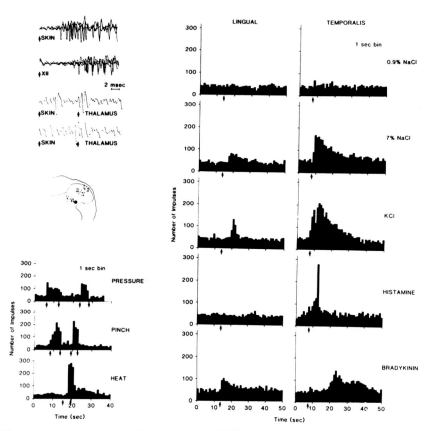

FIG. 2. Responses of a wide dynamic range (WDR) neuron in trigeminal subnucleus caudalis. *Upper left:* Neuronal responses to three or four successive electrical stimuli delivered (at 1 Hz) to its facial receptive field and to the hypoglossal (XIIth) nerve, as well as its histologically verified recording locus and antidromic response evoked by contralateral thalamic stimulation (third trace), which could be blocked as a result of collision produced by a preceding orthodromically evoked spike (fourth trace). *Arrowheads* indicate time of onset of the skin, XIIth nerve, or thalamic stimulus. *Lower left:* Histograms illustrate distribution of the number of neuronal impulses evoked by two pressure, two pinch, and one noxious heat-stimulation trials applied to the neuron's facial receptive field. *Arrowheads* indicate time of stimulus onset and offset. *Right:* Histograms showing the responses of this same WDR neuron to algesic chemical stimulation. Data were obtained from the same WDR neuron illustrated on the left. Histograms show distribution of the number of neuronal impulses evoked by the four algesic chemicals indicated; these chemicals were injected into small branches of the lingual and temporalis arteries. The lack of responses to control injections of 0.9% NaCl are also clearly seen. *Arrowheads* indicate time of onset of injection that lasted 8 to 10 sec. (From Amano et al., ref. 41, with permission.)

We have recently completed a study of the rat subnucleus caudalis and similarly found that a considerable proportion of neurons could be activated by electrical stimulation of high-threshold jaw XIIth nerve muscle afferents and that these deep inputs were preferentially directed at *cutaneous* nociceptive (WDR and NS) neurons (43). While only a few WDR and NS neurons in the cat caudalis were shown to receive C fiber muscle afferent inputs, a much higher proportion (60%) of rat caudalis nociceptive neurons tested showed C fiber, excitatory inputs from the XIIth nerve.

The muscle afferent-evoked responses were considered to reflect predominantly nociceptive afferent inputs in view of (a) the long latency and high threshold of most neuronal responses evoked by the electrical stimulation; (b) the predominance of afferents of small diameter in the muscle nerves stimulated (9); (c) the preferential input to neurons functionally classified as cutaneous nociceptive neurons; (d) the additional activation of most (80%) of these WDR and NS neurons, which are excited by electrical stimulation of muscle afferents, by noxious mechanical or thermal stimulation of muscle; and (e) their additional activation by algesic chemicals (7% NaCl, KCl, bradykinin, histamine, 5-HT) injected intraarterially into the small arteries supplying the jaw-closing and tongue muscles (e.g., Fig. 2). Furthermore, their muscle afferent-evoked responses could be depressed (Amano, Hu, and Sessle, unpublished observations) by conditioning electrical stimulation applied to central neural structures (e.g., nucleus raphe magnus), implicated in central mechanisms of analgesia (44,45). Stimulation of raphe magnus, in which serotonin and other neurochemicals are localized, induced inhibition in all 16 WDR and 19 NS neurons tested (e.g., Fig. 3); nine LTM neurons also showed depression. Figure 3 further shows that certain afferent inputs could depress neuronal responses to deep as well as cutaneous afferent inputs. In addition, it is to be noted that these various properties are consistent with those documented for neurons in the superficial and deep layers of the spinal dorsal horn that receive inputs from muscle nociceptive afferents (see above). These same mechanical, thermal, and algesic chemical stimuli also induced deep pain in man (3,46), and so we believe that these caudalis neurons represent neural elements critically involved in the transmission of acute myofascial pain in the craniofacial region. As pointed out below, additional evidence suggests their involvement also in referred pain and other pathophysiological conditions manifesting muscle pain. Their receipt of deep afferent inputs as well as superficial inputs also has led us to question (2) the common use of terminology and classifications of somatosensory neurons solely on the basis of their cutaneous receptive field properties.

Similar mechanisms appear to be involved in the transmission of acute pain from the TMJ. We have recently documented in studies of over 200 single neurons in the cat or rat subnucleus caudalis that a substantial population of caudalis neurons receive TMJ nociceptive inputs (47,48). As with

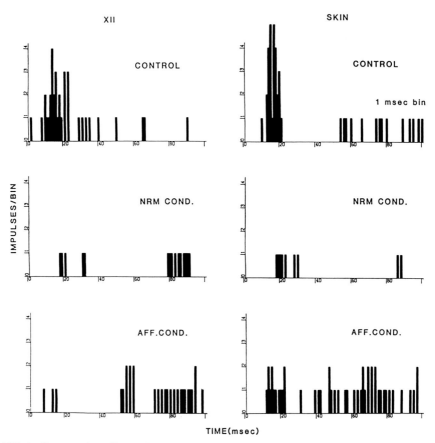

FIG. 3. Suppressive effects of conditioning stimulation of nucleus raphe magnus (NRM) and orofacial afferents on the excitatory responses of a WDR neuron evoked by XIIth nerve stimulation (*left*) or electrical stimulation of its facial (maxillary) mechanoreceptive field (*right*). The NRM conditioning stimulus (20-msec train of 0.2-msec pulses at 400 Hz) was delivered 50 msec prior to the delivery of the test stimulation of the XIIth nerve or maxillary facial skin. The orofacial afferent conditioning stimulus involved a continuous tactile stimulus applied to the supraorbital skin immediately preceding and during the delivery of the test stimulus. Each of the six histograms represents five superimposed responses to five successive XIIth nerve or skin test stimuli delivered at 1 Hz in a control (i.e., no conditioning stimulation) or conditioning paradigm; time 0 reflects the time of delivery of the XIIth nerve or skin test stimulus. (From Amano, Hu, and Sessle, unpublished.)

the muscle afferent inputs, electrical, noxious mechanical, or algesic chemical stimulation of TMJ afferents preferentially excited *cutaneous* nociceptive (WDR and NS) neurons. In a small sample ($N = 10$) of these WDR and NS neurons tested in cats, most ($N = 9$) could also be activated by masticatory muscle afferent inputs as well as by cutaneous (or intraoral) and TMJ afferent stimulation. Visceral afferent convergence may also occur

(Table 1). For reasons similar to those expressed above for the muscle afferent–activated WDR and NS neurons, we consider that these TMJ-evoked responses reflect predominantly TMJ nociceptive afferent inputs, and that they represent the first evidence of central trigeminal neural elements involved in TMJ pain mechanisms.

It should be pointed out that so far our studies have been limited to the subnucleus caudalis. In view of findings by ourselves and others (33) that cutaneous or intraoral nociceptive neurons also exist in more rostral components of the trigeminal brainstem complex, some of which receive jaw muscle afferent inputs (38,39), it is likely that rostral neurons also contribute to brainstem mechanisms underlying deep craniofacial pain. Indeed, recent preliminary evidence suggests that nociceptive inputs from jaw muscle exert facilitatory effects on cutaneous nociceptive neurons in the subnucleus oralis (see below).

Thalamus and Cortex

While properties related to inputs from low-threshold deep receptors are reasonably well documented in the thalamus and somatosensory cerebral cortex (49 – 51), only limited information is available on the thalamocortical processing of deep nociceptive information. Mallart (52) described groups II– and/or III-related activity in the ventrobasal and medial thalamus of the cat evoked by stimulation of forelimb and hindlimb afferents, and, more recently, single neurons driven by noxious mechanical or algesic chemical stimulation of limb muscles as well as by cutaneous noxious stimuli have been reported in the ventrobasal thalamus and immediately surrounding regions (53,54) and in SI somatosensory cortex (55,56). Thalamic and SI cortical neurons driven by deep stimuli in pathophysiological conditions (e.g., arthritis) are described below.

With respect to deep inputs from the craniofacial region, low-threshold XIIth nerve muscle afferent-evoked responses have been recorded in the primate ventrobasal thalamus and SI area of the somatosensory cortex and MI area of the motor cortex (57–60). SI neurons in cats receive jaw muscle afferent inputs (61,62), and low-threshold jaw and facial muscle afferent inputs have been shown to excite neurons in MI and SI cortex areas of monkeys (58–60). Except for a recent brief description of high-threshold XIIth nerve afferent inputs to SII cortex of the cat (63), there appears to be no detailed account of the projection sites and neuronal properties related to the thalamocortical processing of nociceptive messages from craniofacial muscular and articular tissues.

REFLEX RESPONSES

While the research focus has been primarily directed at CNS mechanisms related to the processing of ascending nociceptive information from deep tissues and its relevance to pain perception, a few studies have clearly documented that deep inputs to the CNS are also involved in sensorimotor and autonomic integration. For a detailed consideration of the role in sensorimotor control of these inputs specifically to higher brain centers (e.g., thalamus, cortex), the interested reader is referred to refs. 9, 49, 50, and 51. In terms of the somatic and autonomic reflex changes that can be induced by noxious stimulation of deep stimuli, it has been demonstrated that noxious stimulation of muscle or articular tissues can reflexly evoke cardiovascular and respiratory changes, and that some of these alterations appear to be important in the reflex cardiopulmonary adjustments that occur during physical exercise (3,64). A limb flexion reflex can also be evoked by noxious mechanical, algesic chemical, or high-threshold electrical stimulation of muscular or articular tissues of the limbs (7,65). More recent studies have shown that deep noxious stimuli generally activate alpha motoneurons supplying limb flexor muscles and inhibit alpha motoneurons innervating limb extensors; gamma motoneurons of both extensors and flexors may also be influenced by these group III and IV afferent inputs (3,66). These effects have been viewed as nociceptive reflex responses that serve to protect the limb from further noxious stimulation and as mechanisms counteracting excessive movement so as to prevent further damage to the muscular or articular tissues of the limb (3,66,67). It is also to be noted that high-intensity stimulation of limb muscle afferents can indeed produce a prolonged facilitation of the flexion reflex (68), and this effect may be related to pathophysiological mechanisms occurring in response to injury or inflammation (see below).

In the craniofacial region, stimulation of high-threshold afferents in Vth, VIIth, and XIIth cranial nerves can elicit reflex responses in the jaw, tongue, and facial muscles (69,70,71,72); these reflex effects appear to be due, at least in part, to activation of nociceptive afferents supplying the craniofacial musculature (9). In view of the lack of clear evidence documenting that deep noxious stimuli do indeed induce alterations in craniofacial muscle activity and of implications of such reflex effects as integral mechanisms associated with temporomandibular/myofascial pain and dysfunction (9,73–75), we have recently investigated reflex effects of deep noxious stimuli on craniofacial muscle activity in cats. While we primarily focused on the effects of TMJ stimulation (76), some of the observed reflex changes could also be induced by algesic chemical stimulation of the masticatory muscles. Injection into the TMJ of algesic chemicals (7% NaCl, KCl, histamine) resulted in a sustained (30-sec or more) reflex increase in electromyographic activity of tongue and jaw-opening muscles (Fig. 4); excitatory effects were also seen in the jaw-closing (middle temporalis) musculature but were generally weaker. These findings suggest that trauma or noxious stimulation of deep craniofacial tissues can produce a sustained excitation of several masticatory muscles that may serve to protect the masticatory system from potentially

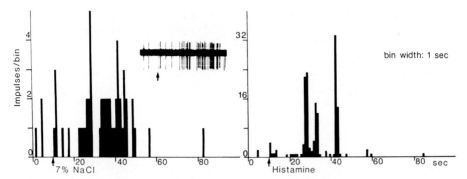

FIG. 4. Excitatory effects of algesic chemical stimulation of the TMJ on the activity of a single motor unit recorded in the anterior digastric muscle. Each histogram shows the distribution of the number of motor unit impulses (bin width 1 sec) evoked by the single appliclation of 7% NaCl (*left*) or histamine (*right*); note the difference in the scale of the ordinates of the histograms. Each *arrow* indicates the time of onset of the application. **Inset:** Trace (duration 50 sec) of the unit's response evoked by 7% NaCl. (From Broton and Sessle, ref. 76, with permission.)

damaging movements and stimuli; such effects may be related to clinically based concepts of myofascial dysfunction, such as splinting, myospastic activity, and trigger points, which Drs. Simons, Travell, and others in this volume discuss.

SOME PATHOPHYSIOLOGICAL CONSIDERATIONS

Reference has already been made above to the involvement of the spinal and trigeminal CNS mechanisms processing deep nociceptive information in acute myofascial and articular pain and in the muscle dysfunction that may accompany deep pain. While Dr. Awad and others in this volume consider at length the pathophysiology of deep pain, I will briefly consider how these acute pain mechanisms might be related to pathophysiological processes associated with deep pain.

Whereas pain from cutaneous tissues or from articular tissues situated directly beneath the skin (e.g., knee joint) is usually well localized, pain originating in muscle or more deeply situated joints is often poorly localized, diffuse, and frequently referred (3,46) (see other chapters in this volume). Some of the neuronal properties described above, as well as additional properties outlined below, may indeed reflect CNS neural correlates of the poor localization and referral of deep pain. As pointed out elsewhere (1,4,30,37,42), it is unlikely that peripheral branching of individual primary afferents contributes significantly to such sensory phenomena; instead, central convergence of afferents is considered to be the more likely substrate for referral of pain. The recent CNS studies reviewed above support such a viewpoint since considerable convergence of cutaneous, visceral, muscle, or joint afferents earmarks the properties of spinal and trigeminal somatosensory neurons transmitting deep nociceptive information. In the trigeminal subnucleus caudalis, for example, many neurons appear to receive exclusively nociceptive information from cutaneous tissues (42) and these are well suited to code the intensity and spatial localization of superficial noxious stimuli (33,77). However, as noted above, many of the WDR and NS caudalis neurons receiving *cutaneous* nociceptive information also receive convergent afferent inputs from one or more other sources (Table 1), including craniofacial muscles and the TMJ. Indeed, few neurons receive exclusively deep nociceptive inputs. Thus, there appears to be only a limited neural basis for the localization of deep craniofacial pain, and considerable opportunity does exist through these excitatory convergent mechanisms for the poor localization of deep pain and for referral between deep craniofacial structures and more superficial sites and even cervical regions. Other evidence suggesting the involvement of central convergent mechanisms in the neural basis of pain referral comes from recent studies in the ascending spinal somatosensory system, where the injection of algesic chemicals into muscle or the presence of an acute localized inflammation or a chronic arthritis can result in changes in spinal dorsal horn, thalamic, and SI cortical neurons (2,29,78,79) that reflect an enhanced responsiveness to afferent inputs not only from the site of inflammation but also from other convergent inputs.

Similar mechanisms also probably contribute to the spread of pain from the site of an injury or inflammatory process to adjacent tissues. Peripherally based phenomena associated with the release and spread of endogenous neurochemical substances such as histamine and the kinins have long been considered to underlie such spread of pain, and indeed recent studies reaffirm this view (e.g., experimentally induced inflammation can sensitize and enhance the response of nociceptive afferents supplying deep or superficial tissues, as Dr. Mense has pointed out in Chapter 3, *this volume*). Nonetheless, it is also clear from recent studies that if peripheral phenomena are experimentally bypassed (e.g., by local anesthesia of the inflamed site), the resulting alterations in the responsiveness and receptive field properties of central spinal somatosensory neurons suggest that central factors contribute to the changes initially induced by the inflammation (2,79,80). These central factors have been viewed in terms of an unmasking or strengthening at central somatosensory neuronal relays of convergent afferent inputs that normally are relatively "ineffective" in exciting the central somatosensory neurons (2,22,81), although not all the observations are completely consistent with this view (2). Changes in opioid or protooncogene expression also occur in spinal dorsal horn neurons after inflammation or small fiber stimulation (e.g., with mustard oil), but the question of whether peripheral and/or central mechanisms contribute to these changes awaits further study (82,83).

These central changes related to the application of inflammatory agents into deep tissues or to the presence of a chronic inflammation (e.g., arthritis), and their association with peripheral sensitization and/or central convergent phenomena, are also of interest because of their effect on the cutaneous receptive field properties of central somatosensory neurons. Many of the spinal dorsal horn or thalamic neurons become not only more responsive (compared to neurons in normal animals) to gentle movement of the inflamed site, but some also show marked sensitivity and prolonged responses to light, brief mechanical stimulation of the skin or bursting patterns of background activity (2,28,29,84,85). The injection into a limb muscle of the algesic chemical bradykinin also induces prolonged changes in receptive field size as well as a lowering of mechanical threshold of cat spinal dorsal horn neurons (78), and Wall and colleagues (68,80,81,86) have documented prolonged facilitatory effects of muscle afferent stimulation on the cutaneous receptive field properties of neurons in the ventral as well as dorsal horn of rat spinal cord. Electrical stimulation of muscle afferents as well as muscle tetany produce an enhanced central excitability of the neurons that may last up to 60 min or more; C fibers particularly appear to be involved in these effects. While activation of cutaneous C fibers by electrical stimulation or the small-fiber irritant mustard oil also induces the facilitation, the effects are not as dramatic as those elicited by stimulation of muscle afferents.

We have found complementary data in recent studies of functionally identified cutaneous nociceptive neurons in the trigeminal brainstem complex of the rat (43). High-intensity stimulation of hypoglossal nerve muscle afferents markedly enhanced the excitability to especially C fiber cutaneous afferent inputs of 55% of 33 WDR and NS neurons tested in the subnucleus caudalis; this effect often lasted for 15 to 30 min. We were also interested to see if a similar facilitatory effect of muscle afferent inputs could be induced in the cutaneous afferent inputs of caudalis nociceptive neurons by a more natural activation of the muscle afferents. We used the small-fiber irritant mustard oil, which has been shown to induce facilitatory effects on spinal cord neurons. The injection of 5% mustard oil into the deep masseter muscle also induced an enhancement of the *cutaneous* afferent inputs to 40% of 25 WDR and NS neurons tested (Fig. 5C). This effect lasted for 3 to 20 min and was reversible. Furthermore, a reversible expansion of the cutaneous mechanoreceptive field of many of these nociceptive neurons was also seen (Fig. 5B). This spatial change could involve both the tactile (in WDR neurons) and the nociceptive (in WDR and NS neurons) components of the field. We have also recently observed a similar facilitation of the cutaneous mechanoreceptive field properties of functionally identified WDR and NS brainstem neurons recorded more rostrally in the trigeminal subnucleus oralis of the rat (Dallel, Raboisson, Woda, and Sessle, unpublished observations).

These remarkable effects of muscle afferent inputs on the *cutaneous* mechanoreceptive properties of trigeminal nociceptive neurons suggest mechanisms that may relate to those neural processes outlined above that may

33. Sessle BJ. *J Dent Res* 1987;66:962–981.
34. Gobel S, Hockfield S, Ruda MA In: Kawamura Y, Dubner R, eds. *Oral-facial sensory and motor functions.* Tokyo: Quintessence, 1981;211–223.
35. Hoffman DS, Dubner R, Hayes RL, Medline TP. *J Neurophysiol* 1981;46:409–427.
36. Hu JW, Dostrovsky JO, Sessle BJ. *J Neurophysiol* 1981;45:173–192.
37. Sessle BJ. In: Fromm GH, Sessle BJ, eds. *Trigeminal neuralgia: Current concepts of pathogenesis and treatment.* Stoneham: Butterworths, (in press).
38. Hayashi H, Sumino R, Sessle BJ. *J Neurophysiol* 1984;51:890–905.
39. Sessle BJ, Greenwood LF. *Brain Res* 1976;117:211–226.
40. Olsson KA, Landgren S, Westberg KG. *Exp Brain Res* 1986;65:83–97.
41. Amano N, Hu JW, Sessle BJ. *J Neurophysiol* 1986;55:227–243.
42. Sessle BJ, Hu JW, Amano N, Zhong G. *Pain* 1986;27:219–235.
43. Hu JW, Chen X, Sessle BJ. *Neurosci Abstr* 1988;14:563.
44. Basbaum AI, Fields HL. *Annu Rev Neurosci* 1984;7:309–338.
45. Willis WD. In: Fields HL, Besson J-M, eds. *Pain modulation* (Progress in Brain Research, Vol 77. Amsterdam: Elsevier, 1988;1–29.
46. Lewis, T. *Pain* (facsimilie ed). London: Macmillan, 1981.
47. Broton JG, Hu JW, Sessle BJ. *J Neurophysiol* 1988;59:1575–1589.
48. Hu JW, Sharav Y, Sessle BJ. *Neurosci Abstr* 1989;15:1190.
49. Jones EG, Porter R. *Brain Res* 1980;2:1–43.
50. Landgren S, Silfvenius H, Olsson KA *Exp Brain Res* 1984;9:(suppl):359–375.
51. Wiesendanger M, Miles TS. *Physiol Rev* 1982;62:1234–1270.
52. Mallart A. *J Physiol (Lond)* 1968;194:337–353.
53. Honda CN, Mense S, Perl ER. *J Neurophysiol* 1983;49:662–673.
54. Kniffki K-D, Mizumura K. *J Neurophysiol* 1983;49:649–661.
55. Iwamura Y, Kniffki K-D, Mizumura K, Wilberg K. *Pain* 1981;1(suppl):S213.
56. Lamour Y, Willer JC, Guilbaud G. *Exp Brain Res* 1983;49:35–45.
57. Bowman JP. *The muscle spindle and neural control of the tongue.* Springfield, IL: Charles C Thomas, 1971.
58. Huang C-S, Hiraba H, Sessle BJ. *J Neurophysiol* 1989;61:350–362.
59. Huang C-S, Sirisko M, Hiraba H, Murray GM, Sessle BJ. *J Neurophysiol* 1988;59:796–818.
60. Sirisko MA, Sessle BJ. *Exp Neurol* 1983;82:716–720.
61. Iwata K, Itoga H, Ikukawa A, Hanashima N, Sumino R. *Brain Res* 1985;342:179–182.
62. Lund JP, Sessle BJ. *Exp Neurol* 1974;45:314–331.
63. Hanson J. *Arch Ital Biol* 1985;123:63–68.
64. Mitchell JH, Schmidt RF. In: Shepherd JT, Abboud FM, eds. *Handbook of physiology, section 2: The cardiovascular system, vol III: Peripheral circulation and organ blood flow, part 2.* Bethesda, MD: American Physiological Society, 1983;623–658.
65. Gardner E. *Am J Physiol* 1950;161:133–141.
66. He X, Proske U, Schaible H-G, Schmidt RF. *J Neurophysiol* 1988;59:326–340.
67. Schaible HG, Schmidt RF. *Exp Brain Res* 1984;9(suppl 9):284–297.
68. Wall PD, Woolf CJ. *J Physiol (Lond)* 1984;356:443–458.
69. Hanson J, Widen L. *Acta Physiol Scand* 1970;79:24–36.
70. Lindquist C, Martensson A. *Acta Physiol Scand* 1970;80:149–159.
71. Sessle BJ. *Exp Neurol* 1977;54:323–339.
72. Willer JC, Lamour Y. *CR Soc Biol (Paris)* 1975;169:1177–1185.
73. Bell WE. *Temporomandibular disorders: Classification, diagnosis, management,* 2nd ed. Boca Raton, FL: CRC Press, 1987
74. Laskin D, Greenfield W, Gale E, Rugh J, Neff P, Alling C, Ayer WA. *The president's conference on the examination, diagnosis and management of temporomandibular disorders.* Chicago: American Dental Association, 1983.
75. Moller E. In: Klineberg I, Sessle BJ, eds. *Oro-facial pain and neuromuscular dysfunction: Mechanisms and clinical correlates.* Oxford: Pergamon Press, 1985;69–92.
76. Broton JG, Sessle BJ. *Arch Oral Biol* 1988;33:741–747.
77. Dubner R. In: Klineberg I, Sessle B, eds. *Oro-facial pain and neuromuscular dysfunction: Mechanisms and clinical correlates.* Oxford: Pergamon, 1985;3–19.
78. Hoheisel U, Mense S. *Pain* 1989;36:239–247.

79. Hylden JL, Nahin RL, Traub RJ, Dubner R. *Pain* 1989;37:229–244.
80. Wall PD. In: Goldberger ME, Gorio A, Murray M, eds. *Development and plasticity of the mammalian spinal cord*. Padova: Liviana, 1986;101–110.
81. Woolf CJ. In: Fields HL, Dubner R, Cervero F, eds. *Advances in pain research and therapy*, vol 9. New York: Raven, 1985;193–201.
82. Hunt SP, Pini A, Evan G. *Nature* 1987;328:632–634.
83. Iadarola MJ, Brady LS, Draisci G, Dubner R. *Pain* 1988;35:313–326.
84. Calvino B, Villanueva L, Le Bars D. *Pain* 1987;28(1):81–98.
85. Menetrey D, Besson JM. *Pain* 1982;13:343–364.
86. Cook AJ, Woolf CJ, Wall PD, McMahon SB. *Nature* 1987;325:151–153.

Advances in Pain Research and Therapy, Vol. 17,
edited by James R. Fricton and Essam Awad.
Raven Press, Ltd., New York © 1990.

5

Myofascial Pain Syndrome

Characteristics and Epidemiology

James R. Fricton

*Department of Diagnostic and Surgical Sciences, University of Minnesota,
School of Dentistry, Minneapolis, Minnesota 55455*

Myofascial pain syndrome (MPS) continues to be regarded by some as a specific disease entity, by others as a wastebasket term for soft tissue complaints, and by others as simply nonexistent (1–6). Confusion regarding this syndrome may stem from lack of obvious organic findings, the lack of a unified theory to explain it, and the inconsistencies in the literature defining the syndrome.

However, recent studies have identified myofascial pain as the most common cause of chronic pain, is involved in most workers' compensation cases involving pain, and is often a source of litigation in the disability determination process (7–10). Although recent research is beginning to shed light on objective characteristics of MPS, its prevalence, pathophysiology, and many other questions remain unanswered. The purpose of this chapter is to describe the state of clinical knowledge of MPS and identify the areas that need further study.

Myofascial pain syndrome is defined as a muscular pain disorder involving regional pain referred by trigger points within the myofascial structures local or distant from the pain (5,11–14). The clinical characteristics include trigger points in muscles, pain in a zone of reference, occasional associated symptoms, and the presence of contributing factors (Table 1) (5,15–17). A trigger point is defined as a localized deep tenderness in a taut band of skeletal muscle that is responsible for pain in the zone of reference and, if treated, will resolve the pain problem (5,9,14,18). The zone of reference is defined as the area of perceived pain referred by the irritable trigger point. Palpation of active trigger points will alter the referred pain (intensify or reduce) or cause radiation of pain toward the zone of reference.

The characteristics may long outlast the precipitating events, setting up

TABLE 1. *Clinical characteristics of myofascial pain syndrome*

Trigger points	Zone of reference
Ropelike band of muscle	Constant dull ache
Tenderness on palpation	Fluctuates in intensity
Palpation alters pain	Consistent patterns of referral
Consistent points of tenderness	Local or distant trigger points
	Alleviation with extinction of trigger point
Associated symptoms	Contributing factors
Otological symptoms	Physical disorders
Paresthesias	Parafunctional habits
GI distress	Postural strains
Visual disturbances	Disuse
Dermal flushing	Nutritional
	Sleep disturbance
	Stress

a self-generating pain cycle that is perpetuated through lack of proper treatment, sustained muscle tension, distorted muscle posture, pain-reinforcing behavior, and failure to reduce other contributing factors such as muscle bracing and lack of sleep. There are generally no neurologic deficits associated with the syndrome unless a nerve entrapment syndrome with weakness and diminished sensation coincides with the muscle trigger points (16). Routine blood and urine studies are generally normal unless caused by a concomitant disorder (19).

Proposed diagnostic criteria used to confirm a diagnosis of MPS include (9):

1. Regional pain complaints.
2. Trigger points in taut bands of skeletal muscle that correspond to the pattern of pain and are consistent with previous reports.
3. Reproducible alteration of the pain complaints with specific palpation of the responsible trigger points. This third criterion is found only in muscles that are readily palpable.

Although these diagnostic criteria have been used in research and clinical practice, to date there has been no testing of its sensitivity or specificity in diagnosing MPS compared to normals subjects, patients with joint disorder, or patients with other muscle disorders.

The regional pain found with MPS needs to be distinguished from the systemic muscular pain associated with fibromyalgia (20–22). However, the various other terms used in the past for the broad category of muscle pain syndromes, including "fibrositis," "myofascial pain dysfunction" [of the temporomandibular joint (TMJ)], "myelogelosen," "interstitial myofibrositis," "musculofascial pain dysfunction," "TMJ dysfunction," "nonarticular rheumatism," and "myalgia," can confuse the reader considerably (21,23–30). In a recent multisite study of fibromyalgia, Wolfe and colleagues (31) established diagnostic criteria for fibromyalgia that included:

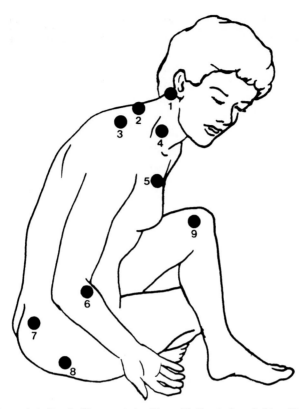

FIG. 1. Tender point sites in fibromyalgia. (From Wolfe et al., ref. 31, with permission.)

1. Generalized aches or stiffness involving three or more anatomical sites for at least months.
2. Exclusion of other conditions that may cause similar symptoms.
3. The presence of reproducible tenderness in 11 of 18 prespecified reproducible sites (Fig. 1).

These two disorders have many similar characteristics and may represent two ends of a continuous spectrum. For example, as Simons points out in Chapter 1, 16 of the 18 tender point sites in fibromyalgia lie at well-known trigger point sites. Many of the clinical characteristics of fibromyalgia, such as fatigue, morning stiffness, and sleep disorders, can also accompany MPS. In Chapter 3 (*this volume*), Bennett compares these two disorders and concludes that these are two distinct disorders but they may have the same underlying pathophysiology. The clinical significance of distinguishing between them lies in the potentially better prognosis in treatment of MPS as compared to fibromyalgia.

The lack of diagnostic criteria for both MPS and fibromyalgia that do not rely on patient report is currently hindering the widespread recognition of these disorders, particularly in the area of disability determination. Monsein, in Chapter 10 (*this volume*), points out that some studies have suggested that musculoskeletal pain, and particularly myofascial pain, is the most common diagnosis associated with injured workers receiving compensation (32,33). Since guidelines involved in disability determination rely heavily on objective findings such as imaging and laboratory tests, patients with MPS are often neglected, causing considerable controversy, confusion, and litigation. Two questions arise regarding the issue of disability compensation for patients with MPS: (a) Can these patients be diagnosed without relying on patient pain complaints? and (b) Can pain associated with MPS be permanently disabling? The answers to these questions are complex and the state of research is still inconclusive. However, a basic understanding can be gained from examining the research associated with the individual components of MPS: trigger points, referred pain, and associated problems.

TRIGGER POINTS

Trigger points can range from 2 to 5 mm in diameter and are found within hard, palpable bands of skeletal muscle and fascial structure of tendons and ligaments (5,9,12,14). The trigger points may be active or latent (5,16). Active trigger points are hypersensitive to palpation and give rise to pain in the zone of reference. Latent trigger points displayed only hypersensitivity. This tenderness has been studied to determine its reliability, its presence in normal subjects, and its association with presenting symptoms. In a study of the interrater and intrarater reliability of a manual palpation technique to determine the scope of tenderness (number of tender sites) in 44 head and neck muscles, Fricton and Schiffman found intraclass correlations of .86 and .84, respectively (34). The high reliability was explained based on the standardization of the palpation technique described in Figure 2. Tenderness of MPS using pressure algometry has also been studied by numerous investigators. Reeves et al. (35) and Schiffman et al. (36) both have established the reliability and validity of pressure algometry in documenting myofascial trigger points. Reeves used a spring loaded algometer and found interrater reliability to be acceptable. Schiffman et al. (36) studied the interrater reliability of tenderness at individual muscle sites and made a comparison of tenderness between normal and MPS subjects. They found that by using the pressure algometer, tenderness scores at individual trigger points had moderate to good reliability at 13 of 15 head and neck sites tested. The strain gauge pressure algometer was used because it afforded more sensitive measurements, good clinical agility, and better consistency between multiple instruments (Fig. 3). In addition, they found MPS patients had significantly

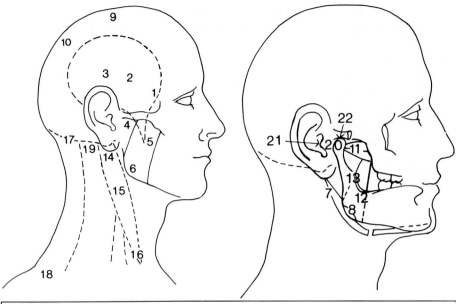

STRUCTURE

Muscle: Extra-oral	Muscle: Neck
1. Anterior Temporalis	14. Superior Sternocleidomastoid
2. Deep Temporalis	15. Middle Sternocleidomastoid
3. Middle Temporalis	16. Inferior Sternocleidomastoid
4. Deep Masseter	17. Insertion of Trapezius
5. Anterior Masseter	18. Upper Trapezius
6. Inferior Masseter	19. Splenius Capitis
7. Posterior Digastric	
8. Medial Pterygoid	TMJ
9. Vertex	20. Lateral Capsule
10. Reference Point	21. Posterior Capsule
Muscle: Intra-oral	22. Superior Capsule
11. Lateral Pterygoid Site	
12. Medial Pterygoid	
13. Temporalis Insertion	

DESCRIPTION

Palpation is performed by first locating the distinct muscle band or part of joint and then palpating using the sensitive spade-like pad at the end of the distal phalanx of the index finger using firm pressure (approximately 1 lb per square inch). The patient is asked, "Does it hurt or is it just pressure?" The response is positive if palpation produces a clear reaction from the patient: *i.e.*, palpebral response, or if patient stated that the palpation "hurt", indicating that the site was clearly more tender than surrounding structures or contralateral structure. Any equivocal response by the patient would be scored as negative. Site #10 can be used as a reference site to demonstrate to the patient what "pressure" feels like. Due to poor accessibility of lateral pterygoid site, the fifth finger should be used to palpate with the patient's jaw in laterotrusion to the ipsilateral side. Palpation of the lateral and superior aspects of the TMJ is accomplished with full mouth opening. The deep masseter is palpated immediately below the notch in the zygomatic arch with the mouth closed.

FIG. 2. Manual palpation technique for myofascial pain syndrome. (From Fricton and Schiffman, ref. 34, with permission.)

more tenderness at all sites as compared to normal. Again, they cited the importance of training and use of a standardized technique to maintain good reliability.

Palpating the active trigger point with sustained, deep, single-finger pressure alters the pain in the zone of reference (area of pain complaint), which can be distant from the muscle with the trigger point. This can occur immediately or be delayed a few seconds.

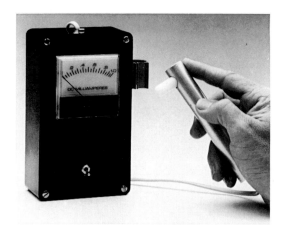

FIG. 3. A strain gauge–based pressure algometer. (From Schiffman, et al., ref. 36, with permission.)

The patterns of referral are reproducible and consistent with patterns of other patients with similar trigger points. This enables a clinician to use the zone of reference as a guide to locate the irritable trigger point for purposes of treatment. There are few reports of the patterns of referred pain that can occur with individual trigger points. Travell and Simons presented the most definitive descriptions of these patterns in their textbook (5) (Fig. 4A through 4D). These patterns appear to be based on clinical expertise and are difficult to study empirically because of the frequent presence of multiple active

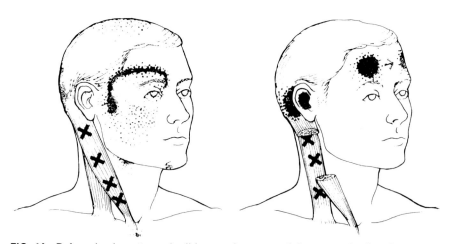

FIG. 4A. Referred pain patterns (*solid* areas show essential zones; *stippling* shows spill-over areas) with location of corresponding trigger points (**X**s) in right sternocleidomastoid. *Left:* Sternal (superficial) division. *Right:* Clavicular (deep) division. (From Travell and Simons, ref. 5, with permission.)

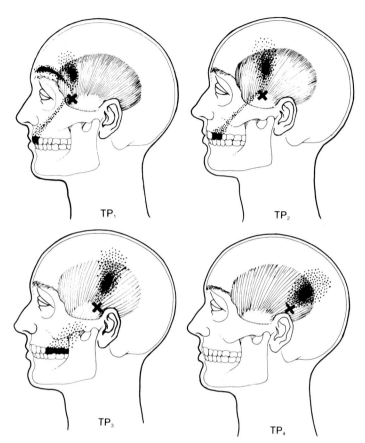

FIG. 4B. Referred pain patterns from trigger points in left temporalis muscle (see Fig. 4A for key). *Upper left:* Anterior "spokes" of pain arising from anterior fibers (trigger point 1 region). *Upper right:* Middle "spokes (trigger point 2). *Lower left:* Middle "spokes" (trigger point 3). *Lower right:* Posterior supraauricular "spokes" (trigger point 4). (From Travell and Simons, ref. 5, with permission.)

trigger points with overlapping referral patterns that do not follow traditional dermatomal or myotomal patterns. An area of future research involves the reproducibility of these referral patterns. Methods include studying single muscle syndromes, studying the effects of local anesthetic injections on the referral patterns, or studying experimental models of trigger points using repetitive muscle strain or muscle injections of noxious substances.

The patterns of pain that the patient describes can change, suggesting that trigger points can shift between active and latent. This occurs frequently during treatment when some specific trigger points are reduced, leaving others to continue causing pain. A study examining the changes in pain and tenderness in response to treatment for head and neck pain demonstrated a

with overlapping areas of pain referral and changes in pain patterns as trigger points are inactivated.

Although routine clinical electromyographic (EMG) studies show no significant abnormalities associated with trigger points, some specialized EMG studies reveal differences (38). A burst of electrical activity is found with needle insertion into the trigger point and not in adjacent muscle fibers (39,40). In an experimental EMG study of trigger points, Simons (41) and Fricton et al. (42) found abnormal electrical activity associated with the local muscle twitch response when specifically snapping the tense muscle band containing a myofascial trigger point. Increases in EMG associated with, but not necessarily at, the trigger point in acute conditions is continuous and is abolished by local anesthetics, spinal anesthesia, and obliteration of the trigger point (16,43). The consistency of soft tissues over the trigger points has been found to be more than that over adjacent muscles (44–46). Skin overlying trigger points in the masseter muscle was also warmer as measured by infrared emission (47,48). Measurement of skin resistance with an exploratory probe showed marked reduction at the skin above the trigger point as compared to adjacent overlying skin (49). Although each of these findings represents primarily solitary studies, they do provide preliminary evidence of a broad range of objective characteristics that may prove important in diagnosis of MPS.

The nature of the localized intramuscular pathological process of the trigger point is still not fully understood. A number of histological and biochemical studies have been completed on biopsies of tender points in patients diagnosed as having fibrositis. In many studies, this diagnosis was used for both generalized and regional muscle complaints. The findings of these studies have demonstrated nonspecific changes in the muscle and may shed light on changes occurring in trigger points because of the similarities in sites between fibrositis and MPS. Histological studies usually show fatty infiltration and sometimes show increases in fibrocytic and sarcolemmal nuclei, as well as loss of cross-striation (36,50,51). Other studies reveal myofibrillar degeneration, accumulation of acid mucopolysaccharides, and occasional local inflammatory responses with lymphocytic infiltration (23). Ultramicroscopic analysis revealed a progressive degeneration of the muscles with disruption of the mitochondria, increase in glycogen, and I band (actin) lysis that progressed to eventual disintegration of contractile fibers and breakdown into granular ground substance with long-standing trigger points (50,52–55).

Interestingly, light microscopy revealed no evidence of inflammation (51). Bengtsson et al. (54) reported on 77 biopsies from 57 patients. Moth-eaten fibers were found in 35 and ragged red fibers in 15 of 41 trapezius biopsies. In another study, Bengtsson et al. (56) studied the muscle energy metabolism by chemical analysis of biopsy samples from 15 patients. They found a decrease in the levels of adenosine triphosphate (ATP), adenosine diphosphate

(ADP), and phosphocreatine, and an increase in the levels of adenosine monophosphate (AMP) and creatine. Lund et al. (57) recently found evidence of abnormal tissue oxygenation in muscles with tender points, suggesting hypoxia in the painful muscle. Biochemical studies reveal localized increases of fluid water and chloride (50,58). Ibraham and colleagues (59) found decreased serum lactate dehydrogenase (LDH) fraction LD_1, and increased serum LDH fractions LD_3, LD_4, and LD_5. Along with this were found increased muscle LD_1 and LD_2 levels, decreased muscle LD_3 and LD_4 levels, and normal levels of LD_5. Increased aldolase in muscles was also observed. These findings suggest that increases in metabolism occur during early phases of trigger point development.

It has been hypothesized that these changes represent localized progressive increases in oxidative metabolism and depleted energy supply with resultant progressive abnormal muscle changes that include initially reactive dysfunctional changes and then fibrotic changes occurring within the muscle and surrounding connective tissue (3). This is substantiated by Lund and associates' (57) studies showing abnormally low subcutaneous oxygen tension in trigger points consistent with a region of increased metabolism. Bengtsson and associates (56) showed a decrease in high-energy phosphates and an increase in low-energy phosphate that is consistent with trigger points being an area of energy depletion. Electromyographic evidence also suggests that some increased background irritability of the alpha motor units at a trigger point makes them more responsive to stimuli. Localized tenderness and pain in the muscle appears to involve groups III and IV muscle nociceptors (60,61). However, the specific noxious stimuli responsible for pain in MPS can only be speculated upon. Many substances, including potassium, lactate, substance P, and bradykinin, as well as pressure and sustained contraction will stimulate muscle nociceptors in cats (62,63).

REFERRED PAIN

In acute cases of MPS, pain generally occurs only over the trigger point, but as the syndrome becomes chronic the trigger point can refer pain to a distant area (16). As mentioned earlier, this area is termed the "zone of reference." As in most visceral structures, myofascial structures refer pain in predictable, reproducible patterns that may not follow dermatomal, myotomal, or sclerotomal patterns but are specific for each myofascial trigger point (64,65) (Fig. 4). However, patterns can occasionally follow the meridian pathways of the acupuncture system (66–69). This consistency of the pain patterns enables clinicians to use the area of pain complaint to locate the trigger points that give rise to the pain.

In most cases of MPS, the pain description may range from a localized steady, dull ache to a diffuse soreness, tightness, or pressure. In some acute cases in small muscles, such as the digastric or lateral pterygoid, the pain may be described as a severe sharp or stabbing spasm. The severity of pain can vary from mild and bothersome to severe and excruciating and may fluctuate over long periods of time. Vasoconstriction, pallor, sweating, coldness, or decreased sensation of the skin over the zone of reference may be present in severe cases. Slightly higher clinical EMG levels in muscles within the zone of reference have also been reported (16).

Patients report aggravating factors to include fatigue, cold temperatures, a cool breeze over the area, weather changes, sustained tension on affected muscles (as in excess chewing, clenching, bruxism, and shoulder shrugging), excess strengthening exercise, immobility, emotional and physical strain, systemic disease such as viral infections or connective tissue disease, and trauma. They report alleviating factors to include heat (such as hot baths), massage, relaxation, muscle stretching, aerobic exercise, and a good night's sleep.

In examining the basic concept of MPS, namely referred pain from trigger points, there must be evidence that supports the notion that the referred pain is related to and generated by the trigger point, particularly if it is distant from the trigger point. This evidence primarily stems from clinical observation and needs to be studied more rigorously in clinical trials. First, the last diagnostic criterion for MPS demonstrates that in accessible muscles, palpation of the active trigger points will alter the referred pain. In addition, injections of local anesthetic into the active trigger point will reduce or eliminate the referred pain and the tenderness (70). Treatment such as spray and stretch or exercises directed at the muscle with the trigger point will also predictably reduce the referred pain (25,71,72). Other evidence to confirm the relationship includes the use of pressure algometry to show a positive correlation between both the scope of tenderness and the severity of pain (Fricton and Schiffman, unpublished data). In addition, the change in scope of tenderness in response to treatment correlates positively with the change in symptom severity ($r = .54$) (73). Although the relationship between the pain and trigger points has good support for its existence, there are many associated problems that have traditionally confused the clinician and complicated diagnosis.

ASSOCIATED PROBLEMS

Myofascial pain syndrome, particularly in the head and neck, is often accompanied by signs and symptoms in addition to pain, coincidental pathology conditions, and frequent behavioral and psychosocial problems. Table 2 lists many of the signs and symptoms noted by 164 patients with MPS in the head and neck. In addition, other symptoms may include scratchy sensations, hyperesthesia, tooth sensitivity, and increased salivation (74). Ad-

TABLE 2. *Additional signs, symptoms, and disorders that have been found with MPS of the head and neck*

	N	%
Neurological		
Tingling	45	27.4
Numbness	43	26.2
Blurred vision	23	14.0
Twitches	20	12.2
Trembling	13	7.9
Excess lacrimation	12	7.3
Gastrointestinal		
Nausea	40	24.5
Constipation	24	14.6
Indigestion	22	13.4
Diarrhea	11	6.7
Vomiting	8	4.9
Musculoskeletal		
Fatigue	65	39.6
Tension	60	36.6
Stiff joints	32	19.5
Swelling	20	12.2
Otological		
Tinnitus	69	42.1
Ear pain	68	41.5
Dizziness	38	23.1
Diminished hearing	29	17.7

From Fricton et al., ref. 9, with permission.

ditional signs such as excessive sweating, skin flushing, muscle twitching, and swelling have also been seen (5,9). Numerous otological symptoms, such as ear pain, tinnitus, diminished hearing, dizziness, vertigo, and fullness in the ear, have been reported despite negative examinations of the ear (48,75,76). These signs and symptoms may appear to mimic many other conditions, including migraine headaches, neuralgias of the head and neck, temporal arteritis, causalgia, TMJ disorders, arthritis, spinal disc disease, sinusitis, tooth pathology, and other common pain-producing pathological conditions (74,77).

In addition, multiple overlapping diagnoses often exist in chronic head and neck pain, confusing the diagnosis further. It is unclear whether MPS develops in response to other pathological conditions or coincidentally. For example, trigger points often develop in association with joint pathology such as osteoarthritis, subluxation, and disc disease (9,78,79). In a study of 164 patients with head and neck MPS (9), joint problems were the most frequent codiagnosis at 42%. It has been postulated that MPS develops as a result of reflex muscle splinting in an effort to protect the dysfunctional joint from aggravating movement. Trigger points have also been found with systemic or local infections of viral or bacterial origin, with lupus erythematosus, with scleroderma, with rheumatoid arthritis, and along segmental distribution of nerve injury, nerve root compression, or neuralgias (9,64). Pathology of specific viscera have been observed to coincide with the development of specific trigger points and patterns of pain referral, such as trigger points in the pectoralis major found with acute myocardial infarction (64). Metabolic disturbances such as hypothyroidism, hyperuricemia, increased creatinine levels, estrogen deficiency, mild iron-deficiency anemia, chronic alcoholism, and low potassium or calcium reserves have also been cited as coinciding with the presence of trigger points (5). Nutritional imbalances such as sustained low blood levels of ascorbic acid, decreased plasma levels of free tryptophan and ascorbic acid and low levels of vitamins E, B_1, B_6, and B_{12}, and folic acid (as occurs with alcoholism) have also been found associated with MPS (5). Research needs to be done to determine the exact relationship that these conditions have with MPS.

As with many chronic pain conditions, one will also see concomitant social, behavioral, and psychological disturbances that may precede or follow the development of pain. Patients report psychological symptoms such as frustration, anxiety, depression, hypochondriasis, and anger if acute cases become chronic through inadequate treatment (80–83). Maladaptive behaviors such as pain verbalization, poor sleep and dietary habits, lack of exercise, poor posture, bruxism, and medication dependencies can also be seen when pain becomes prolonged (5,9,84–87). Each of these may complicate the clinical picture by perpetuating the pain, preventing compliance, and causing self-perpetuating chronic pain cycles to develop.

Parafunctional muscle habits such as bruxism, clenching, and shoulder shrugging can be generated as a form of tension release as well as a learned behavioral response (32,33,88–90). One hypothesis suggests that some patients show difficulty in verbalizing anger, hostility, or anxiety and, as stress increases, an increase in contraction of musculature through these habits produces trigger points and pain (80,81,86,91–93). However, the relationship between stress and MPS is difficult to assess because stress is difficult to define and as a result the study of stress suffers from major methodological problems. Although no evidence suggests a direct causal relationship between stress and myofascial pain, some studies suggest that a correlation does exist between them. There is a higher than normal incidence of psychophysiological disorders such as migraine headaches, backache, neck pain, nervous asthma, and ulcers in patients with myofascial pain, which suggests similar etiological factors (94,95). Also, higher than normal levels of urinary concentrations of catecholamines and 17-hydroxysteroids commonly associated with a high number of stressful events were found in a group of myofascial pain dysfunction syndrome patients compared to controls (96).

Because trigger points usually develop in adults, others suggest they may result from progressive physical strain placed on certain muscles as we age

TABLE 3. *Postural problems found in 164 patients with MPS of the head and neck*

	N	%
Body		
Poor sitting/standing posture	157	96.0
Forward head tilt	139	84.7
Rounded shoulders	135	82.3
Poor tongue position	111	67.7
Abnormal lordosis	76	46.3
Scoliosis	26	15.9
Occlusion		
Slide from retruded contact position to intercuspal contact position of 1 mm or greater	140	85.5
Unilateral occlusal prematurities in intercuspal contact position	113	68.9
Class II, Division 1	96	58.5
Class II, Division 2	51	31.1
Class III	16	9.8

From Fricton et al., ref. 9, with permission.

(97). This concept is supported by clinical findings such as the strong relationship that lack of exercise and poor muscle posture have with the presence of trigger points (97). For example, many patients with MPS of the masticatory muscles are found to have occlusal prematurities, and experimental long-term hyperactivity of masticatory muscles has been related to the development of muscle pain (32,58,89,98). It has been suggested that occlusal disharmonies contribute to condylar displacement and occlusal avoidance patterns, and both can contribute to abnormal proprioceptive input and sustained muscle contraction in an attempt to correct the poor occlusal relationships and allow harmonious neuromuscular function (98–100). This may also occur in other musculoskeletal systems in the body. For example, poor posture caused by a unilateral short leg, small hemipelvis, increased cervical or lumbar lordosis, noncompensated scoliosis, and poor positioning of the head have been implicated in MPS (5,17,101,102). Table 3 lists postural problems associated with patient having MPS in the head and neck (9). Since the evidence implicating poor posture with MPS is correlational, further research is needed to determine if posture is an etiological or a consequential factor.

PATHOPHYSIOLOGY OF MPS

Whatever etiological factors are involved, it appears that the development of trigger points may be a progressive process, with a stage of neuromuscular dysfunction of muscle hyperactivity and irritability that is sustained by numerous perpetuating factors and then followed by a stage of organic dystrophic changes in the muscle bands with the trigger points (50,103) (Fig. 5).

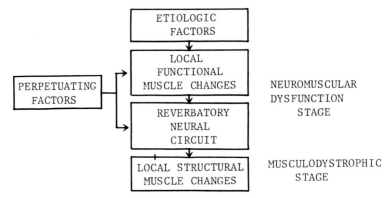

FIG. 5. A proposed mechanism for MPS involves the development of neuromuscular dysfunction characterized by self-sustaining muscle hyperactivity and irritability followed by dystrophic changes involving the muscle bands with trigger points. This process is further sustained by postural, metabolic, systemic, and other perpetuating factors.

The clinical and experimental characteristics coupled with the theories proposed by Awad (1973), Simons (1981), Melzack (1981), and Simons and Travell (1981) assist in understanding the pathophysiology of the neuromuscular dysfunction stage (3,23,103,104). These theories are proposed as only one of many possible explanations for this phenomenon. It is hoped that further research is stimulated to support or refute them.

Etiological factors, including macrotraumatic or microtraumatic events, may disturb the normal or weakened muscle through muscle injury (e.g., whiplash, excess jaw opening) or sustained muscle contraction (e.g., bruxism, muscle tension, postural habits). These traumas release free calcium within the muscle through disruption of the sarcoplasmic reticulum and, with ATP, stimulate actin and myosin interaction and local contractile and metabolic activity, resulting in increases in noxious by-products. Substances such as serotonin, histamine, kinins, and prostaglandins sensitize and fire groups III and IV muscle nociceptors, and a reverberatory neural circuit is established between the nociceptors, the central nervous system, and the motor units (60–62). These afferent inputs converge with other visceral and somatic inputs in the cells, such as those of laminae I or V of the dorsal horn, on the way to the cortex, resulting in perception of local and referred pain (105–107). These inputs may be facilitated or inhibited by multiple peripherally or centrally initiated alterations in neural input to this "central biasing mechanism" of the brainstem through various modalities, such as cold, heat, analgesic medications, massage, trigger point injections, and transcutaneous electrical stimulation (104). The cycle may be perpetuated by protective splinting of the painful muscle through distorted muscle posture and by avoiding painful stretching of the muscles. Any other perpetuating factors resulting in further sustained neural activity, such as continued bruxism, poor postural habits, or inputs from pathologic viscera or dysfunctional joints, will support the reverbatory circuit.

With contractile activity sustained, local blood flow decreases, resulting in low oxygen tension, depleted ATP reserves, and diminished calcium pump action. Free calcium continues to interact with ATP to trigger contractile activity, especially if actin and myosin are overlapping within the shortened muscle, and a self-perpetuating cycle is established. Sustained increases in local noxious by-products of oxidative metabolism then contribute to the beginning of the organic musculodystrophic stage, with sensitization of nociceptors within the interstitial connective tissue at the trigger point and further disruption of the calcium pump. If normal muscle length is not restored and pain continues, functional, postural, and behavioral disturbances may further perpetuate the problem. If the process continues, the muscle band initially tries to respond with hypertrophy but later breaks down to granular ground substance, eventually resulting in localized fibrosis.

EPIDEMIOLOGY

Refinement of the characteristics and case definition of MPS enables major advances in the epidemiology of MPS to be made. Since MPS appears to be a major cause of chronic pain and disability in our society, studies examining the prevalence and incidence are essential. Questions regarding risk factors, functional impact, and progression of MPS are also critical to the assessment and prevention of pain and disability.

To date, most of the research on epidemiology of MPS has been completed on clinical populations. Fishbain and colleagues studied 283 consecutive chronic pain patients who were examined independently by a neurosurgeon and physiatrist and found 85% had a primary diagnosis of myofascial pain (8). The majority had either low back pain (73.1%) or cervical (neck) pain (17.1%). Fricton and colleagues used the criteria defined in this chapter on a clinical population of 296 head and neck pain patients and found 54.6% to have a primary diagnosis of MPS (9). Skootsky et al. studied 172 consecutive patients presenting to a general internal medicine clinic and found that 29.6% of the 54 patients presenting with pain had MPS as the diagnosis (10). They also found the intensity of pain from MPS was as high as that of other diagnoses with pain, and physicians rarely recognized MPS previous to their evaluation.

The prevalence of MPS in a general population is difficult to determine because of the methodological constraints of examining and establishing a diagnosis of MPS. Some past studies have examined the presence of chronic pain in selected sites such as headache and back pain, while others have examined for tenderness in selected muscles. For example, prevalence of different pain states in the past year was studied by L. Harris and Associates, who found headache (73%), back pain (56%), muscle pain (53%), and joint pain (51%) were the most common sites of pain (19). A number of studies have found between 9.8% and 16.7% of males and 20.8% and 74.3% of females in adult populations have severe headaches of a muscle contraction/ migrainous nature (108–110). There were no diagnostic criteria used to distinguish the two types. The presence of muscle tenderness was examined in a number of studies. Sola et al. (49) found the prevalence of one or more ''hypersensitive'' points in the shoulder and neck muscles to be 49.5% in 200 adults (100 male and 100 females) from an asymptomatic general population. These points occurred in groups 62.5% of the time and usually involved four muscles: the trapezius, scalenes, infraspinatus, and levator scapulae. Helkimo studied muscle tenderness in the masticatory muscles in 321 adults from a community (111). He found 66% to have at least one tender site in these muscles. Solberg et al. also studied masticatory muscles, but in 739 young adults, and found 34.2% to have at least one muscle site to be tender (112). None of these studies used diagnostic criteria to establish whether the pain or sites of muscles tenderness were due to MPS. Thus, the prevalence of MPS in a general population can only be indirectly estimated. Furthermore, the presence of pain or tenderness does not suggest anything about the need for treatment or the degree of disability resulting from the problem.

However, in a general population study of prevalence and need for treatment in 262 females, Schiffman and colleagues (113) used current epidemiological methods and established diagnostic criteria to define the prevalence of TMJ disorders and masticatory myalgia. The criteria included the first two of three criteria for MPS in this chapter, namely, regional pain with corresponding muscle tenderness. They labeled the disorder ''myalgia'' instead of myofascial pain to avoid confusion regarding the lack of examination for the third criterion (alteration of referred pain with palpation). The prevalence of masticatory myalgia was found to be 50% of the population. The prevalences of joint disorders (internal derangements) and combination joint and muscle disorders were 19% and 27%, respectively.

When the level of symptoms of all subjects was compared to the level of symptoms of patients presenting for treatment to a pain clinic with the same diagnosis, overall only 6% were estimated to be candidates for treatment. When subjects with symptoms were asked if they had had previous treatment for a TMJ problem, 6.7% responded positively. When subjects with symptoms who had not had treatment were asked why they had not sought treatment, the majority responded that it was not a problem or they could live with the symptoms.

This finding that the majority of people with masticatory myalgia (pain with corresponding muscle tenderness) do not have symptoms severe enough to motivate them to seek treatment raises a considerable number of questions. What happens to these people over time? Do most fluctuate between mild and no symptoms over time while a small percentage become more severe as a result of a triggering event such as trauma or stress? Is there an underlying biological factor such as a joint disorder, muscle type I/type II maldistribution, or a skeletal discrepancy that also predisposes to developing more severe symptoms? Is mild pain with muscle tenderness found in all normal individuals and patients with more severe symptoms have disturbances in a central biasing mechanism that increases perception of pain or decreases tolerance? These questions and others need to be examined with further epidemiological investigations if we are to increase our knowledge of this societal problem.

REFERENCES

1. Hadler NM. *Am J Med* 1986;81:26–30.
2. Simons DG. *Am J Phys Med* 1975;54:288–311, 55:15–42.
3. Simons DG. *Arch Phys Med Rehab* 1981;62:97–99.
4. Simons DG. *West J Med* 1978;128:69–71.
5. Travell J, Simons DG. *Myofascial pain and dysfunction: The trigger point manual.* Baltimore: Williams & Wilkins, 1983;63–158.
6. Weinberger LM. *West J Med* 1977;127:99–103.
7. Cunningham LA, Kelsey J. *Am J Pub Health* 1984;74:574–579.
8. Fishbain DA, Goldberg M, Meagher BR, Steele R, Rosomoff H. *Pain* 1986;26:181–197.
9. Fricton J, Kroening R, Haley D. *Oral Surg* 1985;60:615–623.
10. Skootsky SA, Jaeger B, Oye RK. *West J Med* 1989 (in press).
11. Berges PJ. *Postgrad Med* 1973;53(8):161–168.
12. Bonica JJ. *JAMA* 1957;164:732–738.
13. Brown BR. *JAMA* 1978;239:646–648.
14. Simons DG, Travell JG. *Postgrad Med* 1983;73:66–108.
15. Travell J. In: Ragan C, ed. *Connective tissues: Transactions of the 5th Conference.* New York: Josiah Macy, Jr, Foundation, 1954;12–22.
16. Travell J. In: Bonica J, Albe-Fessard D, eds. *Advances in pain research and therapy,* vol 1. New York: Raven Press 1976;919–926.
17. Travell J, Rinzler SH. *Postgrad Med* 1952;11:425–434.
18. Reynolds MD. *Arch Phys Med* 1981;62:111–114.
19. Sternbach RA. *Clin J Pain* 1986;2:49–53.
20. Abel O Jr, Siebert WJ, Earp R. *J Missouri Med Assoc* 1939;36:435–437.
21. Fassbender HG. In: Fassbender HG, ed. *Pathology of rheumatic disease* (Loewi G, transl). New York: Springer-Verlag, 1975;303–314.
22. Kraft GH, Johnson EW, LaBan MM. *Arch Phys Med Rehab* 1968;49:155–162.
23. Awad EA. *Arch Phys Med Rehab* 1973;54:449–453.
24. Gorrell RL. *JAMA* 1950;142:557–561.
25. Greene CS, Laskin DM. *J Am Dent Assoc* 1974;89:1365–1368.
26. Karakasis D. *J Maxillofac. Surg* 1977;5:310–313.
27. Lange F. *Munch Med Wochenschr* 1925;72:1626.
28. Lange F. *Die muskelharten (myogelosen).* Munich: JF Lehmann's Verlag, 1931.
29. Valentine M. *Ann Rheumat Dis* 1947;6:241–250.
30. Yemm R: *Oral Sci Rev* 1976;7:31–53.
31. Wolfe F, Smythe HA, Yunus MB, Bennett RM, Bombardier C, Goldenberg DM, Tugwell P, Multicenter Fibromyalgia Criteria Committee. *Arthritis Rheum* 1989;32:547.
32. Christensen LV. *J Oral Rehab* 1975;2:169–178.
33. Lefer L. *Contemp Psychoanal* 1969;2:135.
34. Fricton J, Schiffman E. *J Dent Res* 1986;65:1359–1364.

35. Reeves JL, Jaeger B, Graff-Radford SB. *Pain* 1988;24:313–321.
36. Schiffman E, Fricton J, Haley D, Tylka D. In: Dubner R, Gebhart GF, Bond, MR, eds. *Proceedings of the Vth World Congress on Pain.* Amsterdam: Elsevier Science Publishers, 1988;407–413.
37. MacDonald AJ. *Pain* 1980;8:197–205.
38. Arroyo P. *J Fla Med Assoc* 1966;53:29–31.
39. Dexter JR, Simons DS. *Arch Phys Med Rehab* 1981;62:521–522.
40. Travell J. *Proc Rudolf Virchow Med Soc* 1957;16:128–136.
41. Simons DG. In: Bonica JJ, Albe-Fessard D, ed. *Advances in pain research and therapy,* vol 1. New York: Raven Press, 1976;913–918.
42. Fricton J, Auvinen M, Dykstra D, Schiffman E. *Arch Phys Med Rehab* 1985;66:314–317.
43. Elliott FA. *Lancet* 1944;1:47–49.
44. Bayer H. *Klin Wochenschr* 1949;27:122–126.
45. Fisher AA. *Arch Phys Med Rehab* 1988;69:286–291.
46. Fisher AA. *Arch Phys Med Rehab* 1987;68:122–125.
47. Berry DC, Yemm R. *J Oral Rehabil* 1974;1:255–264.
48. Berry DC, Yemm R. *Br J Oral Surg* 1971;8:242–247.
49. Sola AE, Rodenberger M, Gettys G. *Am J Phys Med* 1955;34:585–590.
50. Miehlke K, Schulz G. *Internist* 1961;2:447–453.
51. Yunus MD, Kalyan-Raman VP, Masi AT, Aldag JC. *J Rheumatol* 1989;16:97–101.
52. Bendstrup P, Jespersen K, Asboe-Hansen G. *Ann Rheum Dis* 1957;16:438–440.
53. Bengtsson A, Henriksson KG, Jorfeldt L, Kagedal B, Lennmarken C, Lindstrom F. *Scand J Rheumatol* 1986;15:340–347.
54. Bengtsson A, Henriksson KG, Larsson J. *Scand J Rheumatol* 1986;15:1–6.
55. Miehlke K, Schulz G, Eger W. *Z Rheumaforsch* 1960;19:310–330.
56. Bengtsson A, Henriksson KG, Larsson J. *Arthritis Rheum* 1986;29:817–821.
57. Lund N, Bengtsson A, Thorborg P. *Scand J Rheumatol* 1986;15:165–173.
58. Christensen LV. *Arch Oral Biol* 1971;16:1021–1031.
59. Ibraham GA, Awad EA, Kottke FJ. *Arch Phys Med Rehab* 1974;35:23–28.
60. Mense S. *J Physiol (Lond)* 1977;267:75–88.
61. Mense S, Schmidt RF. In: Rose FD, ed. *Physiologic aspects of clinical neurology.* Oxford, England: Blackwell Scientific Publications, 1977;265–278.
62. Kniffki KD, Mense S, Schmidt RF. *Exp Brain Res* 1978;31:511–522.
63. Lim RKS, Guzman F, Rodgers DW. In: Barker D, ed. *Symposium on muscle receptors.* Hong Kong: Honk Kong University Press, 1962;215–219.
64. Kennard MA, Haugen FP. *Anesthesiology* 1955;16:297–311.
65. Travell J, Bigelow NH. *Fed Proc* 1946;5:106.
66. Ghia JN, Mao W, Toomey TC, Gregg JM. *Pain* 1976;2:285–299.
67. Kroening R. In Allen GD, ed. *Dental anesthesia and analgesia: local and general.* Baltimore, Williams, & Wilkins, 1979;1–21.
68. Lee T-N. *Orthop Rev* 1977;6:63–66.
69. Melzack R, Stillwell DM, Fox EJ. *Pain* 1977;3:3–13.
70. Jaeger B, Reeves JL, Graff-Radford S. *Proc Am Pain Soc* 1986;82, abstr CP7.
71. Fricton JR, Hathaway KM, Bromaghim C. *Cranio Dis Fac Oral Pain* 1987;1:115–122.
72. Jaeger B, Reeves JL. *Pain* 1986;87:203–210.
73. Fricton J, Schiffman E. *J Prosthet Dent* 1986;58:222–228.
74. Travell J. *Arch Phys Med Rehab* 1981;62:100–106.
75. Arlen H. *Ear, Nose Throat J* 1977;56:60–63.
76. Bernstein JM, Mohn N, Spiller H. *Trans Am Acad Ophthalmol Otolaryngol* 1969;73:1210.
77. Travell J. *J Prosthet Dent* 1960;745–763.
78. Guralnick W, Kaban LB, Merril RG. *N Engl J Med* 1978;299:123–129.
79. Weinberg LA, Lager LA. *J Prosthet Dent* 1980;44:642–653.
80. Lupton DE, Johnson DL. *J Prosthet Dent* 1973;29:323–329.
81. Lupton DE. *J Am Dent Assoc* 1969;79:131.
82. Moulton R. *Dent Clin North Am* 1966;10:609.
83. Pomp AM. *J Am Dent Assoc* 1974;89:629–632.
84. Fuchs P. *J Oral Rehab* 1975;2:35–48.
85. Moldofsky H, Scarisbrick P, England R, Smythe H. *Psychosom Med* 1975;37:341–351.

86. Moss RA, Garrett J, Chiodo JF. *Psychol Bull* 1982;92:331–346.
87. Rugh JD, Solberg WR. *Oral Sci Rev* 1976;7:3–30.
88. Fowler RS, Kraft GH. *Arch Phys Med Rehab* 1974;35:28–30.
89. Scott DS, Lundeen TF. *Pain* 1980;8:207–215.
90. Vernallis FF. *J Clin Psychol* 1955;11:389–391.
91. Chaco J. *J Oral Med* 1973;28:45–46.
92. Laskin DM. *J Am Dent Assoc* 1969;79:147,
93. Thomas LJ, Tiber N, Schireson S. *Oral Surg* 1973;36:763–768.
94. Berry DC. *Br Dent J* 1967;4:222–226.
95. Gold S, Lipton J, Marbach J, Gurion B. *J Dent Res* 1975;54:165 (abstr).
96. Evaskus DS, Laskin DM. *J Dent Res* 1972;51:1464–1466.
97. Kelly M. *Ann Rheum Dis* 1946;5:69–77.
98. Loiselle RJ. *J Am Dent Assoc* 1969;79:145–146.
99. Brill N, Schubeler S, Tryde G. *J Prosthet Dent* 1962;12:255–261.
100. Perry HT Jr. *J Am Dent Assoc* 79:137–141.
101. Kendall HO, Kendall F, Boynton D. *Posture and pain.* Huntington, NY: RE Krieger Pub Co, Inc, 1970;15–45.
102. Kraus H. *Clinical treatment of back and neck pain.* New York: McGraw-Hill Book Co, 1970.
103. Simons DG, Travell J *Pain* 1981;10:106–109.
104. Melzack R. *Arch Phys Med Rehab* 1981;62:114–117.
105. Kerr FW. In: Bonica JJ, Albe-Fessard D, eds. *Advances in pain research and therapy,* vol 1. New York, Raven Press, 1976;75–90.
106. Pomeranz B, Wall PD, Weber WY. *J Physiol* (*Lond*) 1968;199:511–532.
107. Selzer M, Spencer WA. *Brain Res* 1969;14:331–348.
108. Andrasik F, Holroyd A, Abell T. *Headache* 1979;19:384–387.
109. Nikiforow R, Hokkanen E. *Headache* 1978;18:137–145.
110. Waters WE. *Headache* 1974;14:81–90.
111. Helkimo J. *Oral Sci Rev* 1976;1:54.
112. Solberg WK, Woo MW, Houston JB. *J Am Dent Assoc* 1979;98:25–34.
113. Schiffman E, Fricton J, Haley D, Shapiro BL. *J Am Dent Assoc* 1989;(in press).

Advances in Pain Research and Therapy, Vol. 17,
edited by James R. Fricton and Essam Awad.
Raven Press, Ltd., New York © 1990.

6

Chronic Myofascial Pain Syndromes

Mysteries of the History

Janet G. Travell

*Department of Medicine, The George Washington University,
Washington, DC 20037*

Unraveling the complex problems of a chronic myofascial pain syndrome (MPS) requires special skill in obtaining the history and understanding the patient. Determining the complexity of the case, the muscles involved, and all perpetuating factors requires selective questioning and artful listening (1). Success in managing these patients depends upon the quality of this communication. The purpose of this chapter is to describe the important aspects of history that are specifically relevant to understanding the patient with MPS.

PHASES

Myofascial pain syndrome is a regional muscle pain disorder that is characterized by tender spots in taut bands of muscle that refer pain to areas overlying or distant to the tenderness. The tender spots are termed "trigger points" and can be active, with pain referral, or latent, with only tenderness. The pain history is interpreted in terms of three phases of refractory chronic myofascial pain. In phase 1, there is constant pain. In phase 2, the pain occurs only on motion or effort. In phase 3, the patient does not complain of pain, but experiences referred tenderness, stiffness, and restricted range of motion.

Phase 1 (constant pain): Patients have continuous, deep, aching pain at rest, referred from hyperirritable, active myofascial trigger points, and are usually unaware of the activities that aggravate pain. They already have such intense pain that they do not perceive an increase, and so cannot distinguish what makes it worse.

Phase 2 (pain on motion): These patients generally feel pain only on specific movements, referred from less irritable active trigger points, and have some relatively pain-free days. Thus, patients can identify what activity makes the pain worse. They must learn not to be spartan, not to suffer from the "good sport syndrome," but should become aware of what aggravates the pain and learn to avoid that activity. This phase is ideal for patient education.

Phase 3 (no pain): Patients with only latent trigger points experience referred tenderness and are usually hampered by restricted range of motion, or "stiffness." The shoulder or hip may be sore when bearing weight in the recumbent position, and thus can disrupt sleep. The discomfort disturbs sleep if the patient lies on the tender region, but is not painful enough to cause the patient to see a doctor for relief. Many Phase 1 patients reach this third phase and are 90% better. But why settle for less than 100%?

Patients with chronic MPSs under moderately good control tend to transfer back and forth between phases 2 and 3. The referred pain or tenderness generally recurs in the same distribution, has much the same quality, and depends on a particular physical activity or stress level. The danger is that the latent trigger points of phase 3 can readily be reactivated. Inactivating them and restoring full function and range of motion is good preventive medicine. When the phase 3 residual problems are addressed, full normalization of muscle function is achieved.

Phase 2 is ideal for patient education and communication. If patients are encouraged to pay attention, they usually can recognize when they use a muscle improperly. A delayed onset of pain often occurs, however, even 12 to 20 hours later; thus, the pain may result from activity performed the day before. This lag in onset means that the cause of the recurrence is overlooked unless the patient is taught how to perceive it.

Sometimes patients do realize what they have done wrong, but feel so guilty for appearing stupid that they fail to inform their physicians. In such cases, the doctor should take the blame and remind the patient that the doctor is the teacher and the patient is the student. If the doctor is not a good teacher, the recurrence of pain is the doctor's fault, not the patient's, because pain relief is ultimately dependent on the patient's success in properly using the involved muscles as taught by the doctor.

Conversely, in phase 2, successive pain patterns mapped between visits may tell the story of progressive improvement, with some pain areas disappearing and others not. The patient should keep a pictorial record of pain recurrences on a body form. The patient shades the body form in red to show where the pain occurred, dates the recurrence, and notes with what activity or life situation each episode of pain was associated (2). The patient shades in green any numbness or tingling with the date of the symptoms. This serves as a pain diary.

HISTORY

Preliminary Review

The completeness of the history is increased by a preliminary review of the patient's story and records. Before the first visit, the patient is requested to submit a chronology of life events and a chronology of medical events, and complete lists of current and previous medications and nutritional supplements.

The *chronology of life events* should give dates for locations of living, education, marriages, children living (age and where they live), sports activities, travel, and employment (what kind, where, for whom).

The *chronology of medical events* should include illnesses, infections, accidents (fractures, falls, etc.), surgical procedures, dental procedures, pregnancies and miscarriages, allergies (tests and hyposensitizations), and vaccinations. The patient may deny an accident if no fracture occurred, but further interrogation will elicit the full history.

Myofascial trigger points are aggravated by high histamine levels and active allergies. Marking the skin to test for dermatographia is a simple way of identifying high histamine levels. The patient is generally aware of inhalant allergies, but special care must be taken to check for food allergies and what foods cause symptoms.

For inhalant allergies, reducing exposure by the use of electrostatic air cleaners is helpful. However, the fact that the patient has an electrostatic air cleaner may not be sufficient. One patient assured me that she was using it every night, but when I inquired further, it turned out that she also opened her bedroom windows every night. She liked fresh air and did not realize that her air cleaner had no chance of eliminating all the pollens that were coming in from outdoors.

The *list of medications* should include all medications currently being taken, including vitamin and mineral supplements. The patient is asked to bring a bottle of every medication so that the actual dosage can be established. This includes prescription and over-the-counter drugs, as well as nutritional supplements. A *list of the medications* taken in the past that caused side effects or did not relieve the pain is also important.

The patient is asked to send, in advance, a copy of all medical records in his or her possession and to request any others to be sent by consulting physicians. These are carefully reviewed before the patient's initial visit.

Interview with Patient

To effectively understand the history, it is important to empathize but not to identify with the patient. Empathy is established by putting oneself in the patients' shoes, objectively seeing their life problems from their point of view, understanding their jobs, their personal relationships, and their emotional stresses. Identification with the patient often results in emotional involvement that is destructive to the doctor-patient relationship and can be damaging to the doctor's own mental health.

Pain Distribution

If the pain is constant (phase 1), the patient is likely either to say, "I hurt all over," or to focus on the most intense pain, not mentioning other pains until that severe pain is relieved.

Learning to discriminate where it really does hurt is essential. One patient said she had pain in her "TMJ." She had received temporomandibular joint arthrograms and multiple tests and treatments by many dentists and physicians for her "TMJ pain." When asked to point to where the pain was located, she said, "In my TMJ." When again asked to point to where it hurt, she put her finger on the mastoid process behind the ear. She never had any pain in the TMJ region. This lack of anatomical knowledge causes similar problems for the shoulder, buttock, low back, and other parts of the body.

When the patient complains of "pain all over," the doctor must ask, "Do you have pain in the nose? The earlobe? The knee?" When the patient says "no" to one or more of these questions, the lesson is learned that pain is not felt all over and that the physician needs to know the precise distribution of pain. Only by mapping the specific pain patterns can one begin to identify the likely locations of the trigger points responsible for the pain complaints.

An accurate picture of all the areas of pain is very important. After completing the pain distribution on a body form that has each pain shaded in red (the same body form used for the pain diary between visits can be used for this purpose), the patient may be asked, "Are these all the areas where you have pain?"

> "Yes."
> "Do your feet hurt?"
> "Why, yes! All my life."
> "Why didn't you mention them?"
> "Don't everyone's feet hurt?"

Another patient may fail to mention headaches, and then reply to a specific question, "They're normal. I've had them as long as I can remember."

Another helpful question is, "What do you do to get relief?" One woman, when asked how she relieved her backache (interscapular), confided that she lay on a hot iron and rubbed the pain away.

> "Oh, dear, I never told anyone else that before. You will think I'm crazy."
> "No, that is exactly what I would expect you to do to help relieve the pain from those muscles in your upper back."

It is important to reassure the patient that whatever the pain history, it is believable to you.

Some patients are afraid of being labeled hypochondriacs or psychological cripples if they reveal all the places where they hurt. Some have been convinced by psychologists and psychiatrists that they really are crazy to think that they have so much pain.

Also, patients should be assured that you do not think they are "doctor shopping" because they have seen so many physicians for their long-standing severe pain problem. Rather, they are to be commended for their determination to get well.

Review of Body Systems

A brief review of the major body systems helps to ensure that a significant medical problem is not being overlooked. In reviewing the gastrointestinal tract, the history should be explored for diarrhea, constipation, nausea, heartburn, abdominal pain, hemorrhoids, blood in the stools, and the like. When a patient is low in folate, diarrhea is likey to occur intermittently with explosive, watery stools. Constipation often is associated with low thyroid function and/or vitamin B_1 inadequacy. Excessive flatus may be dietary or due to loss of normal intestinal bacterial flora.

Simple questionnaires are easily misleading. When one patient was asked if she had diarrhea, she answered, "Oh, no." As she was leaving the office, she asked for a prescription for paregoric. When queried, she replied, "Oh, I'm going to the theater tonight and, if I didn't take the paregoric, during the performance I probably would have to rush out to the bathroom." She did not have diarrhea; she took paregoric regularly as a preventive.

Sleep

If patients report that they "sleep poorly," further questioning is in order. Is it because they cannot fall asleep or because sleep is interrupted repeatedly during the night? Do they wake up early and are unable to go back to sleep? Most important, what disturbs their sleep? In what position do they sleep? (There may be a mechanical cause of pain that interferes with sleep.) Do they have "restless legs" (folic acid deficiency)? Do they have a chronic urinary tract infection and nocturia so that they have to get up at night to empty the bladder?

I asked one patient if he had to get up at night to urinate.

"Oh, no."
"Was there ever a time when you did have to urinate at night?"
"Yes. Now, all the time, several times every night."
"But I thought you said you didn't have to get up at night."
"That's right, I don't. I use a bedside urinal."

Many times, the cause of sleep disturbance is specifically identifiable and correctable. The baby may cry at night because it doesn't have enough blankets and is cold. Body warmth is also important for myofascial pain patients. When the muscles become cool at night, they contract to generate heat, and this tension can activate latent trigger points. An electric blanket is most helpful, even during the summer in an air-conditioned, cool room. Often, only the spouse is aware of the painless jerking of "restless legs" at night. A supplement of folic acid, several milligrams daily, frequently resolves this source of sleep disturbance.

Diet

Questions regarding what foods the patient avoids may be as informative as those regarding what foods they eat. Patients may assure you that they eat a well-balanced, normal diet. When I questioned one man about his diet, he replied, "I have a wonderful appetite!" I repeated my question as to what he ate, and he smiled and said, "I'm always hungry." I changed my question:

> "Are there any foods that you avoid?"
> "Oh, yes, I'm a complete vegetarian."

In his previous medical questionnaire, his doctor had marked his diet as normal. His myofascial pain had started insidiously soon after he stopped eating meat, fowl, fish, and dairy products. He took no vitamin or other nutritional supplements.

The history should also determine whether meals are prepared ahead of time and placed on heated trays under fluorescent lighting, as in a doctors'/nurses' dining room, a home for the elderly, school cafeterias, or even at a first-class hotel buffet. This exposure of food to heat and fluorescent light causes rapid degradation and loss of vitamin C and some B vitamins. Even the exposure of a newborn baby's skin to fluorescent light in the nursery may produce a vitamin B_2 (riboflavin) deficiency with ensuing anemia, convulsions, and death, preventable by adequate supplementation of riboflavin.

The quality of the diet is determined not only by what the patient eats but by how this food is prepared. Are the potatoes fried or peeled and boiled? If boiled, are they cut into pieces to cook faster, which permits the water-soluble vitamins and minerals to leach out? If the raw spinach leaves are soaked in water to wash them well, this leaches out folic acid. Thus raw/green salads, fruits, milk, vegetables, and the like do not always provide an adequate, balanced diet.

Work Situation

A careful history of precisely what the patient ordinarily does at work (or at home) is fundamentally important. Many times, if the patient is in phase

2, it is helpful for the patient to keep a written record of any onset of pain throughout the day and to relate it to activities at the time. The many sources of strain include: awkward positioning of a keyboard or reading and writing material; visitors seated at one side requiring patients to turn the head and neck to face the individual with whom they are talking; holding a telephone receiver between chin and shoulder; or abuse of the muscles in housework (3).

A common source of overlooked muscle strain is long-standing loss of range of motion in one arm, requiring the opposite afflicted extremity to be overworked. One patient, a dentist, had myofascial pain in the left arm and a painless middle finger of the dominant right hand that he could not flex beyond 90 degrees. When asked why, the patient said, "I broke the finger when I was a youngster, 50 years ago, and the joint has been locked ever since."

While talking to the patient, I gently examined the finger and discovered that, indeed, it did bend. I concluded that the middle finger's long extensor muscle harbored latent trigger points that restricted stretch but caused no pain. His muscles had learned to guard that part of the body; I taught them differently. One brief application of the vapocoolant spray–passive stretch procedure promptly restored the full range of finger flexion (4). The dysfunction of the dominant right hand had caused compensatory overload and myofascial pain syndromes of the nondominant extremity.

Patient Education

When the patient is ready to leave the office and has been instructed what to do in order to improve muscle function, he or she is given a pad and asked to write down these recommendations without prompting. Patients rarely can complete the list unaided; with prompting, they can remember and write down the items. This helps to fix in the patient's mind what needs to be done and provides a ready reference at home, a reminder of what to do. We found that our earlier system of simply handing the patient the written list had resulted in spotty compliance. Also, having the patient write down the recommendations *during* the visit, as the items came up for discussion, had not proven as effective as the recall review just before leaving the office.

CONCLUSION

Ultimately, the accuracy and completeness of the history depend on the quality of communication between doctor and patient. This, in turn, requires an unhurried allotment of time. The art of communication is one of the health professional's most valuable skills. Both verbal and nonverbal communication, or body language, play an important role.

REFERENCES

1. Travell JG, Simons DG. *Myofascial pain and dysfunction: The trigger point manual*. Baltimore: Williams & Wilkins, 1983.
2. Travell J. In: Bonica JJ, Albe-Fessard D, eds. *Advances in Pain Research and Therapy*, vol 1. New York: Raven Press, 1976;919–926.
3. Travell J. *Am Med Wom Assoc* 1963;18:159–162.
4. Travell J. *Arch Phys Med* 1952;33:291–298.

CHRONOLOGICAL BIBLIOGRAPHY ON MYOFASCIAL PAIN

Travell W, Travell J. *Arch Phys Ther* 1941;22:486–489.
Travell J, Rinzler SH, Herman M. *JAMA* 1942;120:417–422.
Travell W, Travell J. *Arch Phys Ther* 1942;23:222–246.
Travell J, Berry C, Bigelow NH. *Fed Proc* 1944;3:49 (abstr).
Travell J, Bigelow NH. *Fed Proc* 1946;5:106 (abstr).
Travell J, Travell W. *Arch Phys Med* 1946;27:537–547.
Travell J, Bigelow NH. *Psychosom Med* 1947;9:353–363.
Travell J, Bobb AL. *Fed Proc* 1947;6:378 (abstr).
Travell J, Rinzler SH. *Can Med Assoc J* 1948;59:333–338.
Rinzler SH, Travell J. *Am Heart J* 1948;35:248–268.
Travell J. *J Am Med Wom Assoc* 1949;4:89–95.
Travell J. *Mississippi Valley Med J* 1949;71:13–21.
Travell J, Rinzler SH. *Fed Proc* 1949;8:339 (abstr).
Travell J. *Bull NY Acad Med* 1950;26:284–287.
Travell J. *Circulation* 1951;3:120–124.
Travell J. *Arch Phys Med* 1952;33:291–298.
Travell J. In: Ferrer MI, ed. *Connective tissues, transactions of the second conference*. New York: Josiah Macy, Jr Foundation, 1952;86–125.
Travell J, Rinzler SH. *Postgrad Med* 1952;11:425–434.
Rinzler SH, Stein I, Bakst H, Weinstein J, Gittler R, Travell J. *Proc Soc Exp Biol Med* 1954;85:329–333.
Travell J. *NY State J Med* 1955;55:331–339.
Weeks VD, Travell J. *J Pediatr* 1955;47:315–327.
Travell J. *House Beautiful* 1955;Oct:140–193. (Reprinted 1961;July:80–83, 104–105.)
Travell J. *JAMA* 1955;158:368–371.
Weeks VD, Travell J. In: *AMA Scientific exhibits volume*. New York: Grune & Stratton, 1957;318–322.
Travell J. *Proc Rudolf Virchow Med Soc* 1959;16:128–135.
Travell J. *J Prosthet Dent* 1960;10:745–763.
Travell J. *J Am Med Wom Assoc* 1963;18:159–162.
Travell J. *Headache* 1967;7:23–29.
Travell J. *Office Hours Day and Night: The autobiography of Janet Travell, MD* New York: World Publishing Company; Cleveland, OH: New American Library (Signet), 1968.
Travell J. In: Bonica JJ, Albe-Fessard D, eds. *Advances in pain research and therapy*, vol 1. New York: Raven Press, 1976;919–926.
Travell J. *J Am Osteopath Assoc* 1977;77:308–312.
Travell J. *Arch Phys Med Rehabil* 1981;62:100–106.
Travell JG, Simons DG. *Myofascial pain and dysfunction: The trigger point manual*. Baltimore: Williams & Wilkins, 1983.
Simons DG, Travell JG. *Postgrad Med* 1983;73:66–108.
Travell JG. *JAMA* 1983;249:591–592 (letter).
Travell JG. *JAMA* 1984;251:216 (letter).
Travell J. *J Craniomandib Pract* 1984;2:109–110.

Simons DG, Travell JG. In: Wall PD, Melzack R, eds. *Textbook of pain*. London: Churchill Livingstone, 1984;263–276.

Travell JG. *Dental Management,* 1985;25(June):44–53.

Travell JG. *Dental Management* 1986;26(Dec):28–34.

Travell JG. In: Tollison CD, ed. *Handbook of chronic pain management*. Baltimore: Williams & Wilkins 1989;vii.

TABLE 1. *Previously proposed diagnostic criteria for fibromyalgia*

Major (mandatory)
    Generalized aches or stiffness involving three or more anatomical sites for at least 3 months
    Exclusion of other conditions that may cause similar symptoms
    At least eight typical and reproducible tender points (out of 14)
Minor
    Generalized fatigue
    Chronic headache
    Sleep disturbances
    Anxiety
    Subjective swelling
    Numbness
    Irritable bowel syndrome
    Modulation of symptoms by activity, weather, or stress

that enrolled 293 patients with fibromyalgia and 265 controls who had disorders, such as chronic shoulder and neck pain, that could be confused with fibromyalgia (7). Patients thought to have ''secondary,'' as well as primary, fibromyalgia were enrolled in the study. More than 300 variables were evaluated, including manual and dolorimeter tender point examinations. The combination of widespread pain, defined as axial plus upper and lower segment plus left- and right-sided pain, and tenderness in 11 or more of 18 tender point sites (Table 2; Fig. 1) yielded a sensitivity of 88.4% and a specificity of 81.1%. Symptoms such as fatigue, sleep disturbances, and paresthesias were more common in fibromyalgia patients than controls, but combinations of symptoms and tender poins did not provide greater diagnostic specificity or sensitivity. The study also found no differences in symptoms and signs

TABLE 2. *New criteria proposed for fibromyalgia*

A) **Widespread pain**—widespread defined as axial, upper and lower, and right and left sides of body
B) **Tenderness** in at least 11 of the following 18 bilateral locations (as illustrated in Fig. 1):
    1. Occiput: bilateral, at the suboccipital muscle insertions.
    2. Low cervical: bilateral, at the anterior aspects of the intertransverse spaces at C5–7.
    3. Trapezius: bilateral, at the midpoint of the upper border.
    4. Supraspinus: bilateral, at origins, above the scapula spine near the medial border.
    5. Second rib: bilateral, actually at the second costochondral junctions, maximum just lateral to the junctions on upper surfaces.
    6. Lateral epicondyl: bilateral, 2 cm distal to the epicondyle.
    7. Gluteal: bilateral, in upper outer quadrants of buttocks in anterior fold of muscle.
    8. Greater trochanter: bilateral, posterior to the trochanteric prominence.
    9. Knees: bilateral, at the medial fat pad proximal to the joint line.

Adapted from Wolfe et al., ref. 7, with permission.

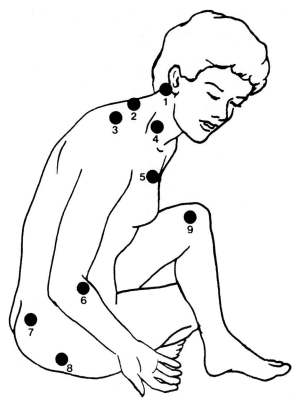

FIG. 1. Sites of examination for tenderness in the new criteria for fibromyalgia as described in Table 2. (From Wolfe et al., ref. 7, with permission.)

in primary versus "secondary" fibromyalgia and recommended that, for diagnostic purposes, this distinction should be abandoned.

The "unexplained" nature of the pain and other symptoms of fibromyalgia is implied in this or any poorly understood syndrome. However, the term "a diagnosis of exclusion" is misleading. It simply means that the pain, fatigue, and other symptoms of this syndrome are not readily explained by another chronic medical disorder. This does not mean that every possible diagnosis imaginable must be excluded by costly and invasive tests. Rather, a complete history and physical examination, with special emphasis on certain symptoms and a tender point evaluation, will almost always provide an accurate diagnosis. One of the most important outcomes of accurate descriptions and better recognition of this condition has been to save many patients undue frustration, cost, and toxicity from unnecessary extensive evaluations or inappropriate treatment. Note that in the new recommended diagnostic criteria, there is no mention of "exclusions."

MANDATORY DIAGNOSTIC FEATURES

The first mandatory diagnostic feature is chronic diffuse pain. The pain is characteristically symmetrical, that is, right and left sided, and above and below the waist. However, not uncommonly the pain will begin in a more localized area and seems to "spread" over time. Some patients continue to manifest a more "localized fibrositis," but otherwise meet criteria for the full-blown syndrome. Over 90% of patients report pain in the low back, neck, and shoulders (8–10). Other commonly involved areas are the hips, knees, chest wall, and hands. The severity of the pain has been as being as great or greater than that in rheumatoid arthritis, and patients use more adjectives when describing the pain, especially "radiating," "burning," and "tingling" (10). Although the pain intensity varies, patients generally always have some pain.

The other mandatory diagnostic feature is diffuse soft tissue tenderness at characteristic anatomical locations, termed "tender points." These points are generally found in muscle or at muscle-tendon insertions (Table 2) and are more tender than other areas in the patient and more tender at these specific points in the patients than in controls. As noted, Smythe was the first to describe the diagnostic utility of palpating for excessive tenderness at these anatomical locations (5), and Yunus et al. (6) were the first group to compare the frequency of excessive tenderness in fibromyalgia patients to that in normal controls. Campbell et al. (8) used a dolorimeter to demonstrate that patients with historical symptoms consistent with fibromyalgia had significantly more tenderness than normal controls at suspected tender points, such as over the mid-upper trapezius muscle, just distal to the lateral epicondyle, and over the medial fat pad of the knee, but there was no difference in patients versus controls at "nontender points" such as over the forehead or shin. The recent multiclinic criteria study suggests that a simple set of nine tender points, each palpated bilaterally, will provide excellent sensitivity and specificity (Table 2).

TENDER POINTS AND TRIGGER POINTS

More important issues in the tender point evaluation include: (a) Are all points around muscle and tendons more tender in fibromyalgia patients than in controls? (b) What is the relationship of tender points and trigger points? and (c) What do tender points pathophysiologically represent? Our study of 75 anatomical locations from head to toe on the right side indicated that many muscle and tendon sites, especially away from the midline, were more tender in fibromyalgia patients than controls and many of these sites clustered together in certain locations (11). Scudds et al. (12) also noted more tenderness in fibromyalgia patients compared to rheumatoid arthritis patients and normal controls when they applied the dolorimeter to "nontender points." The chapters in this text should be helpful in evaluating the relationship of trigger points and tender points as well as the clinical syndromes of myofascial pain syndrome and fibromyalgia. There is as yet no obvious pathophysiological explanation of tender points, and further clinical, electrophysiological, and histochemical studies will be necessary to shed light on this key area.

OTHER CLINICAL FEATURES

A number of other clinical features are very common in fibromyalgia, and the two most discussed are fatigue and sleep disturbances. Some clinicians will not diagnose fibromyalgia if these symptoms are not prominent. Historically, the sleep disturbances are characterized by frequent awakenings and not feeling refreshed in the morning. Moldofsky (Chapter 13, *this volume*) discusses the significance of these symptoms. The fatigue is generally described as "being exhausted" all the time, but the relationship of sleep disturbances, depression, and muscle fatigue following exercise has not been determined. Depressed mood is very common in fibromyalgia, but active, clinically significant depression is present in only 10 to 20% of patients (13). Similarly, anxiety, stress, and excess concern with health have been reported commonly but a psychiatric diagnosis of current major anxiety disorder, obsessive-compulsive disorder, or somatization disorder has been noted in less than 10% of patients (13). Although most patients report muscle pain and soreness following minimal exercise, the possible role of exercise-related metabolic changes in muscle is just being evaluated (14).

Other helpful clinical features present in the vast majority of patients include paresthesias, headaches, symptoms suggestive of irritable bowel syndrome, and functional disability. We noted that 88% of fibromyalgia patients have chronic or recurrent numbness and tingling, usually involving the upper and lower extremities (15). However, there is no evidence for a specific neuropathy in most of these patients, and they should not be subjected to extensive neurological tests or neurosurgical intervention. Headaches are typically frontal-occipital, so-called "muscular" or "tension" headaches, and a minority of patients have migraine headaches. We noted that approximately one third of fibromyalgia patients have Raynaud's phenomenon and that such patients more often have dry eyes and mouth as well as abnormal serological test results, such as low titers of antinuclear antibody, suggestive of an autoimmune disease (16). Caro has noted immunoglobulin deposition in the skin of fibromyalgia patients (17). We do not know the significance of these immune-related findings, but in a 3- to 5-year longitudinal follow-up, fibromyalgia patients rarely developed a specific connective tissue disease. However, all too often an inappropriate diagnosis of systemic lupus erythematosus (SLE), scleroderma, or another autoimmune condition is made in such patients based on such nonspecific findings.

TRIGGERING FACTORS AND CONCOMITANT CONDITIONS

We have found that approximately 50% of patients identify a specific factor that may have triggered their fibromyalgia symptoms (8). The most common factors are physical trauma, emotional trauma, or a medical illness, especially a flulike syndrome. In Chapter 10 (*this volume*) Monsein reviews the possible role of trauma and its medical-legal implications in disability determination for fibromyalgia. The association with a flulike onset has prompted us to evaluate the relationship of fibromyalgia to what has been previously termed "benign myalgic encephalomyelitis" and more recently the "chronic fatigue syndrome" (18). There is convincing evidence that the majority of patients with such chronic fatigue syndromes have fibromyalgia (19). Medications, especially withdrawal of corticosteroids, may also be capable of triggering a fibromyalgia syndrome.

Indeed, most patients with fibromyalgia probably can identify a concomitant condition that may be important in precipitating or perpetuating their condition. This may include a preexisting rheumatic disorder such as chronic low back pain, temporomandibular joint syndrome, or rheumatoid arthritis, a past or current history of depression or anxiety, a recent flulike illness, or physical trauma. However, such associations have not been demonstrated to cause fibromyalgia and therefore the concept of primary versus secondary fibromyalgia is not helpful and should be discarded (7). Rather, it is important to study concomitant disorders and factors in hopes of better understanding and treating fibromyalgia. Current studies demonstrate that fibromyalgia is common, with a prevalence of 2 to 8% in general medical clinics and 4 to 20% in rheumatology clinics (20) (Table 3). No prospective, community-based studies have been reported but two are in progress. Adequate ethnic, social, and economic data from various patient populations have not been reported.

As noted, patients classically present with an insidious onset of diffuse pain, but many have a history of chronic regional pain, such as neck or low back pain. Many such patients undergo needless diagnostic evaluation, hospitalization, and surgical intervention prior to the diagnosis of fibromyalgia (9). Bengtsson et al. noted that 87% of patients had initially localized symptoms and about one third had a sudden onset of symptoms (21).

TABLE 3. *Criteria sets used in the diagnosis of fibromyalgia*

Author	Year	Pain	Tender points required	Tender points examined	Required symptoms
Smythe	1979	Widespread	12	14	Sleep, fatigue, stiffness
Yunus	1981	Widespread	(3–4)–5	40	–
Bennett	1981	Widespread	10	25	Sleep, fatigue
Wolfe	1983	Widespread	7	14	–
"Generic"	1988	Widespread	>50%	14–19	+/–

From Wolfe, ref. 20, with permission.

[a] –, None or not specified; +, some (unspecified here).

LONG-TERM FEATURES

Although no long-term longitudinal studies have been reported, a 3-year and a 1-year prospective study each demonstrated a remarkable stability of symptoms over time and a major impact of fibromyalgia on functional status (22,23). Such stability over time, yet marked individual variability of symptoms, speaks against a stereotypical chronic pain disorder or a psychogenic, hysterical reaction. We noted that, despite treatment, more than 60% of patients had moderate or severe symptoms 3 years after their initial diagnostic evaluation (23). Hawley et al. reported that 23% of their fibromyalgia patients had a complete remission (no pain for at least 2 months) during a mean disease duration of 13 years, and the median duration of remission was 12 months (22). Functional ability and work status have been affected significantly in three recent studies (20).

CONCLUSION

Fibromyalgia is a common, internally consistent syndrome. The characteristic patient is a woman, age 20 to 50 years, who presents with generalized, chronic pain, but on physical examination has no obvious explanation for the pain other than tender points, which occur at uniform anatomical locations. Most patients have associated fatigue and sleep disturbances. The pathogenesis of these symptoms is unclear, but recent research suggests possible central nervous system as well as peripheral abnormalities. There are many explanations for the confusion and controversy surrounding this condition, including the initial descriptions of muscle inflammation and the confusing terminology applied to fibrositis syndromes. However, the most pressing problem in acceptance and understanding of fibromyalgia and myofascial pain syndromes is the absence of any obvious pathophysiological explanation for the soft tissue pain and our inherent bias that such conditions are "psychosomatic."

REFERENCES

1. Valleix F. *Traite des neuralgies au affections douloureuses des nerfs*. Paris: JB Bailliere, 1841;654.
2. Stockman R. *Edinburgh Med J* 1904;15:107–116.
3. Moldofsky H, Scarisbrick P, England R, et al. *Psychosom Med* 1975;37:341–351.
4. Moldofsky H, Scarisbrick P. *Psychosom Med* 1976;38:35–44.
5. Smythe H. In: McCarty D, ed. *Arthritis and allied conditions,* ed 10. Philadelphia: Lea & Febiger 1985;1083–1093.
6. Yunus M, Masi AT, Calabro JJ, et al. *Semin Arthritis Rheum* 1981;11:151–172.
7. Wolfe F, Smythe HA, Yunus MB, et al. *Arthritis Rheum* 1989 (in press).
8. Campbell SM, Clark S, Tindall EA, et al. *Arthritis Rheum* 1983;26:817–824.
9. Goldenberg D. *JAMA* 1987;257:2782–2787.
10. Leavitt F, Katz RS, Golden HE, et al. *Arthritis Rheum* 1986;29:775–781.
11. Simms RW, Goldenberg DL, Felson DT, et al. *Arthritis Rheum* 1988;31:182–187.
12. Scudds RA, Rollman GB, Harth M, et al. *J Rheumatol* 1987;14:563–569.
13. Goldenberg DL. *J Rheumatol* 1988;15:992–996.
14. Bennett RB, Clark SR, Goldberg L, et al. *Arthritis Rheum* 1989;32:454–460.
15. Simms RW, Goldenberg DL. *J Rheumatol* 1988;15:1271–1273.
16. Dinerman H, Goldenberg DL, Felson DT. *J Rheumatol* 1986;13:368–373.
17. Caro XJ. *Arthritis Rheum* 1984;27:1174–1179.
18. Goldenberg DL. *Semin Arthritis Rheum* 1988;18:111–120.
19. Goldenberg DL, Simms RW, Geiger A, Komaroff AK. *Arthritis Rheum* 1989;32:S47 (abstr).
20. Wolfe F. *Rheum Dis Clin North Am* 1989;15:1–18.
21. Bengtsson A, Henriksson KG, Jorfeldt L, et al. *Scand J Rheumatol* 1986;15:340–347.
22. Hawley DJ, Wolfe F, Cathey MA. *J Rheumatol* 1988;15:1551–1556.
23. Felson DT, Goldenberg DL. *Arthritis Rheum* 1986;29:1522–1526.

Advances in Pain Research and Therapy, Vol. 17,
edited by James R. Fricton and Essam Awad.
Raven Press, Ltd., New York © 1990.

8

Methodological and Statistical Problems in the Epidemiology of Fibromyalgia

Frederick Wolfe

*Department of Medicine, University of Kansas School of Medicine,
Wichita, Kansas 67214*

Wovon man nicht sprechen kann daruber muss man schweigen
Ludwig Wittgenstein

PROBLEMS IN DEFINITION AND NOMENCLATURE

Recent Development of Diagnostic Criteria

It is paradoxical that although the fibromyalgia syndrome must have afflicted mankind for centuries and was described in the Book of Job, it has just begun to be recognized plainly within the last two decades (1–6). The causes attendant on this delay in recognition in modern times are important in their influence on our understanding of the syndrome's epidemiology. First, until the Smythe and Moldofsky paper of 1977 (3) there was no reliable way to diagnose the syndrome. Smythe and Moldofsky were not the first within the last 25 years to describe fibromyalgia as we now accept it. For example, Graham, from whom Smythe inherited the chapter in the Hollander textbook of rheumatology (7) and Traut both described fibromyalgia in most of its important details (8,9). However, until the development of reliable and testable criteria, researchers and the syndrome remained locked into innumerable arbitrary, parochial, or idiosyncratic definitions upon which few agreed. Fibromyalgia was anything and everything you wanted it to be (10). In attempting to piece together the epidemiology of the syndrome and to review its literature we run into this problem of imprecise, confused, and contradictory definitions repeatedly.

Confusion with Myofascial Pain Syndromes

A second problem in fibromyalgia epidemiology derives from the century-old syndrome of myofascial pain and its extensive literature. This syndrome

TABLE 1. *Biases in fibromyalgia research*

Selection bias
   Disease toleration bias (self-referral bias)
   Referral filter bias
   Clinic characteristic bias
   Diagnostic access bias
   Diagnostic purity bias
Ascertainment bias
   Diagnostic suspicion bias
   Information bias
   Diagnosis bias

has been exhaustively reviewed by Reynolds (11) and Simons (12,13). The overlap between the myofascial pain syndromes and fibromyalgia has caused and still causes major confusion among clinicians, and in our understanding of fibromyalgia and its epidemiology. One important factor in this confusion is that both syndromes had the same name, "fibrositis," so that even during the last 25 years one could not always be sure to which syndrome authors and clinicians were referring. It has been suggested that myofascial pain should be called just that (the myofascial pain syndrome) and not fibrositis (14). Yunus emphasized the term "fibromyalgia" for the fibromyalgia syndrome (15). These terms have not been universally accepted, but there is an advantage in accepting such usage since by this nomenclature we can orient and understand definition and thinking.

"Fibrositis" has provided us with additional problems. The recognition of the concept of fibrositis as fibromyalgia clearly followed recognition of fibrositis as myofascial pain (16). Many of the terms in each syndrome are similar, ambiguous, and confusing: trigger points and tender points; fibrositic nodules, tender nodules, and taut bands; jump signs, jump responses, and local twitches; widespread pain, referred pain, and zones of reference. Given such ambiguities and similarities it is hardly surprising that clinicians and researchers have trouble separating the syndromes; and, importantly, given the development of fibromyalgia from the construct of myofascial pain, it is hardly surprising that, in many reports and in the minds of clinicians, features of myofascial pain intrude themselves into the research and clinical concept of fibromyalgia. Even authors who write about fibromyalgia confuse the two syndromes.

BIAS IN THE CONDUCT OF FIBROMYALGIA RESEARCH

Beyond definitional problems, there are critical methodological problems. Chief among these is identification bias, but there are other important problems (biases) in fibromyalgia research as well (Table 1).

Biased Ascertainment and Selection

Diagnostic Suspicion Bias

Since Halliday's paper in 1941, which suggested that there was often an association between psychological problems and musculoskeletal pain (17), there has been a well-recognized link between fibromyalgia and psychological abnormality in the medical literature. That this is not just fortuitous is testified to by the large literature relating to psychological status in fibromyalgia (18–24). One consequence of this interaction between psychological status and fibromyalgia is that the syndrome may be regarded primarily as a psychological illness and that patients may be identified because of the presence of behavioral characteristics and psychological illness and then evaluated for the possibility of having fibromyalgia. For example, Muller from Basel, Switzerland, who appears to have identified the largest series of fibromyalgia patients in the world (867 patients), writes in his review of fibrositis syndrome (25) that *"neurotic disturbances . . ."* are present *"in 90 percent . . .* of appropriately examined fibrositis patients, whereby *patients with pronounced symptoms have always shown such disturbances"* (emphasis added). Rosenhall and coworkers of Goteborg, Sweden, studied eye motility dysfunction and reported that patients describe "symptoms of autonomic dysfunction in terms of psychosomatic symptoms," noting that "Hallucinosis of different types was reported by 55 percent of the patients (26). Hadji-Djilani and Gerster (27) of Lausanne, Switzerland, entitled their report "Menier's Disease and Fibrositis Syndrome (*Psychogenic Rheumatism*) (emphasis added). A similar article by the same authors has appeared in the North American literature in the *Journal of Rheumatology* (28). The observations in the above studies were almost certainly the result of biased ascertainment, including diagnostic suspicion bias.

The other side the diagnostic suspicion bias coin is that "normal" psychological status might lead to the search for "another diagnosis." In addition, identification of another rheumatic problem (e.g., osteoarthritis of the knee) might lead to abandonment of the consideration of the diagnosis of fibromyalgia.

Disease Toleration Bias (Self-Referral Bias)

Biased selection relative to psychological status may occur also because patients with a psychological abnormality may seek medical care more frequently than "normals (29,30). Three studies of medical care utilization indicated that fibromyalgia patients had received more medical and surgical care, even for apparently non-fibromyalgia-associated conditions, than did controls (31–33). The association of psychological status with utilization of medical services in fibromyalgia has not been examined, but might be expected to throw additional light on this bias. The effect of this bias would be to increase the prevalence of psychological abnormality in clinics as opposed to the community in a manner similar to what has been shown in irritable bowel syndrome (29,30). Persons so selected might have different disease characteristics and treatment responses in comparison with persons with fibromyalgia in the community.

Referral Filter Bias

More severely afflicted persons, including those with more psychological disturbances, are seen with increased prevalence in speciality clinics where they may be the subjects of clinical studies. Such selection bias is generally unavoidable in clinical studies, but is often unappreciated, leading to erroneous conclusions about fibromyalgia patients in general rather than to fibromyalgia patients in the (specialty) clinic. This bias is well known in most medical disciplines, but has not been generally considered in fibromyalgia research. As with some other forms of bias noted above, more severely afflicted persons may respond poorly to treatment and have different disease characteristics than those with lesser symptoms.

Clinic Characteristic Bias and Diagnostic Access Bias

Patients studied in fibromyalgia clinics, because of geographical location and/or economic barriers, may not reflect economic and racial characteristics of the community at large. Those receiving care in private practice settings (even within university clinics) may have higher socioeconomic status than persons in the community. In most fibromyalgia studies, where ethnic status is described, minorities appear underrepresented (this is also a general case in clinical trials in the United States) (34). In the United States, those persons with liberal medical insurance may be diagnosed and treated more often than those with inadequate insurance. Similarly, access to care may be available to persons receiving public assistance, but limited for the "working poor" and those without health insurance. The effect of such bias could be to overrepresent insured, white middle-class persons in fibromyalgia studies.

Comments

The biases noted above could (and probably do) seriously affect fibromyalgia research. Some biases, such as referral filter bias, clinic characteristic bias, and diagnostic access bias, are probably difficult to avoid, but with adequate description in methods sections of manuscripts the extent of the bias can at least be estimated. More serious is the problem of biased ascertainment (e.g., diagnostic suspicion bias and information bias), since unlike selection bias, in which the nature and extent of the bias can sometimes be estimated, the rate and extent of ascertainment bias is unknown. Ascertainment bias is clearly important in fibromyalgia. The notion that fibromyalgia patients are psychologically disturbed may (and probably does) lead to the performance of fibromyalgia physical and historical examinations more frequently in those patients with obvious psychological abnormality (*information bias*), and the presence of another clear-cut physical disorder may similarly restrict the consideration of the diagnosis of fibromyalgia. Although there are no studies that attempt to estimate bias in fibromyalgia research, it is likely the differences in Muller's 90 + % psychological abnoramlity in fibromyalgia patients (25) and the absence of any psychological abnormality in the elegant and epidemiologically sound study of Clark and coworkers (35) reflect these biases.

Biased Ascertainment and Selection in Clinical Studies

The biases noted above reflect problems relating to (a) who gets to the clinic and (b) who may be diagnosed as having fibromyalgia. Special problems in ascertainment and selection occur during the performance of clinical trials and observational studies beyond those noted above.

Diagnostic Purity Bias

"When 'pure' diagnostic groups exclude co-morbidity they may become non-representative (36). This is an important problem in fibromyalgia research since distinctions have usually been made between "primary" and "secondary" fibromyalgia (2,3,15). Although it is difficult to judge, the "purest" fibromyalgia group appears to be those patients reported by Yunus et al. (2). However, the ages and clinical characteristics of these patients differ in many respects from patients reported by others (37–39). Subsequent work by the same authors (40) using a more liberalized definition of "primary" demonstrated a study sample with characteristics similar to those reported by others. As indicated above, the effect of this type of bias would be to lead to nonrepresentative samples.

The converse of "purity bias" might be considered "impurity bias." The criteria that separate fibromyalgia into primary and secondary components depend on absence of "other diseases," and absence of laboratory and radiographic abnormalities. No good criteria exist to distinguish radiographic abnoramlities that cause (or are associated with) symptoms from those that do not. The term "age-related radiographic abnormalities" has been used by many authors to side-step the issue of primary and secondary fibromyalgia (38,41,42), but begs the question since the correlation of radiographic abnoramlities to clinical disease is poor (43,44). Recent studies have allowed participation by "primary" fibromyalgia patients with a variety of other medical and rheumatic disorders and laboratory abnormalities provided those abnormalities do not "cause" the fibromyalgia symptoms (40,45,46). The effect of "impurity" is hard to estimate since depending on its extent it might lead to more representative or less representative samples.

Diagnostic Problems

Recent studies examining the diagnosis fibromyalgia have utilized "criteria" to classify patients with the disorder, and at least a half-dozen criteria sets have been proposed (1). The recent Fibromyalgia Multicenter Criteria Study (FMCS) (47), although not specifically designed to test "previous criteria," provided data that allowed some assessments of the sensitivity and specificity of sets.

Criteria Insensitivity

The original criteria set of Smythe and Moldofsky was based on finding at least 12 tender points out of 14 specific sites examined in combination with morning fatigue, disturbed sleep, and morning stiffness (3). These criteria were found to be quite specific but were relatively insensitive. Less than 50% of patients with fibromyalgia as diagnosed by "experts" actually met these criteria. One problem with these criteria was that they required tenderness in almost 90% of examined sites, whereas the level of tenderness that worked best in the FMCS was 60% (11/18). Twelve of 14 tender points were found in only 64.7% of fibromyalgia patients. The FMCS also revealed that while sleep disturbance, fatigue, and morning stiffness were common (>75%), the combination of three of these criteria items was present in only 56.0% of fibromyalgia patients. Thus, as with the Smythe and Moldofsky criteria (3), criteria based on the above combination of symptoms were also insensitive (35,38). It is not known whether fibromyalgia patients excluded by these criteria sets might be different from those included, but it seems likely that they might have less "severe" manifestations of the syndrome since the presence and severity of tender points and the above historical items have been used as severity markers in treatment studies (48–50).

Criteria Nonspecificity

The FMCS study found that the number of tender points was the most important determinant of both sensitivity and specificity of the diagnosis of fibromyalgia. Sixty percent positivity provided the "best" sensitivity and specificity in the separation of patients and controls. Sets that used criteria that relied on less than this 60% figure may have had reduced specificity (47).

The criteria proposed by Yunus et al. (2) were found to be a special case. These criteria are the most commonly cited in the medical literature. The FMCS found that the criteria had an approximate sensitivity and specificity of 83.6% and 76.6%, respectively, when the tender point examination was performed as described in the original article (i.e., when palpation evoked "moderate" to "marked" tenderness) but had poor specificity (63.8%) when mild tenderness was the palpation endpoint. The differences in the number of tender points required in the Yunus et al. criteria (2) and those proposed by others (1) appear to be largely explained by the tenderness endpoint and the palpation pressure. Many studies using the Yunus et al. criteria do not describe the tenderness endpoint. Although there are no data that address this point, it seems quite likely that a number of studies that cited these criteria in their methods section in fact did not adhere strictly to the appropriate methodology. It is not possible to know the consequences of such deviations, but one likely consequence might be to identify patients with regional or local pain syndromes. Indeed, the original methodological difference between the Yunus et al. criteria and most other criteria sets has been ignored or misunderstood by most authors. With the confusion between myofascial pain syndrome and fibromyalgia that we have noted above, patients with the myofascial pain syndrome could have been identified as fibromyalgia patients when criteria were misapplied. A second consequence of this misapplication might be to identify patients with emphasis on symptoms rather than physical findings. Whether such criteria misapplication also might lead to study samples with increased psychological abnormalities is not known, but seems possible.

THE LITERATURE OF FIBROMYALGIA

To investigate bias and diagnostic problems in fibromyalgia research we reviewed 58 studies published after 1977 dealing with clinical trials; case control studies and cohort and observational studies were included in this review (21,23–26,31,35,37–39,41,42,45,46,48–86). We considered the following points.

Selection process: Was the selection process described fully so that one could understand how patients were identified and enrolled into the study?
Exclusions: Were exclusions to study entry described?
Referral status: Was the pattern of referral described, including the proportion of patients referred to the clinic versus patients seen primarily in clinic without referral?
Catchment: Was the catchment area of the clinic described?

Referral bias: From the information available was there *prima facie* evidence of referral bias?

Socioeconomic variables: Were data given so that the following factors could be known: socioeconomic characteristics of the clinic in general, and socioeconomic status, education level, and ethnic origin of patients?

Selection adequacy: Considering all of the factors involved in diagnosis, was the selection process adequate to exclude significant selection bias?

Criteria used: Which of the criteria for fibromyalgia were used in the study and/or were criteria modified for the study?

Correct usage of Yunus criteria: If the criteria used were those of Yunus et al. were the criteria of palpation used correctly?

Reliability: Was reliability for the major study instruments established?

Historical ascertainment: Were the methods of obtaining historical data specified in sufficient detail (e.g., questionnaire(s) versus specific questions)? '

Physical ascertainment: Was the method for obtaining physical examination data specified in sufficient detail (e.g., which tender points were examined and how were the examinations carried out)?

Other study ascertainments: If the study employed other examinations were sufficient data presented to understand the methodology?

Appropriate controls: Were the controls utilized appropriate for the clinical questions?

Control descriptions: Were the controls adequately described?

Blinded assessors: Were the assessors blinded to the diagnosis or treatment?

Blinded ascertainment: Were biopsies and laboratory samples read blindly?

Power calculations: Were power calculations presented?

Study power: Did the study have sufficient statistical power?

Appropriate statistics: Did the statistics appear appropriate?

Multiple comparisons: Were multiple comparisons adequately addressed?

Dropouts: Was the dropout rate described?

Intention to treat: Were dropouts adequately analyzed?

Findings

Selection and Patient Characteristics

Of the 58 studies, we only considered the 20 (34.5%) that fully described the selection process (Table 2). Descriptions of the selection process ran from none at all through complete descriptions of the entire recruitment and selection process, including characteristics of nonparticipants. Typically, we found statements such as "patients were selected from the rheumatology clinic." There was rarely information as to how patients got to the clinic, how they were identified and recruited from the clinic, and how they differed

TABLE 2. *Selection characteristics in 58 fibromyalgia studies[a]*

Complete description of selection process	34.5%
Complete description of referral status	34.5%
Referral bias present	8.6%
Referral bias absent	8.6%
Referral bias undeterminable	82.7%
Description of exclusion criteria	50.0%
Biased selection	5.2%
Unbiased selection	34.5%
Selection bias unknown	60.3%

[a] See text for description of terms.

in number and severity from those who may have met criteria but were not enrolled. Only three of 58 studies described the catchment area of their clinic.

Twenty studies (34.5%) provided information regarding the referral status of patients (Table 2). We had enough information on ten studies to classify them as being biased by referral (8.6%) or being free of referral bias (8.6%). For the other 48 studies (82.7%), we did not have enough information to make a judgment.

Although many studies described their criteria for exclusion (29 of 58; 50%) when the selection method within the clinic was not described (random, consecutive, all), it was impossible to judge what the full extent of exclusions was (Table 2).

In no instance were we able to judge the socioeconomic characteristics of the clinic, and only four of the 58 studies presented information about patient socioeconomic characteristics (Table 3). Ethnic origin was mentioned in only ten studies (17.2%). Similarly, only seven studies (12.1%) presented data concerning educational level (Table 3).

We attempted to take the descriptive details regarding selection into consideration in order to characterize the adequacy of the selection process (Table 2). In doing this, we asked the subjective question, "Is this a relatively unbiased sample given what we know about the study?" In 60.3% of the studies there was not enough information to be able to answer that question. Twenty studies (34.5%) appeared unbiased in their selection, and three studies (5%) were clearly biased.

TABLE 3. *Socioeconomic data in 58 fibromyalgia studies*

Description of socioeconomic characteristics of clinic	0.0%
Description of socioeconomic characteristics of patients	6.8%
Description of ethnic origin of patients	17.2%
Description of educational level of patients	12.2%

TABLE 4. *Diagnostic criteria in 58 fibromyalgia studies*

Criteria	Reference	Percentage
Smythe and Moldofsky	3	25.8
Wolfe and Cathey	76	17.2
Bennett	6, 87	10.3
Yunus et al.[a]	2	34.5
Other[b]		27.6

[a] Twenty percent of studies used proper Yunus et al. methodology, 60% could not be determined, and 20% used improper methodology.
[b] Includes six studies modifying criteria of Yunus et al.

Diagnostic Criteria

Fifteen of the studies (25.8%) (Table 4) used the criteria of Smythe and Moldofsky (3). Ten studies (17.2%) used criteria of Wolfe and Cathey (76). The criteria of Bennett (6,87) were used in six reports (10.3%). Twenty (34.5%) used the Yunus et al. criteria (2). Of these 20 studies, four (three from Dr. Yunus' group) gave indication that they used the correct methodology to determine tenderness, including the presence of "verbal response to pain ('oh, it *really* hurts'), physical withdrawal of the part [palpated], or the characteristic recoil out of proportion to the amount of pressure exerted by the examiner, i.e., the 'jump sign' (2). In 12 of the 20 studies, we were unable to determine if the criteria had been used correctly. In four of the 20, the description of how the criteria were used indicated improper usage. Five reports from the Boston University group modified the Yunus et al. criteria to require additional tender points. Various other criteria were used (16 studies, including the five from Boston, used criteria that were different from those noted above), based on changes in the number of tender points, various historical criteria, and exclusions. One study used dolorimetry in place of the Yunus et al. palpation criteria. One study used myofascial pain syndrome criteria. Three studies (5%) failed to describe criteria used. In general, it is not possible to predict the effect on the characteristics of patients and controls that the different criteria may have had. As indicated above, the Smythe and Moldofsky criteria probably select for more severe fibromyalgia and the Yunus et al. criteria select for patients with "other diseases (including myofascial pain)" when they are improperly employed.

In studies that employed controls we found that 72.7% adequately described the selection process or diagnostic process used for control patients. In making this determination we decided that a statement like "controls were normal volunteers" was an inadequate description of controls.

Clinical Studies

Eight of the studies were randomized controlled clinical trials, 41 were case control studies, and 14 were observational trials (Table 5). Several studies

TABLE 5. *Study designs in 58 fibromyalgia studies*[a]

Randomized controlled clinical trials	8
Case control studies	41
Observational studies	14

[a] Some studies included more than one design.

described more than one study method. We identified 42 studies where blinding might have been appropriate. We found blinded observation in 45.2% of these and no blinding in 35.7%, and were unable to determine the blinding status in the other reports.

Except for a few studies that used dolorimetry, no reports used physical examination techniques or historical measures of diagnosis for which reliability data were available.

Although a review of the full statistical methodology was beyond the scope of this report, we noted that only five of the 54 reports (9.2%) performed power calculations (Table 6). Except where studies showed significant difference in patients and controls for most or all of the variables studied, it was often (70% of 54 cases) impossible to judge if the study had adequate power from the description in the report. A number of studies had small samples. Type II errors may have been important in the conclusions of several reports.

In studies where it might have been appropriate to take into account multiple comparisons, only four of 30 reports (13.3%) did so. Type I error may have been important in a number of reports.

Several (three of four) controlled clinical trials did not take into account dropouts with intention to treat analyses or similar techniques, although all treatment trials described dropout rates.

Few studies described how they obtained historical information (questionnaire versus interview); and almost no studies presented data as to the reliability and validity of the historical and physical examination techniques. Blinding was used in all "double-blind" controlled clinical trials, but rarely in observational or case control studies.

Discussion

Figure 1 ("the fibromyalgia funnel") describes the hypothetical course of fibromyalgia patients as they find their way from the community toward

TABLE 6. *Statistical problems in 58 fibromyalgia studies*

Power calculations performed	9.2%
Sample size adequacy not determinable	70.0%
Control for multiple comparisons	13.3%

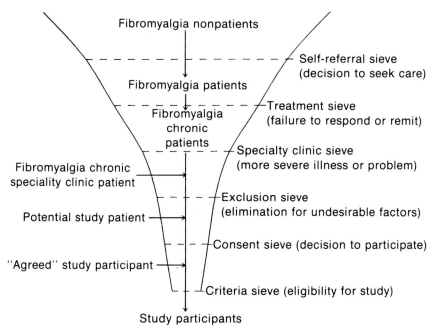

Fibromyalgia nonpatients

Self-referral sieve
(decision to seek care)

Fibromyalgia patients

Treatment sieve
(failure to respond or remit)

Fibromyalgia chronic patients

Specialty clinic sieve
(more severe illness or problem)

Fibromyalgia chronic speciality clinic patient

Exclusion sieve
(elimination for undesirable factors)

Potential study patient

Consent sieve (decision to participate)

"Agreed" study participant

Criteria sieve (eligibility for study)

Study participants

FIG. 1. The fibromyalgia funnel. Hypothetical model describing the course of fibromyalgia patients in their passage from community nonpatients to study subjects.

enrollment as study subjects. Nothing is known about fibromyalgia non-patients in the community, but if we may draw conclusions from irritable bowel syndrome nonpatients (29,30), they may be psychologically normal, and they may rarely see physicians for their fibromyalgia symptoms. The closest glimpse we have of this group is from the studies of Campbell, Clark, Bennett, and coworkers (35,38) in which persons attending a general medical clinic for other medical problems were identified as having fibromyalgia (fibromyalgia nonpatients). These patients were psychologically normal (35).

All other studies started, instead, with "patients" who were self-selected for their symptoms. Hartz and Kirchdoerfer reported on the prevalence of fibromyalgia in a family practice clinic, but not on the patients themselves, in their initial report (68). Hadler emphasized that the decision to become a patient separates the patient from the person in the community (88), but the decision to become a chronic patient separates him even further. Most patients reported in fibromyalgia studies are "chronic" patients (in this designation I include patients who may be seen for the first time in the clinic making the report, but who have consulted other clinics concerning their problems).

What happens to the patient at this stage or just before the "chronic" stage is actually unknown. Some patients seen in a primary care setting (or even, given some sophistication, in a rheumatology clinic) may receive appropriate advice or treatment and retire to the community. Some may go into remission. Those who remain (to be reported on in our studies) are usually referred to the specialty clinic. Their referral out of the clinic, however, could be based on factors such as severity, the presumed presence of an "orthopedic problem," the identification of psychological factors, the suspicion of systemic lupus erythematosus, or other patient characteristics. They are our potential study sample.

These patients are not diagnostically "clean." Most can be identified as having some other rheumatic (and other) condition of variable severity. We then apply diagnostic criteria to this group (and sometimes to others in our clinics) and make some sort of decision as to whom to exclude or include based not only on our criteria but on our perceptions of the significance of the other medical conditions that may be present. Our biases vis-à-vis psychological factors and myofascial pain may be a factor in our diagnostic classification.

When it comes time to do studies, those patients who return to the clinic most frequently (i.e., those seen most recently) are more likely to be selected than those seen years previously. Of this group only some may choose to participate. Participation may be influenced by the perceived severity of the illness to the patient, employment status, education level, and the like. Thus, at the selection funnel, the patients who come out to be studied by us may be far different from the ones that entered.

Murphy [modified in Sackett, (36)] described bias as "a process at any stage of inference which tends to produce results or conclusions that differ systematically from the truth (89). This is not always the case since in some instances the bias may be unrelated to the study outcome. In many instances the effect of bias cannot be known. For example, biased ascertainment might lead in one clinic to inclusion of more psychologically disturbed patients, in another clinic to inclusion of those with myofascial pain, and in another to inclusion of those with severe disease, and in still others it have no effect at all.

It is almost certain that biased ascertainment led to conclusions of the almost universal prevalence of psychological abnormality in one study (25) or to the fact that "Hallucinosis of different types was reported by 55 percent of the patients" in another (26). Selection bias might be responsible for the differences in psychological status of fibromyalgia patients noted in different clinics (21,23,24,33,35,72). Selection of patients with more severe disease via the selection funnel or by selective admission criteria might give a false picture of the rate of response to our therapies. For example, amitriptyline and cyclobenzaprine could be far more effective therapies in less severe patients than in the potentially more recalcitrant patients seen in our clinics and studies. A comparison might be made between studies of rheumatoid arthritis in which patients with disease of 1 year or less in duration are entered and those that enter rheumatoid arthritis patients with 10 years' duration who have failed on second-line drugs. Although most often we were not given enough information to judge the selection process in the studies described in this report, it is likely selection bias (at the level of the clinic) was present and may have influenced study results.

The FMCS suggests that the different fibromyalgia criteria sets may have identified different subsets of fibromyalgia patients, including those with more severe disease and perhaps some who should not have been classified as having fibromyalgia.

Finally, inadequate sample size may have led to type II errors in a number of fibromyalgia studies.

SUGGESTIONS FOR FUTURE RESEARCH

Fibromyalgia research is less than 15 years old, and it is not surprizing to find epidemiological and statistical errors in this young area of investigation. Unfortunately, one finds similar errors in most studies in the rheumatological literature. Questions concerning the nature of fibromyalgia and the patients who have the illness cannot be answered accurately until bias is minimized. We suggest the following guidelines in two areas.

Studies Required

1. Studies of fibromyalgia in the community are desperately needed. We are at the wrong end of the selection funnel. Critical information regarding etiology, patient characteristics, and treatment can be obtained from the community.
2. Longitudinal, prospective studies of the syndrome are essential to proper understanding.

Study Requirements

1. The most important step in improving clinical epidemiological research is a full description of the methods used in recruitment, selection, and diagnosis. Descriptions of clinic catchment and patient socioeconomic mix are required. Poor-quality research frequently hides behind inadequate description.
2. Objective ascertainment is critical. Questionnaire instruments are less

biased than interview by clinicians, and should be used frequently. Blinded assessment of physical examination features is important, particularly when a hypothesis that relates to diagnostic or physical features is being tested. Biased ascertainment with a short comment in the limitations section of the manuscript is not good research. Few readers remember the limitations as well as they remember the "results."

3. Reliability measurements are required for historical and physical examination data, but are almost never performed. Unreliable data aquisition results in negative studies. Although the psychological instruments used in fibromyalgia research are reliable, the reliability of other study measures remains unknown.

4. The use of the new FMCS criteria (47) will lead to uniform diagnostic selection, and these criteria should be adopted widely.

5. Power and sample size calculations are essential, but are rarely performed. Type II errors are frequent in fibromyalgia research. Studies that are concerned with more than one outcome variable have almost never performed power calculations for more than one measure, with the result that some conclusions represent, in fact, type II errors. Multiple comparisons are rampant in fibromyalgia research, leading to frequent type I errors.

REFERENCES

1. Wolfe F. *Am J Med* 1986;81:99–104.
2. Yunus MB, Masi AT, Calabro JJ, Miller KA, Feigenbaum SL. *Semin Arthritis Rheum* 1981;11:151–171.
3. Smythe HA, Moldofsky H: *Bull Rheum Dis* 1977;28:928–931.
4. Smythe HA. In: Kelley WN, Harris ED Jr, Ruddy S, Sledge C, eds. *Textbook of rheumatology.* Philadelphia: WB Saunders, 1985;481–489.
5. Goldenberg DL. *JAMA* 1987;257:2782–2787.
6. Bennett RM. *West J Med* 1981;134:405–413.
7. Smythe HA. In: Hollander JL, ed. *Arthritis and allied conditions.* Philadelphia: Lea & Febiger, 1972;965–968.
8. Graham W. *Bull Rheum Dis* 1953;3:33–34.
9. Traut EF. *J Am Geriatr Soc* 1968;16:531–538.
10. Pigg JS, Driscoll PW, Caniff R. *Rheumatology nursing: A problem-oriented approach.* New York: John Wiley & Sons, 1985;56–57.
11. Reynolds MD. *J Hist Med Allied Sci* 1983;38:5–35.
12. Simons DG. *Am J Phys Med* 1975;54:289–311.
13. Simons DG. *Am J Phys Med* 1976;55:15–42.
14. Simons DG. *Arch Phys Med Rehabil* 1988;69:207–212.
15. Yunus MB. *J Rheumatol* 1983;10:841–844 (editorial).
16. Reynolds MD. *Arthritis Rheum* 1982;25:1506–1507.
17. Halliday JL. *Ann Intern Med* 1941;15:666–677.
18. Ahles TA, Yunus MB, Riley SD, Bradley JM, Masi AT. *Arthritis Rheum* 1984;27:1101–1106.
19. Goldenberg DL. *Am J Med* 1986;81:67–70.
20. Hawley DJ, Wolfe F, Cathey MA. *J Rheumatol* 1988;15:1551–1556.
21. Hudson JI, Hudson MS, Pliner LF, Goldenberg DL, Pope HG Jr. *Am J Psychiatry* 1985;142:441–446.

22. Murphy S, Creed F, Jayson MI. *Br J Rheumatol* 1988;27:357–363.
23. Payne TC, Leavitt DC, Garron DC, et al. *Arthritis Rheum* 1982;25:213–217.
24. Wolfe F, Cathey MA, Kleinheksel SM, et al. *J Rheumatol* 1984;11:500–506.
25. Muller W. *Scand J Rheumatol [Suppl]* 1987;65:40–53.
26. Rosenhall U, Johansson G, Orndahl G. *Scand J Rehabil Med* 1987;19:139–145.
27. Hadj Djilani A, Gerster JC. *Acta Otolaryngol [Suppl]* 1984;406:67–71.
28. Gerster JC, Hadj Djilani A. *J Rheumatol* 1984;11:678–680.
29. Drossman DA, McKee DC, Sandler RS, Mitchell CM, Lowman BC, Burger AL. *Gastroenterology* 1988;95:701–708.
30. Whitehead WE, Bosmajian L, Zonderman AB, Costa Jr PG, Schuster MM. *Gastroenterology* 1988;95:709–714.
31. Cathey MA, Wolfe F, Kleinheksel SM, Hawley DJ. *Am J Med* 1986;81:78–84.
32. Caro XJ, Kinsted NA, Russell IJ, Wolfe F. *Arthritis Rheum* 1987;30:S63 (abstr).
33. Kirmayer LJ, Robbins JM, Kapusta MA. *Am J Psychiatry* 1988;145:950–954.
34. Svensson CK. *JAMA* 1989;261:263–265.
35. Clark S, Campbell SM, Forehand ME, Tindall EA, Bennett RM. *Arthritis Rheum* 1985;28:132–137.
36. Sackett DL. *J Chron Dis* 1979;32:51–63.
37. Wolfe F, Cathey MA. *J Rheumatol* 1983;10:965–968.
38. Campbell SM, Clark S, Tindall EA, Forehand ME, Bennett RM. *Arthritis Rheum* 1983;26:817–824.
39. Bengtsson A, Henriksson KG, Jorfeldt L, Kagedal B, Lennmarken C, Lindstrom F. *Scand J Rheumatol* 1986;15:340–347.
40. Yunus MB, Holt GS, Masi AT, Aldag JC. *J Am Geriatr Soc* 1988;36:987–995.
41. Burckhardt CS, Clark S, Nelson DL. *Arthritis Care Res* 1988;1:38–44.
42. Scudds RA, Rollman GB, Harth M, McCain GA. *J Rheumatol* 1987;14:563–569.
43. Witt I, Vestergaard A, Rosenklint A. *Spine* 1984;9:298–300.
44. Gehweiler Jr JA, Daffner RH. *AJR* 1983;140:109–112.
45. Dinerman H, Goldenberg DL, Felson DT. *J Rheumatol* 1986;13:368–373.
46. Wolfe F, Hawley DJ, Cathey MA, Caro X, Russell IJ. *J Rheumatol* 1985;12:1159–1163.
47. Wolfe F, Smythe HA, Yunus MB, et al. *Arthritis Rheum* 1990 (in press).
48. Carette S, McCain GA, Bell DA, Fam AG. *Arthritis Rheum* 1986;29:655–659.
49. Goldenberg DL, Felson DT, Dinerman H. *Arthritis Rheum* 1986;29:1371–1377.
50. Bennett RM, Gatter RA, Campbell SM, Andrews RP, Clark SR, Scarola JA. *Arthritis Rheum* 1988;31:1535–1542.
51. Backman E, Bengtsson A, Bengtsson M, Lennmarken C, Henriksson KG. *Acta Neurol Scand* 1988;77:187–191.
52. Bengtsson A, Henriksson KG, Larsson J. *Scand J Rheumatol* 1986;15:1–6.
53. Eriksson PO, Lindman R, Stal P, Bengtsson A. *Swed Dent J* 1988;12:141–149.
54. Clark S, Tindall E, Bennett RM. *J Rheumatol* 1985;12:980–983.
55. Yunus MB, Denko CW, Masi AT. *J Rheumatol* 1986;13:183–186.
56. Caro XJ, Wolfe F, Johnston WH, Smith AL. *J Rheumatol* 1986;13:1086–1092.
57. Carette S, Lefranois L. *J Rheumatol* 1988;15:1418–1421.
58. Hawley DJ, Wolfe F, Cathey MA. *J Rheumatol* 1988;15:1551–1556.
59. Cathey MA, Wolfe F, Kleinheksel SM, Miller S, Pitetti KH. *Arthritis Care Res* 1988;1(2):85–98.
60. Pellegrino MJ, Waylonis GW, Sommer A. *Arch Phys Med Rehabil* 1989;70:61–63.
61. McCain GA, Bell DA, Mai FM, Halliday PD. *Arthritis Rheum* 1988;31:1135–1141.
62. Quimby LG, Block SR, Gratwick GM. *J Rheumatol* 1988;15:1264–1270.
63. Reynolds WJ, Chiu B, Inman RD. *J Rheumatol* 1988;15:1802–1803.
64. Romano TJ. *W Va Med J* 1988;84:16–18.
65. Simms RW, Goldenberg DL, Felson DT, Mason JH. *Arthritis Rheum* 1988;31:182–187.
66. Simms RW, Goldenberg DL. *J Rheumatol* 1988;15:1271–1273.
67. Ferraccioli G, Ghirelli L, Scita F, et al. *J Rheumatol* 1987;14:820–825.
68. Hartz A, Kirchdoerfer E. *J Fam Pract* 1987;25:365–369.
69. Jacobsen S, Danneskiold Samsøe B. *Scand J Rheumatol* 1987;16:61–65.
70. Rosenhall U, Johansson G, Orndahl G. *Scand J Rehabil Med* 1987;19:147–152.
71. Hadler NM. *Am J Med* 1986;81:26–30.

72. Ahles TA, Yunus MB, Gaulier B, Riley SD, Masi AT. *Pain* 1986;24:159–163.
73. Bengtsson A, Henriksson KG, Larsson J. *Arthritis Rheum* 1986;29:817–821.
74. Felson DT, Goldenberg DL. *Arthritis Rheum* 1986;29:1522–1526.
75. Leavitt F, Katz RS, Golden HE, Glickman PB, Layfer LF. *Arthritis Rheum* 1986;29:775–781.
76. Wolfe F, Cathey MA. *J Rheumatol* 1985;12:1164–1168.
77. Caro XJ. *Arthritis Rheum* 1984;27:1174–1179.
78. Hench PK. *Am J Med* 1986;81:60–62.
79. Wolfe F, Cathey MA, Kleinheksel SM. *J Rheumatol* 1984;11:814–818.
80. Moldofsky H, Lue FA. *Electroencephalogr Clin Neurophysiol* 1980;50:71–80.
81. Wysenbeek AJ, Mor F, Lurie Y, Weinberger A. *Ann Rheum Dis* 1985;44:752–753.
82. Vaeroy H, Helle R, Frre O, Kass E, Terenius L. *Pain* 1988;32:21–26.
83. Moldofsky H, Tullis C, Lue FA, Quance G, Davidson J. *Psychosom Med* 1984;46:145–151.
84. Moldofsky H, Saskin P, Lue FA. *J Rheumatol* 1988;15:1701–1704.
85. Moldofsky H, Lue FA, Smythe HA. *J Rheumatol* 1983;10:373–379.
86. Gupta MA, Moldofsky H. *Can J Psychiatry* 1986;31:608–616.
87. Bennett RM. *Physi Cli Financ Wor* 1984;1–9.
88. Hadler NM. In: Hadler NM, ed. *Clinical concepts in regional musculoskeletal illness.* Orlando: Grune & Stratton, 1987;7–21.
89. Murphy E. *The logic of medicine.* Baltimore: John Hopkins University Press, 1976.

Advances in Pain Research and Therapy, Vol. 17,
edited by James R. Fricton and Essam Awad.
Raven Press, Ltd., New York © 1990.

9

Quantification of Tenderness by Palpation and Use of Pressure Algometers

Kai Jensen

Department of Neurology, Gentofte Hospital, University of Copenhagen, Copenhagen, Denmark

Tenderness may be defined as the increased pain sensitivity to pressure resulting from a lowered pressure-pain threshold, a stronger response to pressures in the noxious range (as illustrated by a steeper stimulus-response curve), or a combination of both (Fig. 1). At present the pathophysiological mechanisms underlying focal as well as generalized tenderness are largely unknown. Possible explanations are:

1. Sensitization of nociceptors in the tissues under pressure, which is readily explicable in inflammatory conditions.
2. Sensitization/dysmodulation of segmental second-order neurons in the dorsal horn of the spinal cord.
3. A general dysmodulation of pain signals in the CNS leading to a universal increase in pain sensitivity.

Tenderness as a clinical sign must, therefore, be evaluated in context with other clinical observations before it can be ascribed a pathophysiological significance in a particular patient.

Manual palpation, with the purpose of searching for tenderness, is part of the clinical examination of patients in almost any medical specialty. Most often, focal tenderness signals pathology of the underlying tissues, such as an inflamed appendix, a fractured wrist, or a skeletal muscle 1 to 2 days after unusually strenuous exercise. However, the pressure exerted on the superficial tissues influences the resulting sensation, and referral of pain and tenderness in the absence of any local pathology may be misleading. In many instances tenderness serves the purpose of protection of the affected tissues by leading to immobilization, whereas in other instances, such as fibromyalgia and other chronic pain conditions, pain and tenderness seem irrelevant to the preservation of health in the individual. This apparent lack of purpose adds to the frustration of patients and clinicians alike. The number

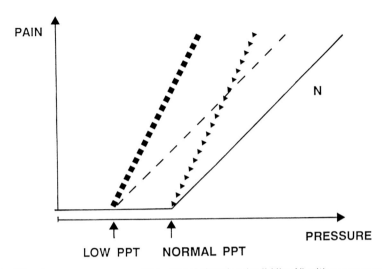

FIG. 1. Stimulus-response curves. The normal situation (*solid line* N) with a pressure-pain threshold at "Normal PPT." In the hyperalgesic state (*arrowheads*), the response to a given stimulus is increased. A situation of reduced PPT ("Low PPT") but otherwise normal stimulus-response relationship is shown by the dashed line. A combination of a lowered PPT and an increased response to a given stimulus is shown by *solid squares*.

of people suffering from pain and tenderness of this kind makes it imperative that we improve our understanding of the pathophysiology of these conditions. Quantification of pain and tenderness is a prerequisite for such improvements to take place. Methods for quantification of tenderness will be discussed with emphasis on the reliability and application of pressure algometers and the factors that may influence the results.

MANUAL PALPATION

Manual palpation for tenderness as part of the clinical examination needs no special introduction. However, it may be relevant to observe that palpation is a four-step procedure: (a) instruction of the patient and the circumstances under which palpation takes place, (b) the technical aspects of using the fingers, (c) the scoring of tenderness, and (d) evaluation of results. All four steps should be considered in the attempt to systematize and standardize the procedure.

The Palpation Procedure

Instruction and Circumstances

Identical verbal or written instructions, neutral behavior by the investigator, the same position of the patients whether sitting or supine, and the same undisturbed room allowing both investigator and patients to concentrate on the procedure are but a few of the items to consider. Anxiety will increase the pain rating by the the patients (1,2), and it has been shown that pain thresholds may be experimentally manipulated by the type of instructions given to the subjects (3,4).

Palpation Techniques

A number of different techniques have been employed. Libman's test consisted of pressure against the styloid process by the tip of the thumb (5). The most detailed description of palpation technique has been given by Travell and Simons (6), who use the tip of an index finger to move the superficial tissues over the fascia of the underlying muscle or a pincer palpation between thumb and index/third finger for particular muscles (e.g., the sternocleidomastoid). A similar technique appears to be used by MacDonald (7) and Fricton and Schiffman (8). Lous and Olesen (9) with simultaneous bilateral palpation and Langemark and Olesen (10) with unilateral palpation applied rotating movements of the index and third fingers. The degree of tension of the muscle being palpated as well as the degree of pressure naturally influences the findings and, in one study, subjects identified one observer as having used a higher pressure than the other, contrary to the intention of the two observers (11).

As expected, there is no consensus on palpation techniques. This naturally makes it very difficult to compare studies from different clinics or laboratories. If more than one investigator is to palpate patients in one particular study, a calibration period is required during which the different investigators can reach a reasonably high interobserver reliability, that is, a very low difference in scores between observers for each patient. The recommended position of the patient and the anatomical region of interest, together with the placement and movements of the palpating hand, should ideally be published in the form of videotapes in order to teach, standardize, improve, and document palpation techniques.

Scoring of Tenderness

A variety of scoring scales are available:

1. Behavioral scales, by which the reaction of the patient is recorded (e.g., grimacing, withdrawal).
2. Verbal scales, by which the patients' verbal expressions are recorded— either their spontaneous comments or terms selected from a systematic list of pain descriptors (e.g., slight pain, excruciating pain).

3. Numerical scales, by which the patient rates the tenderness by a number from a list (e.g., 0: no pain; 3: worst pain imaginable).
4. Visual analogue scales (VASs), by which the patient marks his present pain on a continuous line in the interval between the endpoints "no pain" and "worst imaginable pain," the score then being the number of millimeters from the "no pain" end.

Often, however, clinicians as well as researchers tend to use more than one scale at a time (8–10,12,13).

Some investigators record whether a particular spot is tender or not tender (8,9,11). Others have recorded up to three different intensities of tenderness (10,12,14). Tenderness is not easily scored by manual palpation in more than three levels of intensity if VASs are not used. However, the latter are the most cumbersome in clinical practice and also impractical for research if more than a few points are to be evaluated.

Evaluation of Tenderness

The evaluation of tenderness is difficult not only because of the various technical aspects and different scoring systems, but also because two aspects of tenderness are being evaluated in the same procedure. A lowered pressure-pain threshold as well as an increased response to a given stimulus are both likely to be involved (Fig. 1). Furthermore, results should be compared to data from normal subjects matched for age, sex, ethnic, educational, and socioeconomic background, and, preferably, factors related to the individual clinic—data that are often nonexistent! Even with such data, differences in previous pain experience among the patients might still influence the evaluation of the individual case.

Of course, the significance of focal or generalized tenderness is dependent on other clinical findings. Only rarely is tenderness the only sign of pathology. However, in a number of conditions, such as fibromyalgia and various other myofascial pain conditions, tenderness is the major finding. With a lack of knowledge of the specific pathology of these clinical entities, tenderness must be considered with some caution with regard to its true clinical significance.

Test-Retest Reliability

Only a few authors have studied test-retest reliability of their palpation procedure. In 50 chronic headache patients, Langemark et al. (12) found that with a few weeks' interval, the difference in tenderness scores obtained from 10 bilateral head and neck muscles varied with a standard deviation of nine score points, which should be compared to a mean tenderness score of 30 points. Kopp and Wenneberg (11), however, found a marked variation in tenderness scores of masticatory muscles with only a few hours' interval between palpations. Tenderness scores obtained on two occasions by one observer were positively correlated (8,12).

Inter-observer Difference

Fricton and Schiffman (8) reported a positive correlation between observer ratings of tenderness in 40 patients with craniomandibular dysfunction. Only Kopp and Wenneberg (11) considered the variation specifically and found it to be unacceptably high in asymptomatic subjects.

Application in Diagnosis and Treatment Evaluation

A systematic palpation method is mandatory for the diagnosis of fibromyalgia (13,15). Langemark and Olesen (10) showed in a blind study that tension headache patients had significantly higher tenderness scores than a matched control group, and it is of interest that in the recently published "Classification and Diagnostic Criteria of Headache Disorders, Cranial Neuralgias and Facial Pain" (16), tension-type headache may be divided into two subgroups by the presence or absence of pericranial myofascial tenderness as indicated by manual palpation or by the use of pressure algometers. Apart from these conditions, palpatory determination of tender trigger points in a range of pain conditions serves to locate the site for injection therapy or other local treatments. For the evaluation of treatment effects, palpation scores are obvious parameters to monitor. A significant decrease in palpation scores of craniomandibular dysfunction patients in the course of treatment was reported by Fricton and Schiffman (17).

Manual palpation is liable to subject bias as well as to observer bias, and is difficult to grade and to interpret. The development of pressure algometers was an attempt to improve quantification of tenderness at several points by standardizing the technique of pressure application, simplifying the response (scoring) and thereby simplifying the interpretation.

PRESSURE ALGOMETERS

A pressure algometer is an instrument that, when pressed against the body surface, measures pressure only (Fig. 2). It may indicate pressure in different units, including kilograms, pounds, or newtons per area unit, and knowing the size of the contact area, these may be transformed to appropriate pressure units (kilopascals, newtons per square centimeter, or kilograms per square centimeter). When the investigator increases the pressure, the sen-

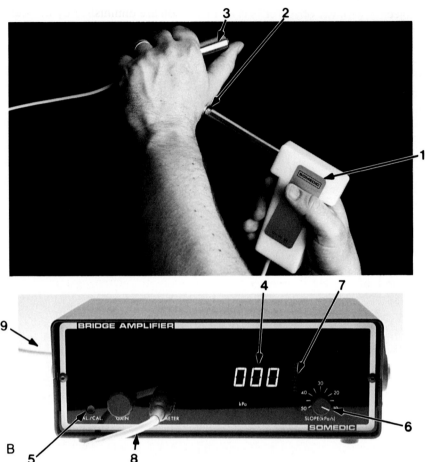

FIG. 2. Pressure algometer (Somedic, box 141 62, S-104 41 Stockholm, Sweden). **A:** Stimulator unit. 1, Pressure-sensitive strain gauge built into the handle; 2, exchangable tips for different areas of pressure application; 3, push button for the subject to signal that the pressure-pain threshold has been reached. **B:** Read-out unit. 4, On-line pressure measurements, calibrated to units of kilopascals; 5, internal calibration; 6, adjustable rate of application (kilopascals per second); 7, display for visual feedback to ensure a constant rate of application; 8, connection to stimulator unit; 9, connection to pen recorder and main switch at the back.

sation of pressure will at some point include pain. The subject is instructed (in a standardized way) to signal that the pain threshold has been reached either verbally or by pressing a push button (Fig. 2). The pressure at this moment is then read from the instrument and taken as the pressure-pain threshold (PPT). By applying a pressure algometer, only one parameter (the PPT) is measured, in contrast to manual palpation, where the responses are more complex (Fig. 1). This would tend to reduce the variation among the subjects. Also, the observer bias and variation are diminished by the standardization of the pressure application.

Pain is a subjective experience, and the instruments should perhaps rightly be called pressure meters and not algometers or dolorimeters. However, in this review they will be referred to as pressure algometers. These instruments were introduced in medical literature in 1911 by Maloney and Kennedy (18), who documented higher PPTs on denervated sides of the face in patients who had undergone trigeminal surgery for neuralgia and patients with facial palsies. The first generation of pressure algometers, in the 1930s to 1960s, were rather crude instruments working on a spring load principle (18–30). More recent models working on mechanical force gauges include those of Fischer (31), Schiffman et al. (32), Tunks et al. (33), and Yamagata et al. (34). Electronic pressure algometers working on a strain gauge principle have also been developed (35,36) (Fig. 2).

A number of factors influence the results obtained by the use of these instruments, as emphasized by Jensen et al. (35). These factors include the size of the contact area and the rate of application. The PPT increases as the area of contact decreases and increases with increasing rate of application (35). At present, only one model permits recording of the rate of pressure application (35,37) (Fig. 2). The rate of application should be fast enough to avoid prolonged pressures to the tissues and fatigue of the investigator and slow enough to allow the investigator to apply the pressure with a constant rate and to allow sufficient time before the PPT is reached so that the reaction time of the individual (and of the observer in case the response is verbal) does not lead to an unnecessary overestimation of the true PPT.

The instrument should be held vertically to the body surface to avoid sharp edges cutting into or stretching superficial tissues, and the material should not evoke other modalities of sensation (e.g., cold from metal surfaces). Hard rubber or similar material seem adequate. The sensation of pressure and pain is the result of stimulation of nerve endings in superficial as well as deeper tissues. This was demonstrated by subcutaneous infiltration with lidocaine, leading to a marked increase in PPT in the temporal region (35). When recording tenderness of myofascial tissues, the state of the overlying superficial tissues therefore must also be considered. The sensation of pressure and/or pain arising from the superficial tissues would theoretically reduce the chances for observation of small changes in myofascial sensitivity to pressure.

Test-Retest Reliability

In the study by Jensen et al. (35), with 50 repeated PPT measurements at the temporal region of one individual with a few seconds' interval, the mean

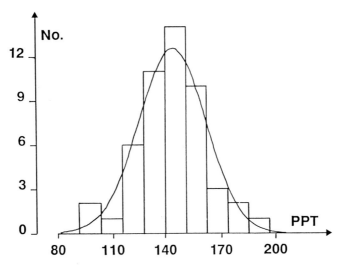

FIG. 3. Distribution of PPT values (N = 50) of the temporal region in one healthy subject (5-sec interval; area, 0.5 cm^2; rate of application, 14 kPa/sec). The distribution is not significantly different from the normal distribution, with a mean of 142 kPa and a standard deviation of 19 kPa (13% of the mean PPT); chi square "goodness of fit" test, $p > .4$. (Data from Jensen et al., ref. 35.)

coefficient of variation was 12% (range 9 to 15%, N = 6) (Fig. 3). This intraindividual coefficient of variation for PPT measurements does not appear to have been calculated by others. However, Dundee and Moore (22) found that for PPT at the tibia, 95% of 1,190 measurements in 300 subjects showed a difference from the individual mean PPT of 10% or less. Differences between two measurements in one individual show a Gaussian distribution (25,35) (Fig. 4). This permits the use of standard statistical tests in paired studies provided a sufficient number of subjects are studied. With a 3-week interval between measurements of PPT in the temporal region of 11 subjects, the mean difference from the mean PPT was -1%, with a standard deviation of 25% of mean PPT (35). With measurements of PPT at the tibia, Dundee and Moore (22) observed that 95% of their 21 subjects differed less than 35% from the mean PPT with a similar time interval. In the fingers and toes, Brennum et al. (37) found the standard deviation of differences between two PPT measurements with 1 week's interval to be 14% of the mean PPT. Within the individual, the variation of PPT at a given region is, thus, acceptable.

A positive correlation between two consecutive PPT measurements was found, as expected, by several authors (28,36,38,39). However, tests of correlation are not suitable as measures of reliability (40).

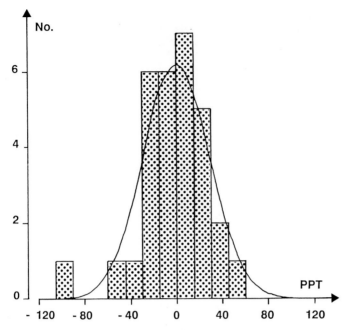

FIG. 4. Distribution of test-retest differences of PPT in the temporal region (N = 30) (45-min interval; area, 0.5 cm^2; rate of application, 14 kPa/sec). The distribution is not significantly different from the normal distribution, with a mean of 0 kPa and a standard deviation of 29 kPa (15% of the mean PPT); chi square "goodness of fit" test , p > .5. (Data from Jensen et al., ref. 35.)

Interobserver Variation

The variation of PPT measurements was smaller for trained than for untrained observers in one study (22). Reeves et al. (39) and Merskey and Spear (28) found no significant differences in PPT between two observers. Actual figures obtained by different observers have not been published, and the question of interobserver variation of PPT measurements is still unanswered. A positive correlation between PPT values obtained by two investigators was found by several authors (27,28,32,33,39,41), but, as emphasized earlier, a significant variation is not excluded by a statistically significant correlation (40).

Side-to-Side Differences and Correlation

Some have observed a difference in PPT according to the lateral dominance of the individual, that is, a higher PPT value on the right side than on the left (37,38,42), while others did not observe such a difference (31,33,35). The right-left differences of PPT in the temporal region are shown in Fig. 5.

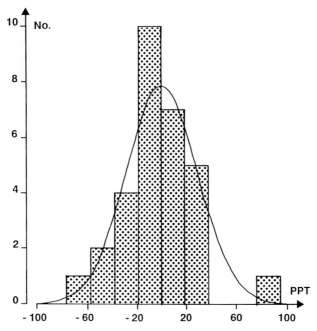

FIG. 5. Distribution of side-to-side differences in PPT of the temporal region ($N = 30$) (1-min interval; area, 0.5 cm²; rate of application, 14 kPa/sec). The distribution is not significantly different from the normal distribution, with a mean of 0 kPa and a standard deviation of 29 kPa (15% of the mean PPT); chi square "goodness of fit" test, $p > .2$). (Data from Jensen et al., ref. 35.)

The variation of PPT between symmetrical sites is therefore also within the acceptable range. As expected, a positive correlation between symmetrical sites of measurements has been observed (4,14,35,37).

PPT Values from Different Anatomical Regions

Certainly, the PPT varies between different anatomical regions (12,31,35, 37,43). In spite of this variation, several authors have observed a significant correlation between PPT values obtained from different anatomical sites in the same individual (12,37). This may reflect that PPT is influenced not only by factors at the site of measurement and the state of the segmental pain modulatory system but also by the pain sensitivity in the individual in general.

Distribution of PPT Within a Group of Subjects

The distribution of PPT values in a group of subjects does not follow a normal distribution (Fig. 6). This was also observed by Fischer (31). The median

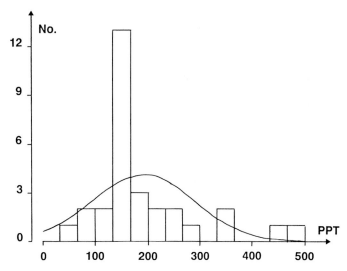

FIG. 6. Distribution of PPT values of the temporal region in 30 healthy subjects (area, 0.5 cm², rate of application, 14 kPa/sec). The distribution is significantly different from the normal distribution, with a mean of 192 kPa and a standard deviation of 98 kPa (51% of the mean PPT); chi square "goodness of fit" test, $p < .01$). (Data from Jensen et al., ref. 35.)

PPT in the temporal region was 161 kPa and the 95% confidence limits for the median 144 to 197 kPa, as opposed to the mean and standard deviation of the same material (Fig. 6). One should, therefore, observe that the mean and standard deviation may not characterize the data correctly and that nonparametric statistical tests should be applied when comparing groups of patients unless very large groups are studied. However, this seems to be considered only rarely. From the observed data, Jensen et al. (35) estimated the number of subjects necessary in a group comparison study to show a moderate difference in PPT with a chosen values of alpha = 0.05 and beta = 0.20 to be 45 in each group.

Age and Sex Differences in PPT

There is no documentation for the influence of age on PPT, but one may suspect PPT to increase with age. Females have lower PPTs than males, as has been consistently demonstrated by Brennum et al. (37), Dundee and Moore (22), Fischer (31), Merskey and Spear (28), and Schiffman et al. (32) and to a lesser extent by Tunks (33). This means that in group comparison studies, the groups should be matched for sex and, until proven otherwise, should also be matched for age.

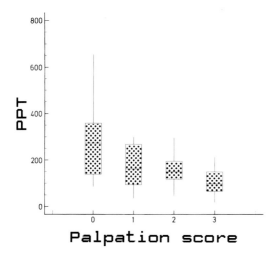

FIG. 7. Pressure-pain threshold values obtained by pressure algometer in the left temporal region of 50 chronic headache patients arranged according to the tenderness score obtained by manual palpation. A significant negative correlation was observed (Spearman's rank correlation test, $p < .01$). (Data from Langemark et al., ref. 12.)

Correlation of PPT with Manual Palpation Scores

Pressure-pain thresholds recorded by use of a pressure algometer correlated well with tenderness scores obtained by manual palpation of 50 tension headache patients (12) (Fig. 7), although this was not found in 25 migraine patients (14). The agreement between manual palpation and PPT recordings was also implied by the lower PPT of tender points found by manual palpation as compared to points not tender to palpation (33,39,44). Earlier tests of pain sensitivity, such as Libman's thumb pressure to the styloid process (5), correlated well with PPT measurements (24) and with observations with another type of an algometer measuring the degree of indentation of the superficial tissues that led to pain sensation (45).

The reliability of the two methods—manual palpation and PPT measurements—has only rarely been studied in the same subjects. Schiffman et al. (32) found PPT measurements to be more reliable than manual palpation. Data on intra- and interindividual variation of both methods obtained from one group of subjects have not been published.

Applications

Diagnostic Purposes

Pressure algometers may document the presence of trigger points in conditions such as fibromyalgia and other myofascial pain dysfunctions. Reeves et al. (39) thus observed a 15 to 20% lower PPT in trigger points when compared to adjacent non–trigger points in the same subjects, and Jaeger and Reeves (44) showed that unilateral trigger points had a significantly lower PPT value than their symmetrical counterparts. By applying the pressure algometer to multiple regions, several authors have demonstrated lower PPT values in patients suffering from fibromyalgia as compared to a control group (32,33,36,43). This may be caused by sensitization of nerve endings in the myofascial tissues or segmental dysmodulation in the CNS, but a lower PPT was also found in the fingers of a similar group of patients (46). The latter finding may indicate that the pain sensitivity of the individual as such was increased. This interpretation is supported by the finding of lower PPT values in tender as well as nontender points in fibromyalgia patients as compared to control subjects (33) and in skinfolds overlying the trapezius muscle (43). However, Campbell et al. (43) did not find any difference in PPT at myofascial control points. Interestingly, Moldofsky et al. (47) observed a decrease in PPT in fibromyalgia patients following sleep deprivation, in contrast to findings in a few control subjects.

Pressure algometers have been applied in other conditions as well, including chronic tension headache (12), migraine (14,38), and rheumatoid arthritis (25,26). Furthermore, Merskey and Evans (41) claimed to be able to discriminate groups with organic causes of pain from those with primarily psychological causes, the latter having lower PPT values. When monitoring the course of diseases such as fibromyalgia or rheumatoid arthritis, treated or untreated, one should observe, however, that there is a tendency for a gradual increase in PPT with time (35).

Evaluation of Treatment

Drugs

Several studies have shown the applicability of pressure-pain threshold measurements in the evaluation of drugs, notably a variety of analgesics. Thus, opioids raise PPT (22,23), as does acetylsalicylic acid (19,25). In rheumatoid arthritis, chloroquine raised the PPT of interphalangeal joints (25). Patients with myofascial pain dysfunction who improved following a range of treatments such as minor tranquilizers, relaxation training, and transcutaneous electrical nerve stimulation had an increase in the PPT on their fingers as opposed to those who did not improve (48). Also, Jiminez and Lane (49) reported an increase in PPT in the course of treatment of chronic pain patients.

Local Treatments of Trigger Points

Specific measurements of changes in trigger point sensitivity following local treatment by vapocoolant spray and passive stretch were carried out by

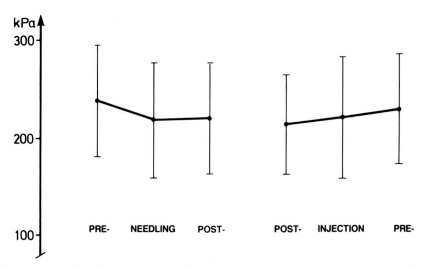

FIG. 8. Mean PPT (95% confidence limit) in the temporal region before, immediately after, and 30 min after needling and injection of 0.2 ml of isotonic saline into the temporal muscle in 15 healthy volunteers, (area 0.5 cm^2, rate of application 14kPa/sec).

Jaeger et al. (44). They were able to show a significant increase in PPT of the treated trigger points, even to values above their symmetrical counterpart on the contralateral side. Fischer (50) also reported cases of decrease in trigger point sensitivity following vapocoolant spray.

Injections

The effect of trigger point injection with local anesthetics on PPT has not been systematically investigated. Fischer (50) reported cases of an increase in PPT. However, needling of the temporal muscle in healthy individuals does not change the PPT and neither does injection of 0.2 ml of isotonic saline (Fig. 8). Furthermore, there was no difference between the effects of the two procedures that were applied in a single-blind manner to 15 healthy subjects. Subcutaneous lidocaine in the temporal region, however, raised PPT significantly more than did saline (35). Thus, the effect of local anesthetics can be documented by the use of pressure algometers. This observation also shows that PPT does not depend solely on the sensitivity of the myofascial tissues but also depends on the sensitivity of the overlying superficial tissues to an unknown degree.

Experimental Studies of Muscle and Pain Physiology and Pathophysiology

In a study of the effect of eccentric exercise on pain, tenderness, and stiffness of skeletal muscle, Jones et al. (51) found PPT to be lowered with a time delay of 24 to 48 hours paralleling the pain to passive muscle stretch, whereas the maximal increase in plasma creatine kinase levels as an index of muscle fiber damage was only maximal after 3 to 5 days. This suggests that PPT measurements have great potential value in experimental muscle pain and sports medicine.

Because the mechanisms of myofascial pain are largely unknown, any method that may be used for the study of pain physiology is welcome. Pressure algometers have long been involved in studies of pain thresholds as such (37). The first studies employing pressure algometers actually concerned the nociceptive innervation of masticatory and facial muscles (18,20). Pressure-pain thresholds have been shown to correlate well with other thresholds for potentially noxious stimuli, such as heat (52), cold (12), ischemia (24) and electrical stimulation (52).

Hyperventilation may raise the PPT (21). Temperature changes influence the PPTs of fingers (53). The influence of anxiety and other psychological factors was observed by Cornwall and Donderi (1) by applying a different type of pressure algometer where a continuous pressure is applied to a finger and the time until development of pain is reported (54).

In some recent studies, Jensen et al. (55) have shown that injection of a mixture of bradykinin and 5-hydroxytryptamine into the temporal muscle lowered the PPT by approximately 10% for a period of 5 to 10 min. Injection of a mixture of bradykinin and substance P lowered the PPT by 15 to 20% for the same length of time (56).

In the laboratory, pressure algometers thus seem to be a valuable tool for the study of experimental pain and nociceptor sensitization.

CONCLUSION

Pressure algometers depend on rather simple technology and are thus relatively inexpensive. They are easy to operate and reliable in test-retest studies. They have shown their potential value in the clinical as well as the experimental situation. Although pressure algometers do not lead to the desired objective measure of pain and although they can never be a substitute for manual palpation in the daily clinic, they constitute a welcome supplement for evaluation of tenderness, allowing a better scoring/scaling and reducing the observer and subject bias. A more widespread use of pressure algometers is recommended.

REFERENCES

1. Cornwall A, Donderi DC. *Pain* 1988;35:105–113.
2. Moldofsky H, Chester WJ. *Psychosom Med* 1970;32:309–318.
3. Blitz B, Dinnerstein AJ. *J Abnorm Psychol* 1968;73:276–280.
4. Wolff BB, Krasnegor NA, Farr RS. *Percept Mot Skills* 1965;21:675–683.

In reviewing the causes for chronic low back pain, Hadler noted that the structural diagnoses responsible for low back pain were usually associated with x-ray changes such as spondylolisthesis, spinal stenosis, and segmental disability. While recognition of myofascial pain syndromes or fibromyalgia was acknowledged, he did point out that this diagnosis is considered to be "controversial" (27).

Other clinicians go further in either disregarding or refuting the concept that chronic low back pain, for example, can even be due to myofascial or muscular pain alone (28; S.D. Kuslich and C.L. Ulstrom, unpublished manuscript). However, there are considerable data in the rehabilitation and rheumatological literature that support the concept of disability and pain secondary to chronic musculoskeletal or soft tissue pathology (29–32). In fact, at a study performed at the University of Miami Pain Clinic, over 85% of 283 consecutive patients were diagnosed as having chronic myofascial pain (33). This is certainly consistent with our experience. Even in individuals with documented bony pathology (i.e., degenerative disc disease, facet joint disease, or radiculopathy), many also demonstrate a component of soft tissue pain.

Much of the controversy surrounding myofascial pain has been the lack of specificity in defining clinical syndromes and clinical findings, (i.e., painful trigger points) as being objective indications of disease. The lack of laboratory findings and questionable correlation with anatomical or histological examination of soft tissues have also produced controversy (34,35). Additionally, it is recognized that in myofascial pain syndromes in particular, anxiety and stress can be major contributing factors. Emotional stress alone can produce an increase in muscular activity (36). It has been postulated, in fact, that it is ongoing muscle tension that produces the majority of the pain. Dr. John Sarno, a physiatrist, has labeled this syndrome "tension myositis" (37). He believes that increased muscle tension leads to constriction of blood vessels, producing a relative anoxia and accumulation of metabolites and pain. The awareness of the pain leads to increased fear and anxiety, producing increased muscle tension (37).

While uncertainty continues as to the pathophysiology of myofascial pain and fibromyalgia, clearly these syndromes exist. As will be discussed in the next sections, current disability assessment models in general do not consider myofascial syndromes as a cause for disability, and therefore evaluation of these syndromes in terms of the impact they have on the patient's ability to function in general, and particularly to maintain gainful employment, is fraught with controversy and ambiguity.

CURRENT METHODS FOR DISABILITY DETERMINATION

While the evaluation of pain is important in all patients with musculoskeletal disorders, it takes on particular importance in those individuals in whom the pain is chronic, particularly if it affects the patient's ability to maintain gainful employment. In the United States, as well as in most western countries, systems are in place to provide financial reimbursement to the disabled individual.

In the United States, the most important disability systems are the Social Security Disability process, workers' compensation, and private disability insurance. In the case of Social Security Disability, a claimant must be unable to "engage in any substantial gainful activity by reason of a medically determinable physical or medical impairment which can be expected to result in death or can be expected to last for a continuous period of less than 12 months." The patient must have evidence of "anatomical, physiological or psychological abnormalities" that can be demonstrated by medically accepted clinical and laboratory diagnostic techniques. The pain is considered as a factor that may prevent an individual from working only when a physical or psychological impairment exists.

In 1982, 1.5 million claimants applied for Social Security Disability. Of these 82,000 patients suffered from what was defined as a "chronic pain syndrome" (1). That is, these individuals claimed that because of their experience of pain they were not able to work, or perform normal physical, social, or emotional fucntions. In these cases, no medically determinal condition could be found that was sufficient to account for the complaints of pain. The implication of this statement becomes extremely important when one considers the issue of myofascial pain syndrome.

For example, in disorders of the spine, conditions considered to represent an impairment include arthritis manifested by ankylosis with x-ray evidence to support this, osteoporosis, or other vertebrogenic disorders (i.e., herniated nucleus pulposus or spinal stenosis) in which the patient presents with pain, muscle spasm, and significant limitation of motion as well as appropriate radicular distribution of significant motor loss and muscle weakness. In addition, acute rheumatoid arthritis and other inflammatory arthritic conditions are considered (2).

Myofascial pain or fibromyalgia is not considered under the present Social Security guidelines to represent an impairment. This is in part due, as mentioned earlier, to the general lack of acceptance of these entities as a disease. Moreover, there is a lack of agreement as to the appropriate clinical findings needed to make the diagnosis, and a total lack of confirming laboratory data. Specifically, tender points, tautness of the muscles, and the like have not been fully accepted by the medical community, and the use of laboratory testing, such as thermography or pressure algometry, is too early in its development to be widespread. Therefore, patients who present with myofascial pain syndromes under the present convention of the Social Security Adminsitration would not fall into the currently defined musculoskeletal impairments and most likely represent the main proportion of the so-called chronic pain syndromes. Since they do not fall into an accepted impairment category it is likely that these individuals will remain most difficult to evaluate, and represent a large proportion of the claimants who must go through a rather complicated and expensive appeals process, if initially denied disability. (For an extremely comprehensive discussion of pain and disability within the Social Security Administration see refs. 1 and 2.)

In workers' compensation systems, a patient must demonstrate that he has been injured on the job. Significant importance, again, is given to the patient's "impairment" as demonstrated by clinical and laboratory findings. Again, the lack of consistent and accepted laboratory findings in the case of myofascial pain disorders makes individuals who have these disorders suspect, and their complaints are often discounted or they are labeled as psychological or psychogenic pain patients, or malingerers. In addition, in the workers' compensation system in many states, patients are given a lump sum settlement that directly relates to the degree of impairment and disability. The lump sum settlement is given in part to compensate the injured worker for his inability to perform certain activities that may limit his ability to obtain gainful employment. In the state of Minnesota, for example, a schedule has been established to rate patients based primarily on x-ray and neurological findings.

For example, in the case of low back pain, if a patient presents with low back pain with normal x-rays and no evidence of loss of motion, spasm, or guarding, his impairment rating is zero. If the patient has clinical findings consistent with decreased range of motion, spasm, or guarding, it is 3.5%. However, if the patient has x-ray findings such as degenerative facet joint changes or a disc bulge, along with the aforementioned clinical signs, the rating goes up to either 7 or 10%, depending on the number of levels involved. Functional limitations are not considered. Patients with soft tissue pain are minimally rewarded in this system, and one could certainly argue that this model discriminates against those with myofascial pain syndromes.

SOFT TISSUE PAIN AS AN IMPAIRMENT

At the present time numerous diagnostic terms to describe myofascial pain syndromes exist, including "sprain," "strain," "lumbago," "fibromyalgia," "sciatica," "soft tissue rheumatism fibrositis," "myofascial pain," "musculoligamentous injury," "myofasciitis," "myositis," "fascitis," "myalgic syndrome," "ligamentitis", and "chronic benign pain syndrome." All of these terms are often used interchangeably to allude to a condition in which an individual experiences pain and the nociceptive origin is believed to be in the soft tissues. For example, there continues to be debate as to whether the syndrome of fibromyalgia, a presumed rheumatological disorder, is a separate entity, a variation, or merely myofascial pain with a different title (12).

In addition, pain of soft tissue origin may produce many of the same characteristics as other conditions. For example, myofascial pain from the back can refer to the leg and mimic symptoms of nerve root compression. Likewise, facial pain of myofascial origin is often confused with the diagnosis of a temporomandibular joint disorder (31).

Until clinical criteria are established, proven valid and reliable, and generally accepted by the majority of the medical community, or a laboratory test, histological findings, or some other objective measurement is firmly established, the confusion surrounding myofascial pain syndromes and the myriad of diagnostic terms used will continue. Certainly, the discovery of objective measurements, as well as universally accepted clinical criteria, would likely lead to the legitimization of myofascial syndromes, shifting them from a well-recognized clinical condition to an accepted cause of a medical impairment.

DEFINING DISABILITY THROUGH SELF-ASSESSMENT

Since a single technique or diagnostic test is not yet available, disability determination for patients with soft tissue injury, as with many other types of impairments, must rely on multidimensional assessments. Disability is a function of many variables. These include not only the degree of tissue pathology but, more importantly, how these nociceptive signals emanating from injured or irritated tissue are modulated by the synaptic pathways in the spinal cord and in the brain and, ultimately, how these signals interface with the patient's consciousness. Thus, the expression of this process is not only the sensation of pain but a whole spectrum of behaviors, emotions, and cognitive beliefs that reflect the patient's limitations. In order to quantify this situation, a biomechanical or disease model that looks only at physical parameters is inadequate.

Rather, a multiaxial or biopsychosocial model is needed to integrate the numerous emotional, psychosocial and environmental variables with the physical findings. (38). As has been pointed out, in most current disability systems the former factors are minimized. Instead, the emphasis has been on rating disability on the basis of physical findings and laboratory tests alone. This is thought to be more "objective" and presumably prevents the patient from misrepresenting himself. Thus, the belief is that the physical examination and laboratory findings are a more accurate representation of function than what the patient reports. However, this is clearly an error in reasoning. X-rays and laboratory findings are measurements of anatomy or physiology, not functioning. Two individuals with the same level of measurable impairment can experience different levels of pain and, in addition, can experience different functional and psychological impacts as a result of that experience.

Traditionally, the clinician has relied on the self-report of the patient to assess his condition in terms of the severity of symptoms and the impact the condition has had on his ability to function. However, rarely is there an attempt to quantify these variables in the same way that laboratory and x-rays attempt to quantify impairment. In order to provide consistency and objectivity in the analysis of the subjective manifestations of pain, the development and integration of scientifically valid and reliable self-report instrumentation and functional assessment testing would fill a necessary function. Utilizing this information, the physician as well as the disability administrator would obtain a far more thorough and comprehensive picture of the respective patient's level of functioning.

The Ideal Instrument

There currently exist a number of valid instruments that measure various aspects of disability (i.e., activities of daily living scales, health status measures, physical symptoms, and cognitive belief scales) and instruments that assess emotional factors and behavioral characteristics. In fact, there are such a number of instruments available that measure the parameters of disability outcome that the U.S. Department of Health has established a separate clearinghouse for health indices (39). At the present time, however, there does not exist a specific instrument that has been established as the gold standard in the assessment of disability and pain (40). If an ideal instrument did exist, in theory, it should meet the following criteria, as proposed by Deyo (39,41):

1. *Practicality:* It should be administered and scored in a reasonable time frame. Self-administration requires the least amount of staff time, but contingencies need to be built in for those individuals with poor or no reading skills, or for those who do not understand the language.

2. *Comprehensiveness:* The instrument should provide information in the various dimensions associated with the disability determination process, that is, social, cognitive, emotional, and behavioral characteristics, as well as functional abilities and activities of daily living.

3. *Reliability:* The instrument should provide consistency over time, assuming stability in the patient's condition. Reliability refers to the reproducibility of results and does not refer to the accuracy of the instrument in measuring the assumed variables.

4. *Validity:* The instrument should quantify in a statistically significant manner and in a consistently predictable direction those variables that the instrument has been designed to measure. Validation of an instrument takes on increasingly more complexity in a manner directly proportional to the number of variables in question. The use of the computer in the development of sophisticated multivariant statistical analysis, however, allows for ac-

TABLE 1. *Measures for assessing chronic pain syndromes in an interdisciplinary pain clinic*

Physical measures
  Location of pain
  Spatial distribution of pain
  Electromyographic activity
  Physical symptoms
  Pressure algometry
Functional measures
  Uptime
  Disability
  Ambulation
  Self-care
  Functional abilities
Behavioral/cognitive measures
  General hypochondriasis, somatic concern, denial
  Number of visits to physicians, hospitalization, surgeries
  Drug usage
  Verbal pain behaviors
  Sleep disturbance
  Coping strategies
  Cognitive processes
  Self-efficacy
Emotional measures
  Depression
  Anxiety
  Anger
Economic factors
  Income
  Expenses
Sociocultural factors
  Living arrangement, independence
  Litigation
  Family involvement
  Quality of life
  Patient goals

Adapted from Williams, ref. 40.

curate discernment of the construct validity of the variables in question. A more challenging issue in terms of assessing validity is the lack of a gold standard or clearly defined objective parameters defining what dimensions should be used to measure disability. Williams suggests a set of physical, functional, behavioral, emotional, economic, and sociocultural parameters (40) for the evaluation of outcome in patients undergoing treatment in a comprehensive pain clinic. Many of these variable are applicable in the assessment of pain and its relationship to disability (Table 1). While this model is indeed comprehensive, it has not gained wide acceptance; moreover, while presently existing instruments are able to measure the various parameters described, utilization of these multiple instruments would be time consuming, expensive, and not practical, except perhaps in the setting of a comprehensive pain management clinic or for research.

5. *Sensitivity/responsiveness:* An instrument should be capable of measuring subtle but important clinical changes over time. This is critical if one is to measure the responsiveness to respective therapeutic interventions and the impact the underlying condition has on the patient over time. In addition, the instrument would require sufficient sensitivity to discriminate subtle differences between patients presenting with similar complaints.

Prototypes of the Ideal Self-Assessment Instrument

While it would not be possible in the limited scope of this chapter to discuss all the various instruments used in the assessment of pain and disability in myofascial syndromes, several instruments and models do serve as prototypes.

Sickness Impact Profile and IMPATH

Of the many self-assessment instruments developed, perhaps the one most thoroughly studied is the Sickness Impact Profile (SIP). The SIP is a 136-item yes/no-formatted questionnaire grouped into 12 categories. Three of the categories—movement, mobility, and ambulation—are combined into a physical dimension (45 items). Four categories—emotional, behavior, social interaction, and alertness and communication—are grouped into a psycho-social dimension (48 items). Five other categories—sleep and rest, home management, recreation, eating, and work—are not aggregated. The test has proven useful in evaluating a wide range of clinical interventions, including bed rest for low back pain (42), epidural stimulation (43), and the use of antidepressants in pain patients (44), and in comparing the results of treatment between a cognitive-behavioral pain program versus relaxation training (45). In addition, the SIP has demonstrated satisfactory internal consistency, good test-retest reliability, and construct validity (41). Moreover, a short version of the SIP has been developed. This 24-item questionnaire specified for low back pain has also demonstrated good reliability, validity, and responsiveness to change in a population of patients with mechanical low back pain (46).

A second assessment instrument, IMPATH, is noteworthy for its integration of systems theory with computer technology (47). It was developed using the 1984 Joint Technical Standards for Educational and Psychological Testing of the American Psychological Association to ensure reliability and validity. The actual instrument consists of approximately 400 yes/no, multiple choice, and visual analog questions. Each question appears on a computer screen and the patient responds by pressing the appropriate key. On completion, the data are automatically stored and analyzed, and a printout is generated.

The information provided by IMPATH includes a medical history, a review of symptoms, and a list of psychological, behavioral, cognitive, and social risk factors that are believed to contribute to the severity of the patient's pain syndrome, life style disruption, and potential for rehabilitation as well as a series of indices that look at life functioning, quality of life, illness impact, and symptom severity. Initial evaluation of IMPATH has shown that it is reliable and that it does accurately measure changes in the patient's clinical condition.

The advantages of a system such as this include:

1. Immediate feedback to the clinician.
2. A comprehensive behavioral and psychosocial assessment that can be used in following the patient in terms of outcome management as well as in terms of disability assessment.
3. An effective way of gathering standardized data on individuals with chronic pain problems.

The disadvantages of a system such as this are:

1. It requires a computer, which not only costs money but also requires space as well as staff time.
2. It takes approximately 1 to 2 hours to complete IMPATH, and some clinicians and patients object to the time consumption.
3. Patients who have difficulty with reading would not be good candidates for IMPATH.

Impath and the SIP represent only two of a number of psychometric instruments currently developed to assess pain. They serve as a prototype, providing objective documentation of information that is necessary to assess the patient's level of functioning and the impact of the pain on his life. These instruments provide quantifiable and statistically valid information about the patient, which allows the clinician or disability examiner to compare the patient's perception of the impact of his problem with that of other pain patients and to develop standards regarding disability status and rehabilitation potential. In general, the information provided by these instruments reflects with more accuracy than the examining physician the extent of distress, the ability or inability to perform activities of daily living, concentration skills, cognitive beliefs, attitudes about rehabilitation, changes in interpersonal relationships, ability to perform and enjoy recreational and social activities, and the patient's perception of his vocational capacities.

However, in the area of self-assessment testing and its relationship to disability determination many questions continue to exist. First, the poor correlation between physical findings and functional status requires reconciliation within the disability determination process. Specifically, how much weight should self-report information be given with respect to information supplied by the physician? Moreover, questions remain as to the optimal length, ease in understanding, and comfort level of both the patient and the physician or disability examiner in interpreting and utilizing this type of information. At the present, no instrument has been universally accepted as the "gold standard" and, therefore, head-to-head comparisons of the various instruments to determine superiority is required (4). Finally, anytime subjective information is requested from the patient for whom potential economic incentives exist, there is the possibility and suspicion that the patient may be exaggerating, receiving coaching from an attorney, or downright lying. Clearly, further research is necessary to assess the validity and reliability of this type of instrument in many types of situations.

Integration of Self-Assessment Data and Clinical Findings

An attempt to integrate self-report data from the patient with their respective clinical findings is that popularized by Waddell and Main (48). Initially a disability index for low back pain was developed looking at nine basic physical activities: lifting, sitting, traveling, standing, walking, sleeping, social life, sex life, and footwear. A factor analysis was performed confirming that these activities were interrelated and, when combined, did provide a good measure of disability. Next, physical impairment was assessed by using a regression analysis to quantify the relative importance and influence of each physical finding for its effect on disability. Redundant items were eliminated and a weighted series of physical factors was developed. The factors included the pain pattern, lumbar flexion, straight leg raising, root compression signs, previous lumbar surgery, time duration, and evidence of fracture. Comparing normal subjects with a low back pain population, and smaller subgroups of patients with spondylolisthesis, fractures, and elective orthopedic procedures, Waddell and Main confirmed the clinical observation that subjective disability can vary significantly from impairment. In addition, they concluded that the physical impairment can be found to account for less than half of the disability, with functional or psychological variables contributing to the rest.

This model has been expanded and refined utilizing discriminatory symptoms (i.e., whole leg pain, whole leg numbness, whole leg "gives way," pain at the tip of the tailbone, and continuous unrelenting pain for the past year); information gathered as part of the history (i.e., intolerance or reactions to treatment, emergency admissions for backache); and nonorganic signs (i.e., superficial, nonanatomical tenderness, pain with simulated rotation, inconsistent straight leg raising, regional weakness or sensory disturbance, or overreaction to the physical examination). Further differentiation between pain due to organic pathology versus functional distress is possible.

In addition, Waddell (49) suggested performing two psychological tests, the modified Zung and the Modified Somatic Perception Questionnaire (MSPQ). The first is a 23-item questionnaire similar to the Beck Depression Inventory. It is a quick screening tool for depressive symptoms. The latter looks at 13 somatic experiences and measure the patient's somatic preoccupation. Utilization of these instruments helps the clinician better understand the patient's underlying beliefs (49).

One major weakness of this model is that it is limited to low back pain specifically, and although it may be relevant to other types of musculoskeletal pain, especially cervical problems, it is not applicable in its present form. However, it does provide a conceptual framework for separating physical from functional factors relating to disability and can therefore suggest appropriate rehabilitation interventions. To quote Waddell, "If physical disease and illness behavior are distinguished, then physical treatment can be directed more appropriately to physical disease, while improved understanding of illness will provide an equally scientific basis for the practice as well as the technology of medicine" (49).

Functional Restoration Model

Mayer and associates have developed a comprehensive model for assessing and treating disability in chronic low back pain based on the concept of functional restoration. Recognizing that the determination of back function depends on complex mechanical interactions between multiple small joints, ligaments, and deep muscles, they have developed a standard battery of physical testing methods to assess spinal function. In addition, several psychological self-report measures are also utilized. In a study published in *JAMA*, 116 patients who were not working at the time of evaluation were randomized and followed for 2 years (50). Of these 116 patients, 87% went back to work. Moreover, in addition to returning to work there was an excellent statistical correlation between clinical improvement and an increase in physical strength and functional capacity testing. In addition, there was also statistically significant improvement in the psychological self-reports for pain and dysfunction.

Mayer has presented a model that measures several physical and psychosocial parameters in patients with chronic low back pain. In addition, he has demonstrated that it is indeed possible to quantify improvement in both physical and psychological terms. While this approach has been shown to be valid, reliable, and responsible, one would question its practicality for myofasical pain syndromes. The cost of the 3-week program is about $8,000 to $9,000 and the initial psychophysiological assessment is also quite expensive. While this in-depth approach has been cost effective for severely disabled and unemployed individuals who are receiving workers' compensation, the methodology is not practical for most primary care settings.

Summary

While the discussion of these models is far from comprehensive, it does provide a sampling of the approaches currently being used in the assessment of pain and disability. The use of psychometric data reported by the patient has been demonstrated to provide reliable and valid information pertaining to the patient's level of functioning. It is now possible to define with accuracy the various parameters associated with disability, to distinguish physical from psychological or functional components, and to measure functional and physical capacities based on standarized testing. Certaintly further research is indicated to see whether this information has predictive value in determining candidates for rehabilitation.

The documentation of symptom severity, analysis of the psychosocial impact of the condition, and objective measurement of function remain critical in determination of disability (51). This will be especially true in myofascial pain syndromes, in which, until a better understanding of the pathophysiology emerges that will permit an attempt at correlating symptoms with impairment, one will have to be satisfied with subjective complaints alone. Moreover, by establishing criteria based on self-report and functional assessment, the discrimination against individuals who claim disability as a result of pain or some other subjective complaint will be minimized. Moreover, by identifying psychosocial contributing factors appropriate intervention can be determined.

CONCLUSIONS AND RECOMMENDATIONS

Pain is best defined as a personal and subjective experience or feeling of discomfort or unpleasantness. Chronic pain is defined as pain lasting for longer than 6 months. In both acute and chronic states, myofascial pain is the most common reason for lost work. The problem has a tremendous economic and human cost. In spite of its recognition from a clinical standpoint, disagreement exists as to its etiology, pathogenesis, and pathophysiology. Like heart disease, rather than suggesting one specific cause, it appears more appropriate to talk about risk factors, be they physical (i.e., trauma, nutritional imbalances), psychological (i.e., depression), social (i.e., secondary gain factors), or others. Furthermore, it appears that from an operational standpoint it is more appropriate to view the problem not from the perspective of a disease but rather from that of an illness. Far more important than the presence or absence of a trigger point is the impact the condition has on the patient's ability to work, socialize, care for himself, and essentially function independently. In order to determine this in a systematic manner, standardized assessment instrumentation that is reliable, accurate, easily administered, and sensitive is required. Several prototypes presently exist. Further research and wider clinical trials are needed.

Moreover, using a medical or disease-based model as the gold standard to assess the extent of disability for the various legal systems (i.e., Social Security, workers' compensation) is terribly inadequate, unfair, and illogical. Clearly, the impact the condition has on a patient's quality of life, psychosocial functioning, and physical abilities depends on the influence of cognitive, cultural, educational, financial, and demographic factors in addition to the underlying physical impairment. These factors must be taken into account to fully comprehend the pathogenesis or expression of myofascial pain syndromes.

Systems that approach the problem from a holistic or biopsychosocial perspective that can be adapted by statute into present legal systems for disability determination and can provide some guidance for appropriate treatment and rehabilitation interventions, as well as predict success, would be ideal.

REFERENCES

1. United States Department of Health and Human Services. *Report of the Commission on the Evaluation of Pain (SSA Pub No 64-031).* Washington, DC: US Government Printing Office, 1987.
2. Osterweis M, Kleinman A, Mechanic D. *Institute of Medicine's Committee on Pain, Disability, and Chronic Illness. Behavior, pain and disability: Clinical, behavioral, and public policy perspectives.* Washington DC: National Academy Press, 1987.
3. Carey TS, Hadler NM, Gillings D, Stinnett S. *J Clin Epidemiol* 1988;41:691–697.
4. Deyo RA, Tsui-Wu Y. *Arthritis Rheum* 1987;30:1247–1253.
5. Hadler NM. *Ann Intern Med* 1982;96:665–669.
6. Powell MC, Wilson M, Szypryt P, Symonds EM, Worthington BS. *Lancet* 1986;2:1366–1367.
7. Wiesel SW, Tsourmas M, Feffer HL, Citrin CM, Patronas N. *Spine* 1984;9:549–551.
8. Nelson MA, Allen P, Clampe SE, De Dombal FT. *Spine* 1979;4:97–101.
9. Waddell G, Main CJ, Morris EW, Venner RM, Rae PS, Sharmy SH, Galloway H. *Br Med J* 1982;284:1519–1523.
10. Clark WL, Haldeman S, Johnson P, Morris J, Schulemberger C, Trauner D, White A. *Spine* 1988;13:332–341.
11. Stone D. In: Albrecht GL, ed. *Cross National rehabilitation policies: A sociological perspective.* Beverly Hills, CA: Sage Publications, 1981;49–64.
12. Bennett RM. *Am J Med* 1986;81(suppl 3A):15–23.
13. American Medical Association. *Guides to the evaluation of permanent impairment.* Chicago: American Medical Association, 1984.
14. Brena SF, Chapman SI, Stegall PG, Chyatte SB. *Arch Phys Med Rehabil* 1979;60:387–389.
15. McGeachy J. *Can Med Assoc J* 1988;139:887–888.
16. Flor H, Turk DC, Scholz OB. *J Psychosom Res* 1987;31:63–71.
17. Fordyce WC. *Am Psychol* 1988;43:276–283.
18. Turk DC, Rudy TE. *J Consult Clin Psychol* 1986;54:760–768.
19. Engel GL. *Am J Med* 1959;26:899–915.
20. Frymoyer JW, Rosen JC, Clements J, Pope MH. *Clin Orthop Rel Res* 1985;195:178–184.
21. Pope MH, Rosen JC, Wilder DG, Frymoyer JW. *Spine* 1980;5:173–178.
22. Greenwood JG. *Spine* 1985;10:773–776.
23. Gatchel RJ, Mayer TG, Capra P, Diamond P, Barnett J. *Spine* 1986;11:36–42.
24. Cunningham LS, Kelsey J. *Am J Publ Health* 1984;74:574–579.
25. Luck JV, Florence DW. *Orthop Clin North Am* 1988;19:839–844.
26. Frymoyer JW. *N Engl J Med* 1988;318:291–299.

27. Hadler NM. *Am J Med* 1986;81(3A):26–30.
28. Lee CK. *Orthop Clin North Am* 1988;19:7–803.
29. Cailliet R. *Soft tissue pain and disability*. Philadelphia: FA Davis Company, 1977.
30. Simons DG, Travell JG. *Postgrad Med* 1983;73:66–108.
31. Travell JG, Simons DG. *Myofascial pain and dysfunction: The trigger point manual*. Baltimore: Williams & Wilkins, 1983.
32. Travell JG, Rinzler SH. *Postgrad Med* 1952;11:425–434.
33. Fishbain AA, Goldberg M, Meagher BR, Steele R, Rosomoff H. *Pain* 1986;26:181–197.
34. Awad EA. *Arch Phys Med Rehab* 1973;54:449–453.
35. Larsson SE, Bengtsson A, Bodegard L, Henriksson KG, Larşson J. *Acta Orthop Scand* 1988;59:552–556.
36. Holmes TH, Wolf HG. *Psychosom Med* 1952;14:18.
37. Sarno JE. *J Nerv Ment Dis* 1981;169:55–59.
38. Turk DC, Rudy TE. *J Consult Clin Psychol* 1988;56:233–238.
39. Deyo RA. *Controlled Clin Trials* 1984;5:223–240.
40. Williams RC. *Pain* 1988;35:239–251.
41. Deyo RA. *Arch Phys Med Rehabil* 1988;69:1044–1053.
42. Deyo RA, Diehl AK, Rosenthal M. *N Engl J Med* 1984;315:1064–1070.
43. Augustinsson LE, Sullivan M. *Spine* 1986;11:111–119.
44. Pilowsky I, Hallett EC, Bassett DC, Thomas PG, Penhall RK. *Pain* 1982;14:169–176.
45. Turner JA. *J Consult Clin Psychol* 1982;50:757–765.
46. Deyo RA. *Spine* 1986;11:951–954.
47. Fricton JR, Nelson A, Monsein M. *J Craniomandib Pract* 1987;5:373–381.
48. Waddell G, Main CJ. *Spine* 1984;9:204–208.
49. Waddell G. In: Jayson M, ed. *Understanding the patient with back pain from the lumbar spine*, 3rd ed. New York: Churchill Livingstone, 1987.
50. Mayer TG, Gatchel RJ, Mayer H, Kishino ND, Keeley J, Mooney V. *JAMA* 1987;258:1763–1766.
51. Million R, Hall W, Haavik Nilsen K, Baker RD, Jayson MIV. *Spine* 1982;7:204–212.

Advances in Pain Research and Therapy, Vol. 17,
edited by James R. Fricton and Essam Awad.
Raven Press, Ltd., New York © 1990.

11

Masticatory Muscle Hyperactivity and Muscle Pain

Glenn T. Clark and Shiro Sakai

Dental Research Institute and School of Dentistry, University of California, Los Angeles, Los Angeles, California 90024

The belief that masticatory muscle hyperactivity is causally related to masticatory muscle pain is commonly held (1–3). The actual evidence for this belief is somewhat limited, however, and it is the purpose of this chapter to review the evidence. Prior to this review, it is essential to define these conditions. Masticatory muscle pain is defined as a dull, aching, continuous but variable pain that increases with function and can be verified as having elevated tenderness by palpation of the involved muscle. Muscle hyperactivity can be broadly defined as abnormally prolonged and/or elevated levels of muscle activity beyond what would normally be required for function and postural maintenance. Considering this definition, there are at least five distinct types of skeletal muscle activity (postural, normal functional, habitual, abnormal sleep state, and protective) and one form of nonskeletal muscle activity (vasomotor) that may occur in the masticatory system.

POSTURAL MUSCLE ACTIVITY OR POSTURAL TONE

Postural muscle activity or "postural tone" can be defined as the normally occurring activity in the jaw-closing muscles required to maintain the mandible in a relaxed and comfortable posture. This definition does not include muscle activity associated with volitional movements such as chewing, talking, or swallowing and excludes habitual activities such as clenching, bracing, or setting of the jaw into maximum intercuspation or in any eccentric mandibular position. The normal postural position of the jaw is a position with the lips very close or touching and the teeth separated 1 to 3 mm in distance (4–6). This position is not the most relaxed position, because most patients achieve their lowest jaw-closing muscle electromyographic (EMG) levels with the teeth separated 5 to 13 mm (7). This more open relaxed position is not a normal postural position for various sociocultural reasons and, therefore, it is more correct to use the term "postural position" rather than "rest position" to describe the usual, near-closed mouth position.

Several factors are likely to influence postural muscle activity levels. First, jaw-closing muscle activity is very strongly dependent on gravitation forces (i.e., head position) (8). Yet the influence that working at a desk, driving a car, or even standing for long periods have on the postural tone in the masticatory muscles is not known. The postural muscle activity levels reported in the literature are traditionally measured in conscious, sitting subjects in an EMG laboratory or doctor's office setting and they usually do not specify the position the mandible was in during the experiment. This recording environment is not entirely natural and it would be valuable to know how much postural tone fluctuates under natural day-to-day environmental circumstances.

A second factor of concern is the relationship between daytime postural tone and the patient's previous night's sleep. For example, if the patient is physically tired or fatigued because of a poor night's sleep, is there an observably different daytime postural muscle tone? It would also be interesting to know if there is a change of baseline nonbruxing muscle activity levels in muscle pain patients at night. Since very little information is available on the baseline jaw muscle activity levels that are maintained in the natural environment and during sleep, these questions cannot be answered.

A third factor that clearly influences masticatory muscle pain is emotional stress or anxiety. The studies on stress and masticatory muscle activity are primarily in the headache literature because stress-induced postural muscle activity has been postulated as the main cause of tension headaches (9–12). Fortunately, because the temporal region is a primary pain site for these headaches, many headache researchers have investigated the temporalis muscle (13–16). Although temporomandibular (TM) dysfunction and tension headaches are arguably different disorders, the overlap between a TM disorder patient with a predominantly muscle pain problem and a chronic recurrent temporal region headache patient is significant (17–20). The distinction between these two conditions may be more related to whether the diagnosis is rendered by a neurologist or a dentist. Disregarding the diagnostic dilemma, the underlying theory for both problems is that muscle hyperactivity leads to muscle pain and, therefore, the tension headache literature is relevant in the review of this theory.

The influence that environmental stress and anxiety have on temporalis postural muscle tone has been documented extensively in the laboratory (21,22). These studies consistently show transient elevations during an induced laboratory stress test in both headache patients and controls. A significant difference in postural tone between pain and nonpain controls in forehead muscles is not evident in the headache literature (23–25).

For the few studies in the temporomandibular joint (TMJ) literature that have shown a slight elevation of postural muscle activity in the jaw-closing muscles in muscle pain patients versus controls, this elevation could be a consequence and not a cause of the pain (26–29). Furthermore, it has never been shown that this small difference between muscle pain patients and controls is clinically important. In other words, is this difference enough to produce a chronically painful jaw muscle condition?

The actual level of prolonged muscle activity that can be tolerated without pain developing in the jaw is not known, but the levels of muscle activity that can be sustained for long periods (up to 60 min) have been established for other muscles. For example, research on human elbow flexors showed that sustained activity levels above 8% of the maximum voluntary contraction level would consistently produce mandatory cessation of effort in less than 60 min (30). Blood flow data from human calf muscles also showed that little or no postcontraction hyperemia resulted following a static contraction for 2 min at the 7.5% level of maximum voluntary contraction (31). Unfortunately, comparison is difficult because only one study on masticatory muscle pain patients normalized the resting masseter and temporalis muscle activity levels to a percentage of their maximum voluntary contraction level. This study reported postural activity levels in pain patients near 3% of maximum for the anterior temporalis and 2% for the masseter muscles (29). It should be noted that this resting EMG level may be artificially high since masticatory muscle pain patients usually have a lower maximum voluntary contraction level because of the pain (32). Even so, this level is still below the 8% threshold required for ischemic pain production in a limb muscle. In theory, if the postural activity levels were to rise significantly above the assumed tolerance levels to a level at or above the 8% level for a significant period of time, this would produce a painful muscle state.

In summary, both the TMJ literature and the headache literature show weak or inconsistent evidence for an elevated postural muscle activity level, especially when controls were utilized as the cause of masticatory muscle pain. This lack of a strong relationship between putative myogenic pain and postural muscle activity levels has in fact led many to question the whole concept of myogenic headaches (33–35). Until more convincing evidence is available regarding the relationship between postural skeletal muscle activity levels in the natural environment and muscle pain, one cannot assume a relationship (either positive or negative).

NORMAL FUNCTIONAL ACTIVITY

The second category of normal functional muscle activity is defined to include all normally occurring volitional activities required for routine function. These behaviors are chewing, talking, and swallowing. Because the perioral, tongue, and pharyngeal muscles are not usually involved in a masticatory muscle pain disorder, abnormal talking and swallowing behaviors are not thought to be a common form of muscle hyperactivity. On the other hand, abnormal chewing has been discussed in the literature as a potential form of muscle hyperactivity (36,37). The theory states that a painful masticatory muscle response can occur if the chewing cycle is altered in such a way as to prevent adequate blood flow between each chewing stroke. Adequate blood flow is essential to continue any repetitive contraction, and if blood flow is inadequate during chewing, even healthy subjects will develop pain after only a few minutes.

A painful ischemic muscle condition has been experimentally produced in subjects by having them rapidly chew their food or by having them chew very tough foods. Researchers have speculated that abnormal chewing patterns develop through an acquired structural abnormality such as the loss of posterior teeth or inadequately restored teeth with poor occlusal contact relationships. Experiments have shown that the ability to efficiently incise and chew food is reduced in patients with a poor occlusion because they require either a longer total time (more chewing strokes) to chew food or a prolonged closing phase with each chewing stroke (37).

Thus inefficient chewing can theoretically produce muscle pain because of the reduced resting period between each chewing stroke. Opponents to this theory say that the cause-and-effect relationship between an assumed abnormal chewing behavior and muscle pain is not clearly demonstrated by the existing research. For example, the total time spent in chewing is probably no more than 1 hour each day (20 min for each meal) or less than 7% of the total waking day. An adequate rest period certainly exists between each meal to allow for a full recovery of the jaw musculature from a function-induced ischemia. Furthermore, even though the experimental chewing research has demonstrated that prolonged vigorous chewing can induce pain in the jaw muscles, patients do not chew at this artificially fast rate (38). Finally, there are innumerable malocclusion patients who have a less than ideal structure and exhibit little or no jaw function impairment.

In summary, the existing evidence has not proven that functional hyperactivity (e.g., chewing inefficiently) is an important form of muscle hyperactivity that causes a chronic muscle pain condition. Conversely, vigorous chewing can clearly make the pain worse when masticatory muscle pain is present.

HABITUAL MUSCLE ACTIVITY

The third form of activity is habitual muscle activity, which is defined as a nonfunctional learned oral motor behavior. One obvious habit of concern is sustained tooth clenching. Other oral habits include positioning or setting the jaw or tongue in an eccentric or abnormal position. Several other perioral behaviors are commonly seen in the jaw, such as lip and cheek biting and bracing and pressing the tongue against the teeth. Although conscious state habits are the primary focus of this category, it is also speculated that these habitual activities can carry over and occur during sleeping states. Sleep state muscle hyperactivity will be discussed further in the next section.

Whether it occurs during sleep or while awake, it is probable that clenching has the greatest potential for a harmful effect. The distinction between a light tooth clenching or tongue bracing habit and an elevated postural activity is difficult to make. The latter implies a nonvolitional, nonlearned change in baseline activity occurring in jaw muscles, whereas the two former habits are learned volitional behaviors that can be stopped immediately by making the patient aware of the behavior. It should be pointed out that patients are typically not consciously aware of their habitual behaviors, so direct questioning of the patient about his or her habits is usually negative.

Much of the dental literature over the years has emphasized that all oral habits are potentially harmful depending on the frequency, duration, and effort involved in the activity (39). Unfortunately, there are no definitive reports that have quantified a level of jaw muscle activity associated with a specific oral habit as it occurs in the natural environment. Oral habits are not easily seen by an observer because patients in an EMG research laboratory do not typically demonstrate these behaviors.

Fortunately, recent advances in ambulatory EMG techniques now allow us to look at mean daytime jaw muscle activity levels at intervals as short as 30 min (40,41) (Fig. 1). By also having the patient monitor pain levels and stress levels in a diary, correlations can be made between behavior and pain (Fig. 2). There are several reports in the literature using these techniques that have shown a clear relationship between increased daytime EMG levels and pain conditions (43). Unfortunately, these data are not detailed enough to correlate specific oral habits with increased EMG activity, and it is also difficult to say whether this type of recording situation produces a completely natural behavior. As these techniques improve and more detailed information is available, ambulatory EMG monitoring may eventually provide a better understanding of the interrelationships between day-to-day events, habitual jaw muscle activity, and muscle pain.

In summary, until more research has been published, it is now only possible to speculate that habitual muscle activity is a likely form of pain-inducing hyperactivity.

ABNORMAL SLEEP STATE MUSCLE ACTIVITY

The fourth category of masticatory muscle activity is abnormal sleep state muscle activity. It can be defined as any abnormal muscle contraction that occurs during a sleeping condition not associated with airway maintenance

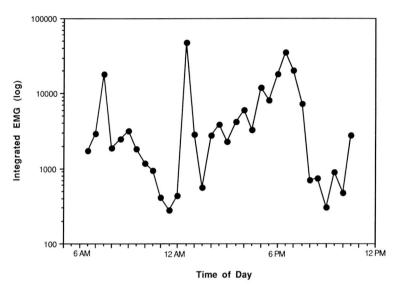

FIG. 1. Integrated temporalis EMG activity was recorded and plotted every 30 min during a single day for a chronic recurrent temporalis region headache subject. The recording was performed with an ambulatory EMG recorder (42). The surface electrodes were applied on the anterior temporalis and the subject carried a 30-min timer and a recording diary. The EMG device accumulated all electrical activity above 10 μV. By pressing the switch every 30 min the subject read the cumulative electrical activity, converted to digital numbers, on the screen of the recorder. The horizontal axis on the graph shows the time of day, and vertical axis shows the cumulative EMG levels in microvolt-seconds per 30 min using a logarithmic scale.

and swallowing. The jaw muscle activities of primary concern are the strong and often rhythmical contractions that result in tooth grinding movements (bruxism) (44). Actual tooth grinding (e.g., rhythmical movements) is not always present. Abnormal jaw muscle activity during sleep has also been reported to occur as a continuous isometric contraction lasting for several seconds to as much as 5 min without any grinding noises being produced (45). These rhythmical or brief, sustained high-level contractions are probably not learned or habitual behaviors and might be best described as uncontrolled patterned outflows of central nervous system activity occurring during sleep. The assumption that they are not learned is based on the fact that true tooth grinding in an adult is a very persistent behavior and it produces extremely high force levels (high enough to crush tooth enamel). It is highly illogical to assume such a behavior is a learned response. Most polysomnographic studies of bruxism provide evidence that it tends to occur under a certain set of brain wave conditions (46). Unfortunately, only a few studies exist and not all agree, but bruxism is most frequently reported to occur during a transition from a deeper stage of sleep to a lighter stage (46).

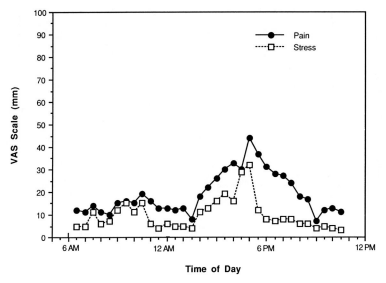

FIG. 2. Visual analogue scale (VAS) for pain and stress levels every 30 min during a single day from same subject as in Fig. 1. These data were gathered by having the subject record his subjective pain and stress levels in the recording diary on a VAS.

These behaviors are typically never seen in the waking state. Bruxism should not be considered a pathological brain dysfunction, but more of a patterned, central nervous system instability that occurs idiopathically in many people.

Rhythmical tooth grinding or brief static isometric contraction of high force is not the only form of nocturnal muscle activity. Many clinicians have described patients who exhibit transient episodes of clenching activity in their sleep during stressful life events (47). These behaviors are different from bruxism in that they are transient behaviors, which are reversible with treatment interventions such as oral appliances and biofeedback, and probably do not occur at such high force levels (Fig. 3). It is easy to speculate that they are a type of habitual or learned behavior that is carried over into the sleep state.

Numerous sleep EMG studies have been performed documenting both masticatory muscle activity in TM disorder patients and the influence various treatments have on this activity (48,49). These studies provide powerful documentation that a certain percentage of TM disorder patients have sleep-state muscle hyperactivity above that of normal nonpain subjects (Fig. 4) (50). Unfortunately, this technique does not provide detailed minute-by-minute EMG data and, therefore, cannot distinguish clenching from grinding. It also does not prove cause and effect, because many bruxism subjects (evidenced by tooth wear) do not have elevated muscle pain.

In summary, even though these recordings do not differentiate the specific

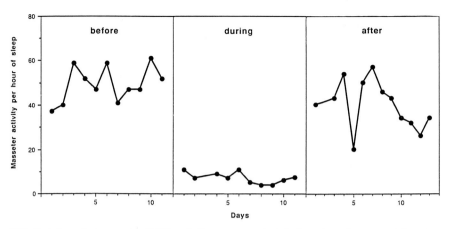

FIG. 3. Integrated masseter EMG activity was recorded during sleep for several days before, during, and after occlusal appliance therapy for one subject. The surface electrodes were applied unilaterally on the subject's masseter muscle and the EMG device recorded all activities above 20 μV during sleep. The subject was a chronic masticatory muscle pain patient (49). The vertical axis is in EMG units per hour of sleep, and 1 EMG unit was equal to the cumulative EMG level produced by a single brief (<1-sec) maximum clench.

nature of the nocturnal muscle activity, they do provide the most reasonable evidence that high levels of nocturnal clenching activity are related to jaw muscle pain disorders.

PROTECTIVE MUSCLE ACTIVITY AND POSITIVE FEEDBACK

The last category of skeletal muscle activity is protective muscle activity, which is defined as involuntary muscle activity that occurs in an effort to prevent or avoid a painful movement. Protective jaw muscle activity, or trismus, can occur for any number of reasons, such as the presence of a painful derangement or arthritic TM joint, a chronically painful jaw muscle, or an oral infection, or even following a traumatic dental surgical treatment (51,52). One example would be a brief abnormal contraction of the jaw-closing muscles during opening as the jaw joint undergoes a painful click or pop (53).

Several investigators over the years have documented these abnormal skeletal muscle activity patterns in the masticatory system (54–56). Distinguishing protective muscle hyperactivity from other patterns of muscle activity is important to treatment since this condition will not usually change until the noxious stimulus causing it is removed (57). One theory is that when a chronically painful tissue injury or pathology exists, such as in a fibromyalgia disorder or chronic painful arthritis, then an almost self-sustaining protective muscle activity pattern can be created. The resulting in-

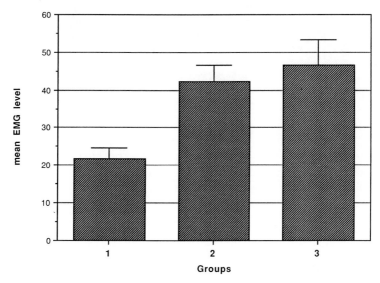

FIG. 4. Mean integrated masseter muscle EMG levels and standard error for subjects grouped according to a clinical index of jaw dysfunction (50). These data show that groups 2 and 3 are significantly different at the 0.05 level from group 1. All EMG levels were recorded from the subjects' masseter muscles unilaterally during sleep for 10 to 14 days. The three groups represent a nonpatient control group (1) with few or no symptoms, and two TMJ clinic patient groups with mild to moderate symptoms (2) and with severe symptoms (3). The vertical axis is in EMG units per hour of sleep, and 1 EMG unit was equal to the cumulative EMG level produced by a single brief (<1-sec) maximum clench.

creased activity from this feedback may cause a cyclical response in which pain causes increased activity and this in turn causes more pain. Although no clear evidence for this cyclical response exists, it has been speculated to contribute to the commonly reported spread of a local muscle pain disorder to a more generalized phenomenon (51).

In summary, the possible role of secondary or protective muscle activity should not be ignored when considering jaw muscle pain. Trismus has been documented to occur in the jaw in a number of situations, and even though additional research is needed to clarify the level and extent of this activity in TM disorder patients, it does provide supportive evidence for the relationship between muscle hyperactivity and muscle pain.

VASOMOTOR ACTIVITY

This final category of muscle activity involves the sympathetic nervous system–controlled smooth muscles that surround the arterial system and regulate blood flow. Abnormality of the vasomotor system could be defined as any sustained contraction that prevents adequate perfusion into the muscle such that normal functional or postural activity levels produce a painful ischemic site. Traditionally, the literature on muscle hyperactivity has almost exclusively dealt with the concept of striated muscle hyperactivity while more or less ignoring the potential of smooth muscle hyperactivity. This focus on skeletal muscle activity has occurred primarily because most quantitative studies on muscle activity have utilized EMG as the measurement tool, and EMG provides a measurement of the activity in skeletal muscles only.

Vasomotor muscle activity levels may also be important and are possibly related to muscle pain problems. For example, the effect of experimental alteration of blood flow has been studied via the blood pressure cuff method (58). This research has been predominantly performed on limb muscle groups, where the occlusion of blood flow is relatively easy (59,60). Fortunately, a few studies on contraction-induced changes in blood flow in the masseter and temporal muscles have been performed (27,61). Both the limb muscle and masticatory muscle studies have demonstrated that when a total blockage of blood flow occurs without any associated skeletal muscle activity, this situation does not produce a painful ischemia state (58). However, if any skeletal activity is present then ischemic muscle pain soon results, and this pain will occur even under conditions of normally nonpainful skeletal muscle function. Unfortunately, experimental proof that a partial occlusion or reduction of blood flow might theoretically occur with increased vasomotor activity is lacking. What is known is that the muscle pain patient has reduced endurance capability and develops a painful ischemia with function more rapidly than do normal subjects.

In summary, even though it is an attractive theory to explore, the relationship between vasomotor activity and chronic muscle pain is not yet known.

CONCLUSIONS

This review has focused on the possible relationship between muscle pain and several masticatory muscle activity patterns. Based on this review, the assumption that masticatory muscle hyperactivity leads to pain and dysfunction cannot be discarded even though little support exists for the concept of elevated postural muscle activity in the tension headache literature. This literature has primarily looked at postural muscle activity in the EMG laboratory and is limited for that reason. Evidence for elevated sleep state masticatory muscle hyperactivity does exist from the nocturnal EMG monitoring studies. Preliminary evidence also exists from a few reports on elevated daytime muscle activity levels (presumably due to habitual behaviors) using ambulatory EMG monitoring. It is likely that in the presence of local pain, protective muscle activity is also a contributing factor to jaw muscle pain disorders. Finally, reduced endurance capacity of painful muscles suggests an altered blood perfusion and implicates an autonomic (possibly vasomotor hyperactivity) dysfunction.

What seems to be called for now is a conceptual reclassification of muscle activity disorders into more specific categories of muscle hyperactivity. This reclassification will help researchers design better studies to test the theories and help the practitioner prescribe more appropriate treatment. Although this review does not make specific treatment recommendations, it is evident that treatment recommended for each category of hyperactivity is likely to be different. Only by accurately defining the specific cause of the pain and dysfunction of the jaw system will it be possible to understand the etiology of a chronically painful muscle disorder and then prescribe the best treatment approach for our patients.

REFERENCES

1. Laskin DM. *J Am Dent Assoc* 1969;79:147–153.
2. Schwartz LL. *J Chronic Dis* 1956;3:284–293.
3. Travell J. *J Prosthet Dent* 1960;10:745–763.
4. Boos RH. *J Prosthet Dent* 1952;16:575–587.
5. Hickey JC, Zarb GA. *Boucher's prosthodontic treatment for edentulous patients.* St. Louis: CV Mosby Company, 1980.
6. Niswonger ME. *J Am Dent Assoc* 1934;21:1572–1582.
7. Rugh JD, Drago CJ. *J Prosthet Dent* 1981;45:671–675.
8. Mohl N. In: Solberg WK, Clark GT, eds. *Abnormal jaw mechanics: Diagnosis and treatment.* Chicago: Quintessence Publishing Co, Inc, 1984;97–111.
9. Ad Hoc Committee on Classification of Headache. *JAMA* 1962;179:717–718.
10. Budzynski T, Stoyva J, Adler C. *J Behav Exp Psychiatry* 1970;1:205–211.
11. Vaughn R, Pall ML, Haynes SN. *Headache* 1977;16:313–317.
12. Wolff HG. *Headache and other head pain.* New York: Oxford University Press, 1963.
13. Philips C. In; Ruchman S, ed. *Contributions to medical psychology*, Vol 1. Oxford, England: Pergamon Press, 1977;91–113.
14. Philips HC, Hunter MS. *Headache* 1982;22:173–179.
15. Tunis MM, Wolff HG. *Arch Neurol Psychiatry* 1954;71:425–434.
16. van Boxtel A, Goudswaard P, Janssen K. *Headache* 1983;23:215–222.
17. Magnusson T, Carlsson GE. *Swed Dent J* 1978;2:85–92.
18. Pincus JH, Tucker GJ. *Behavioral neurology.* New York: Oxford University Press, 1985.
19. Reik L, Hale M. *Headache* 1981;21:151–156.
20. Schokker RP, Hansson TL, Ansink BJJ. *J Craniomandib Disord Facial Oral Pain* 1989;3:71–74.
21. Simons DJ, Day E, Goodell H, Wolff HG. *Res Publ Assoc Res Nerv Ment Dis* 1943;23: 228–244.
22. Yemm R. *Arch Oral Biol* 1971;16:269–273.
23. Bakal DA, Kaganov JA. *Headache* 1977;17:208–215.
24. Martin PR, Mathews AM. *J Psychosom Res* 1978;22:389–399.
25. Sutton EP, Belar CD. *Headache* 1982;22:133–136.
26. Lous I, Sheik-Ol-Eslam A, Møller E. *Scand J Dent Res* 1970;78:404–410.
27. Møller E, Rasmussen OC, Bonde-Petersen F. *Adv Pain Res* 1979;3:271–281.
28. Rugh JD, Montgomery GT. *J Craniomandib Disord Facial Oral Pain* 1987;1:243–250.
29. Sheikholeslam A, Møller E, Lous I. *Scand J Dent Res* 1982;90:37–46.
30. Björksten M, Jonsson B. *Scand J Work Environ Health* 1977;3:23–27.
31. Richardson D. *J Appl Physiol* 1981;51:929–933.

32. Helkimo E, Carlsson GE, Carmeli Y. *J Oral Rehabil* 1975;2:397–406.
33. Haynes SN, Cuevas J, Gannon LR. *Headache* 1982;22:122–132.
34. Pikoff H. *Headache* 1984;24:189–198.
35. Sjaastad O. *Curr Med Res Opin* 1980;6(Suppl 9):4154.
36. Møller E. In: Kawamura Y, Dubner R, eds. *Oral-facial sensory and motor function*. Tokyo: Quintessence Publishing Co, Inc, 1981;225–239.
37. Møller E, Sheikholeslam A, Lous I. *Scand J Dent Res* 1984;92:64–83.
38. Rugh JD. *J Comp Physiol Psychol* 1972;80:169–174.
39. Krogh-Poulsen W. In: Solberg WK, Clark GT, eds. *Temporomandibular joint problems: Biologic diagnosis and treatment*. Chicago: Quintessence Publishing Co, Inc, 1980;93–110.
40. Clark GT, Sakai S. Paper presented at Canadian and American Pain Societies Joint Meeting, 1988.
41. Sakai S, Clark GT, Flack VF. *J Dent Res* 1989;68:224 (abstr).
42. Burgar CG, Rugh JD. *IEEE Trans Biomed Eng* 1983;30:66–69.
43. Finlayson RS, Rugh JD, Dolwick MF. *J Dent Res* 1982;61:277 (abstr).
44. Glaros AG, Rao SM. *Psychol Bull* 1977;84:767–781.
45. Rugh JD, Orbach R. In: Mohl ND, Zarb GA, Carlsson GE, Rugh JD, eds. *A textbook of occlusion*, Chicago: Quintessence Publishing Co, Inc, 1988;249–261.
46. Satoh T, Harada Y. *Electroencephalogr Clin Neurophysiol* 1973;35:267–275.
47. Rugh JD, Solberg WK. *Oral Scien Rev* 1976;7:3–30.
48. Casas JM, Beemsterboer P, Clark GT. *Behav Res Ther* 1982;20:9–15.
49. Clark GT, Beemsterboer PL, Solberg WK, Rugh JD. *J Am Dent Assoc* 1979;99:607–612.
50. Clark GT, Beemsterboer PL, Rugh JD. *J Oral Rehabil* 1981;8:279–286.
51. Bell WE. *Temporomandibular disorders: Classification, diagnosis, management*. Chicago: Year Book Medical Publisher, 1986.
52. Travell JC, Simons DG. *Myofascial pain and dysfunction: The trigger point manual*. Baltimore: Williams & Wilkins, 1983.
53. Stohler C, Yamada Y, Ash MM. *Helv Odontal Acta* 1985;95:13–20.
54. Costen JB. *Ann Otol Rhinol Laryngol* 1939;48:499–514.
55. Steinhardt G. *Quintessence Int* 1978, May:1–10.
56. Tovi F, Zirkin H, Sidi J. *J Oral Maxillofac Surg* 1983;41:466–469.
57. Clark GT. *Int Dent J* 1981;31:216–225.
58. Myers DE, McCall WD. *Headache* 1983;23:113–116.
59. Dorpat TL, Holmes TH. *Arch Neurol Psychiatry* 1955;74:628–640.
60. Rodbard S. *Headache* 1970;10;105–115.
61. Rasmussen OC, Bonde-Petersen F, Christensen LV, Moller E. *Arch Oral Biol* 1977;22: 539–543.

Advances in Pain Research and Therapy, Vol. 17,
edited by James R. Fricton and Essam Awad.
Raven Press, Ltd., New York © 1990.

12

Psychosocial Factors and Muscular Pain

H. Merskey

*Department of Psychiatry, University of Western Ontario, and London
Psychiatric Hospital, London, Ontario N6A 4H1 Canada*

MUSCLE OR MIND?

There is a basic dilemma that has permeated the fields of physical medicine, rheumatology, and neurology, and has involved psychiatry and psychology. It is to distinguish regional or widespread complaints of pain in terms of the different disciplines, and to determine the etiology of such complaints. For at least 60 years there has been a growing trend to identify regional pains with psychological illness (1,2). Most of these pains involved the musculoskeletal system, in which, like psychiatry, clinical techniques were underdeveloped. Perhaps even more importantly, those clinical techniques that were available were undervalued and insufficiently applied. I propose to look first at some of the techniques and problems in investigation of myofascial syndromes and fibromyalgia, comparing them with the same situations in psychiatric illnesses that cause pain. Only then will it make sense to look at the substantial associations between psychological and social factors and pain.

The problems of making observations relating to muscle pain syndromes start from the fact that more impressive diagnostic techniques exist in neighboring disciplines. Angulated broken bones and unchallengeable x-ray portrayals of fractures establish hard data in the clinical practice of orthopedics. The gross disturbances of arthritis and the associated serological patterns that can be studied offer firm points of departure for the rheumatologist. The overt lesions of neurology, with altered reflexes and specific findings in nerve conduction or electromyography (EMG) studies, give confidence in the reliability of neurological examination and the scientific value of neurological diagnoses. By contrast, the examination of muscle pain syndromes is in its infancy. The most-cited work in the field that describes individual myofascial syndromes (3) was published only 6 years ago, and deals only with the upper half of the body. Reliability studies for the multiple myofascial syndromes are few and limited, just as they are for the many chronic pain syndromes, which have been described by the International Association for the Study of Pain (4). It was only in 1978 that Smythe and Moldofsky developed full systematic criteria for a sufficient number of tender points and their locations that would serve to identify fibrositis (fibromyalgia) as a distinct entity (5).

While facet joint syndromes are recognized and other subordinate patterns of spinal arthritis can be identified, the consistency and discriminability of different muscle pain syndromes, even in the hands of experts, either has not been studied or remains unknown to the general medical practitioner. Here again, the lack of reliability studies, the variability of x-ray findings, and the difficulties in establishing an independent "gold standard" for diagnosis still handicap the subject. Even the common and convincing observation by many patients that they anticipate the changes of weather in their joints still lacks adequate scientific demonstration in relation to weather changes. We know that other types of weather forecasting are fallible when matched against the actual barometric fluctuations and measures of precipitation. We tend to think the same about this striking human experience and perhaps are embarrassed by our inability to understand why it occurs.

Besides the matters of posture and atrophy, which often constitute "soft signs," we are dependent upon observations of tenderness and spasm. The former are generally considered to be subjective, the latter often unreliable. An effect corresponding to spasm can be produced voluntarily merely by flexing a muscle. It is true that it is hard to flex localized muscle fibers, consciously or unconsciously, in areas that are not normally under separate individual voluntary control, such as the back muscles. In muscle sprain syndromes, for example acute cervical sprain, such patterns of muscle spasm are often identified at onset but do not persist, even though the subjective complaints of pain and tenderness remain. Furthermore, examination of power depends upon the cooperation of the patient, who may hesitate to exert a painful limb. The investigation of sensation demands scrupulous attention to detail, which is frequently, and often justifiably, neglected in clinical practice because it is both time consuming and unrewarding. Sometimes this lack of attention to detail results in unintentional misleading of the patient, and a suggestion of effects that are not adequately verified by alternative instructions and retesting.

We rely heavily upon the history, and history taking in these syndromes requires a care and specificity that are frequently jettisoned. Clinical reports often describe a patient's headache as "vague." Is it really vague? We may doubt this. The word has a pejorative implication and requires closer examination. Most of us at some time will have had a tension headache or an ache or discomfort in the body. It is hard to be definite about the boundaries of such sensations. We may say ourselves that the limits are vague. However, when the indefinite limits are reinterpreted as a vague description, it becomes a put-down to the patient, whose valid observations tend to be rejected.

Patients often have more than one sensation in the same region, and the sensation fluctuates. Sometimes it is a feeling of partial loss of sensation or numbness; sometimes it is a feeling of heaviness, dullness, or uncertainty in using fingers or a limb. Both types of sensation are described as "numbness" in conventional speech, but they are not identical. Most doctors do not seek to determine which meaning is implied. Sometimes there are two patterns in the headache of one individual. A constant aching pain may be combined with an intermittent throbbing or stabbing sensation. It is surprising how often we fail to determine the duration of each complaint. Patients may be called inconsistent in their description of pain, when the fault really lies with inadequate history taking.

These mistakes are easy to make. They can only be avoided by individuals who can allocate ample time for the examination of each patient. Often the process of obtaining a refined discrimination, which is being recommended implicitly here, cannot be incorporated into routine medical practice.

In these circumstances it is not surprising that feelings of uncertainty attach to the questions of myofascial pain syndrome. There are a few practitioners who have established a record of capable diagnosis and success in treatment. Their skills are at a premium. Many more practitioners function with partial knowledge and partial success, as is the case in any branch of medicine. It is often not clear why some cases respond and others do not. Frequently, the only hard evidence of whether a patient has really improved comes from his or her own report. In consequence, even the good results are uncertain in their interpretation. They are often attributed to placebo responses, a phenomenon that frequently leaves the physician uneasy and with a bad conscience, even when he can appear to be happy with the outcome.

The situation in psychiatry can be described more briefly: It used to be bad in every respect and now is exceptionally good in some respects. Since the introduction of research diagnostic criteria (6,7) and the publication of the *Diagnostic* and *Statistical Manual of Mental Disorders* (3rd edition) (DSM-III) (8), solid evidence of reliability has been attached to many common psychiatric syndromes, such as schizophrenia, phobic anxiety, and major affective disorder. Unfortunately, the section of DSM-III that deals with somatoform disorders is weak in as much as the criteria for conversion syndromes and idiopathic pain syndrome [DSM-III (R)] are still unsatisfactory and promote overdiagnosis of these categories. Personality disorder, which is a pervasive issue in practice, both in psychiatry and other fields of medicine, remains an unreliable category despite serious and well thought out attempts to improve it. Hysterical syndromes affecting bodily regions present particular problems of differential diagnosis that will be discussed in detail later. Meanwhile, we need to consider there are hypotheses about psychiatric illnesses which can result in complaints that could be confused with muscle pain.

PSYCHOLOGICAL MECHANISMS OF PAIN

If it is suggested that the mind gives rise to pain, experienced as a sensation in the body, then we must inevitably try to think of some understandable manner in which that could happen. What is the mechanism? One obvious psychiatric mechanism is hallucination. If patients with schizophrenia have hallucinations of other people speaking their thoughts aloud or talking about them, or feelings that their body is being changed by rays from a distance, then it seems plausible that they might experience hallucinations of pain. This does happen, but only very rarely (9). It is not a practical issue for the great majority of patients with chronic pain. Hallucinations may occur with severe depressive illness as well, but the depression is readily recognizable and treatable by the usual psychiatric measures.

The second theoretical way in which pain might be induced as a result of psychological states is through muscle contraction. This well-recognized mechanism is usually thought to be one of anxiety leading to increased muscle contraction with inadequate disposal of metabolites. Lewis and colleagues observed that excess muscle contraction with inadequate circulation does lead to pain (10). Once anxiety has resulted in pain, the pain perpetuates the anxiety and the cycle continues. This is a direct psychophysiological mechanism and should be distinguished carefully from a hysterical mechanism.

There is a third possible mechanism which may also be related to anxiety in a psychophysiological manner, but without necessarily involving increased muscle contraction. If we assume that nociceptive input will be increased in individuals who are anxious, then a modest or unimportant lesion that causes some mild discomfort in a tranquil individual might promote more troublesome pain in an axious person. Essentially, this constitutes magnification of an existing pain rather than the creation of a pain *de novo*. This may well be the most important of all the clinical mechanisms in which psychological factors involve pain.

Finally, there is the question of the production of pain by a hysterical mechanism. In such a case, we should not suppose that there is any physical change, at least initially, in the peripheral tissue where the pain is located. Instead, the experience is a result of an unconscious emotional conflict due to a thought process that is, at first, unknown to the patient. Evidence that makes this mechanism very likely has been discussed at length elsewhere by the author (11). It has been tempting to explain muscle pain on this basis, because it is well-recognized that so-called muscle contraction pains, such as those found with muscle contraction headache, are not accompanied by proportionate changes in quantitative measures of EMG muscle activity (11,12).

Given that such mechanisms for psychological causes of pain exist, we should next consider whether there is an association between pain and psychiatric illness. If such an association can be found, then it might be at least plausible to suppose that numerous cases of pain in muscle regions might be produced by the foregoing mechanisms. In fact, nobody denies that there is a very strong association between certain types of psychiatric illness and pain. Neurotic or reactive depression, anxiety disorders, and patterns of multiple complaints, often called somatization disorder or hypochondriasis, are well recognized as being associated with chronic pain (2,13). With the resolution of the psychiatric illnesses, the pain may also improve. This provides convincing support for the view that, at least in some instances, the pain is due to psychological causes. However, in other cases, obvious physical disorders are treated successfully, and the depression or other psychiatric syndrome that accompanied them may resolve concomitantly. In these cases it is likely that pain has caused the psychiatric illness rather than vice versa.

THE DISTINCTION FROM HYSTERIA

Although hysteria is a definite cause of pain, the frequency with which this happens is uncertain. We now have reason to believe that hysteria is much less common as a mechanism that initiates pain than we thought it was in the past. There was a peculiar coincidence between psychological theory and physical findings that led for many decades to a misleading emphasis on hysteria as a cause of pain. Although the word has been used for many centuries, with various meanings, hysteria only began to be accurately differentiated from psychophysiological symptoms, depressive symptoms, and other effects of mood upon the body after it was recognized that certain symptoms did not correspond to anatomical patterns. This was particularly clear in the classical hysterical paralyses, astasia, abasia, and so forth. In addition, a loss of sensation that stopped at the midline or did not follow dermatomal distributions, or pain that overlapped the boundaries of nerve distributions, was understood to result from the patient's idea of a symptom rather than from actual physical interference with the nervous system.

Other writers had previously recognized the production of symptoms by idea (14), but it was only in the 19th century that the relationship of hysteria to the patient's idea of a symptom was clearly enunciated. Russell Reynolds (15) identified this relationship and Charcot (16) reinforced the view by demonstrating that hysterical symptoms could be produced by hypnosis, and that they followed the pattern of the idea, rather than the idea of the nervous system. Freud was very impressed by the work of Charcot, taking it as his own point of departure. His explanation served to help us understand why symptoms took particular patterns and how they could be produced by the repression of conflict into the unconscious. Against the background of these concepts, it became customary to suppose that certain phenomena revealed on physical examination were evidence of hysteria. These included non-anatomical sensory boundaries for pain or loss of sensation, sensory changes at the midline, and "giveway weakness."

The first difficulty with such an analysis today is that these displays might be mimicked by patterns of regional muscle change, myotomes, or even sclerotomes. The referral of pain from muscles can be regional, as documented by the work of Travell and Simons (3). Repetition strain syndrome, at least in some cases, must have a physical cause and to reject that viewpoint would defy logic. Diffuse muscle tenderness can result from myxedema. Fibromyalgia, with its consistent pattern of particular tender points, could easily have been overlooked in the past. Such syndromes may not have been traditionally recognized and were probably confused with psychological illness. Indeed, the history of muscle pain syndromes, which even 10 years ago were still being described as "psychogenic rheumatism," is enough, in itself, to identify a problem.

We also know that a finding of reduced strength, or giveway weakness, in a limb might be due as much to inhibition by pain as to a formal pattern of hysteria. Why should the patient cooperate in exactly the way that the examiner intends, when he or she is uneasily aware that it is likely to hurt? Other traditional signs of hysteria have lately been shown to be gravely suspect. Gould et al. (17) examined seven such signs: a history suggestive of hypochondriasis, potential secondary gain, la belle indifference, nonanatomical patchy sensory loss, changing boundaries of hypoalgesia, sensory loss that splits at the midline (on pinprick or vibratory stimulation), and giveway weakness. They looked for these phenomena in 30 patients with acute central nervous system damage, usually stroke. All of the patients had at least one of the signs. Twenty-nine showed at least one feature of a supposedly nonphysiological sensory examination. The mean number of items per patient was 3.4. The authors concluded that hysteria is easily misdiagnosed if these items are accepted as pathognomonic and that the tests that are said to provide absolute evidence of hysteria, lack any validity.

Furthermore, it is known in the psychiatric literature that the diagnosis of hysteria may merely be another way of arriving at the presence of substantial cerebral organic disease. Slater (18) was the first to emphasize this, but it has been confirmed by others (19). There are many syndromes that were previously called hysteria, and are now believed to be organic in origin. They include hemifacial spasm, facial dyskinesia and dystonias, spasmodic torticollis, and painful legs and moving toes (19).

Most of the misdiagnoses of hysteria have resulted from overvaluation of poor signs on physical examination, lack of understanding and recognition of some alternate organic disease that is yet to be well defined, or a misinterpretation of the situation with regard to so-called secondary gain, which will be discussed later. For the moment, let us look at the criteria for the diagnosis of somatoform pain disorder, 307.80 in DSM-III(R). They are:

a. Preoccupation with pain for at least 6 months
b. either (1) or (2):
   1. Appropriate evaluation uncovers no organic pathology or pathophysiologic mechanism (e.g., a physical disorder or the effects of injury) to account for the pain
   2. When there is related organic pathology the complaint of pain or resulting social or occupational impairment is grossly in excess of what would be expected from the physical findings.

This diagnosis as described is not a psychiatric diagnosis, despite the fact that it appears in a psychiatric manual. It is merely a statement that physical explanations are insufficient to account for the symptoms. When knowledge of a physical illness changes, this definition, too, must change. The only benefit of this diagnosis is that it can be made without committing the psychiatrist to explaining the disorder. I think I could find that quite useful. However, it would not be much help to my colleagues or to the patient unless I made it clear that I was really offering a diagnosis of ignorance.

The foregoing may be all very well, but the question as to what is happening with regional pain syndromes is still unresolved. One explanation is that there are taut bands, trigger points, and patterns of muscle pain referral found with myofascial pain that will account for much of the pain. However, this does not explain all of the pain, nor the regional sensory losses often found. In this respect, information of critical importance has emerged from recent neurophysiological research.

In the last 15 years, Wall and his colleagues have conducted a series of studies that have demonstrated that there is enormous plasticity in the function of the nervous system. Thus, it has been shown that the receptive fields of afferent neurons in the dorsal horn of the spinal cord can change and extend (20). In the rat, 3 to 4 days after deafferentation, cells that formerly responded to stimulation within the usual anatomical area begin to respond to stimuli from other areas. A comparable event would occur in man if cells in the area of the spinal cord serving the little finger only responded to local stimulation, but, after damage to the region of the ulnar nerve, began to respond to stimulation in other parts of the upper limb.

Such effects can also result from causing a punctate burn in one part of a limb. The presence of a burn in one area permits excitation of cells throughout the whole region (21). Cook et al. (22) even showed that electrical conditioning stimuli at 1 Hz for 20 sec to C fiber afferents from the gastrocnemius muscle of the rat would more than triple the receptive field of a cutaneous afferent neuron, whether it responded originally to a firm mechanical stimulus or to pinch. Moreover, neurons that originally responded only to pinch would begin to respond to touch about 15 min after the stimulation. Thus, mechanisms exist in the spinal cord that allow regional pain to develop from a localized disturbance, including subcutaneous changes. Perhaps the most striking evidence of this is contained in the paper by Wall and Woolf (23). A train of 20 electrical stimuli at 1 Hz, applied to the gastrocnemius-soleus nerve produced changes in the excitability of reflex responses by motoneurons lasting up to 90 min. Woolf and Wall (24) later pointed out, "Because brief afferent inputs from deep tissue have even more pronounced effects than cutaneous inputs, this may explain the more widespread sensory disturbances that accompany deep injury."

Whether the initial insult is deep injury, local repetition strain, or any other subcutaneous change, the evidence shows that mechanisms exist in the spinal cord that will allow regional pain to develop from a localized disturbance. Nonanatomical pain distributions may well be physiological.

Up to this point I have not presented much evidence on the psychogenesis of muscle pain, or its exacerbation by social factors. I have been spending my time undercutting the diagnosis which I used to make.

MOTIVES FOR PAIN

Many soft tissue syndromes of pain are associated with entitlement to compensation or a claim for compensation of some sort, whether from a workers' insurance policy or a motor vehicle accident. In these circumstances, it is often said that the pain is subjective and, thus, depends upon the word of the individual, and that we might have reason to disbelieve him or her. Indeed, this is true, but it needs to be qualified. In the first place, there are pain syndromes that are free from the problem of compensation, still depend upon the word of the individual, and are accepted quite readily even though they lack physical signs. These include trigeminal neuralgia, cluster headache, and some dental pains. They are accepted because a consistent pattern of symptoms is reproduced and no additional reasons exist for it to be reported, other than that it bothers the patient.

Patterns of pain after motor vehicle accidents, such as cervical sprain with dysphagia, or after industrial injuries are also capable of being consistent. This consistency tends to be denied, however, because it might be produced for the sake of obtaining money. In consequence, it used to be argued that large numbers of individuals would get better as soon as their compensation was stopped. Compensation cases were seen to be, or believed to be, different from those with no claim for compensation. After Miller (25) made the statement that individuals with minor head injury always recovered after settlement, Mendelson (26) reviewed the results of 10 follow-up studies of different forms of pain related to injury and compensation. All ten concurred in finding that a significant number of individuals continued to have symptoms or to be unemployed. Thus, one of the principal motives for pain that had been attributed to individuals must be heavily discounted. Within pain clinics, little difference has been found between patients receiving compensation and those not receiving it (27–30). Where differences have been found [e.g., by Dworkin et al. (31)], they are attributable essentially to unemployability of the group receiving compensation.

PSYCHOLOGICAL CAUSES

It is generally assumed in the literature that psychiatric illness is promoted by stress of one sort or another. Marital difficulties or other interpersonal problems at home, difficulties in relationships at work, bereavement, and the usual categories of psychological stress are probable causes of painful disorders. This is commonplace throughout the psychiatric literature and needs no particular justification. Whenever a recognized psychiatric syndrome is diagnosed with sound evidence from the symptomatology and the state of the individual, it is likely that at least some relevant stresses will be identified. If not, we tend to think of the illness as endogenous or organic and, again, it will conform to appropriate patterns.

With soft tissue syndromes, psychological events clearly aggravate the problem. This is perhaps more evident in a condition such as migraine than with low back pain, but patients who become depressed for other reasons frequently experience exacerbations of their pain from the disorder that they are known to suffer. It is nevertheless surprising how little evidence exists to show, in the absence of a psychiatric diagnosis, that stress is relevant to the etiology of soft tissue syndromes.

Patients in pain clinics have varying amounts of psychiatric illness. Some studies [e.g., Blumer and Heilbronn (32)] found that all the patients have a disorder or condition that the investigator considers to be psychological in origin. Others have found variable proportions, depending on the techniques used to sample the population, the criteria for the illness, the particular sample, and the cutoff points employed on screening tests (33).

In those instances in which psychiatric illness is not evident in patients with pain, stress might be a potential explanation for the pain even without formal psychological evidence. However, no authors have produced evidence that demonstrates that a pain disorder that is not due to a psychiatric illness might be due to environmental stress. Measurements of stress using brief questionnaires are not satisfactory for research purposes, and show poor relationships with psychological illness. More intensive investigations of emotional stress are time consuming and difficult. Marbach et al. (34) completed a careful study of the relationship between stress and facial pain and found no evidence that independent stresses exacerbated or promoted the pain.

Psychological findings in fibromyalgia have been considered elsewhere

(35,36) and will be briefly summarized here. Usually, only some of the patients who have fibromyalgia can be identified as having a recognizable psychological disorder. Even in a well-conducted study by Hudson and colleagues (37) that shows a high rate of psychiatric illness among patients with fibromyalgia, the illness was not always concurrent, and psychological factors were not obligatory causes of the disorder. In general, 30% of patients in most family practices and in hospital departments are likely to have psychological illness (38). This may be because of a primary psychological reason for the illness, selection bias, or psychological effects of physical change. Thus, while psychiatric factors might aggravate some cases of fibromyalgia, they are unlikely to be a cause of the illness. No practicing clinician can ignore the importance of stress in some patients, but it is not an adequate explanation for the common soft tissue pains that do not have proper psychological evidence to account for them.

BEHAVIORAL CONCEPTS

Another approach to muscle pain is to treat it as a subset of the conditions that promote pain behavior. Although the substantial literature dealing with this approach to pain has merit and is very popular, it has significant drawbacks. For example, when the concepts are strictly applied as defined by Fordyce (39), it rejects the patient's experience. Also, the words "pain behavior" or "abnormal illness behavior" are frequently used as a code or euphemism for hysteria. One is often left in doubt as to whether the term "pain behavior" is being applied to hysteria, depression, or any other condition that can be included under the broad term "operant pain." Moreover, the tendency to label a patient who has a motivational or psychological element to his or her pain as displaying "pain behavior" will lead to mistakes in judgment. "Pain behavior" is, first and foremost, linked with organic disease (40). The model for pain behavior is derived directly from physical illness. Difficulties develop only when "pain behavior" is alleged to be disproportionate to the physical state. The application of these ideas to patients with fibromyalgia or myofascial pain syndromes, particularly when the physician does not interpret the situation similarly to the patient's insight based on experience, is potentially disruptive to relations between the health professional and the patient.

The merits of the behavioral approach to pain are, however, twofold. First, it shares with the more traditional psychiatric attitude an interest in looking at environmental circumstances (contingencies, in the language of the psychologist), counseling individuals, and encouraging them to be constructive in a difficult situation. Such approaches are essentially common. The behavioral therapist has had the main role in renewing our recognition that exercise can be highly beneficial to muscle syndromes. Fordyce et al. (41)

demonstrated very clearly that much chronic pain in their populations could be improved by continued activity. This is not, of course, a universal finding with patients in chronic pain. The greatest need that I have in my own practice, one that I suspect is shared by many others, is to learn how to distinguish those patients who would benefit from exercise from the others who would be made worse, even if only temporarily.

SELECTION PHENOMENA

In looking at any group of patients in internal medicine, psychiatry, physical medicine, or any comparable hospital specialty, we see a group of individuals who have been selected to attend either the office of the specialist or the clinic or the inpatient ward of a hospital. The more specialised the center the more highly selected the cases. Even in general practice there is a selection process. The more tranquil, less hypochondriacal, more contented, more energetic people will keep away from the office of their general practitioner, while more hypochondriacal, tenacious people, who are concerned about their bodies, demand answers, and fear any changes they notice, will be present in increased numbers in the office of the family doctor.

In most general practice and hospital populations, 20 to 30% of the patients are said to be there for psychiatric reasons (38). Crook and Tunks (42) have described a number of characteristics of patients with chronic pain who are receiving treatment, compared with patients with chronic pain in the general population. Distinguishing factors in the clinic population included an increased likelihood of being injured, a report of more intense and more constant pain, more difficulties with the activities of daily living, more depression and social withdrawal, and more long-term consequences due to unemployment, litigation, and substance abuse. These clearly comprise a mixture of physical, psychological, and social factors, weighting the clinic patient in the direction of more severity and intensity.

EFFECTS OF PAIN

The effects of muscle pain should be briefly noted. Beside being unpleasant and interfering with the activities of daily living, muscle pain may lead to the need for additional treatment, injections, drug intake, abstention from work, and diffuculty in social and personal relationships, even including difficulty in sexual intercourse. Invisible handicaps are worse than visible handicaps of the same proportion. They attract less sympathy and require more explanation. Patients with chronic pain naturally become irritable (a good biological defensive reaction) and may well become depressed because of the handicaps under which they labor. In fact, a mixture of depression, anxiety, and external irritability is commonplace in chronic pain patients with physical lesions (33). Most patients with chronic pain seem to go through a temporary phase of depression as severe as a major affective disorder in the diagnostic terms of DSM-III. When they encounter social setbacks or increased pain because of increased activity, they may undergo relapse, then regain hope and proceed once more with their attempts at reconstituting their lives normally. However, in explaining the frequency of psychiatric illness in any population with chronic myofascial pain syndromes it should be recognized that not only may the psyche cause pain but pain may disturb the psyche.

CONCLUSIONS

We are left with unresolved issues. Psychiatry does not account for most muscle pain. Important physical considerations are frequently neglected. Without question, motives, emotional stress, and psychological illness will all produce pain syndromes or exacerbate physical conditions. Organic disease causing pain will also produce distress and psychological disorders. The effects of selection must be carefully noted in evaluating all these phenomena.

REFERENCES

1. Walters A. *Brain* 1961:84:1–18.
2. Merskey H, Spear FG. *Pain: Psychological and psychiatric aspects.* London: Bailliere, Tindall & Cassell, 1967.
3. Travell JS, Simons DG. *Myofascial pain and dysfunction: The trigger point manual.* Baltimore: Williams & Wilkins, 1983.
4. International Association for the Study of Pain. *Classification of chronic pain: Descriptions of chronic pain syndromes and definitions of pain terms.* Monograph for the Sub-Committee on Taxonomy, IASP. Pain Supplement 3. Amsterdam: Elsevier Science Publishers, 1986.
5. Smythe HA, Moldofsky H. *Bull Rheum Dis* 1978;28:928–931.
6. Feighner JP, Robins E, Guze SB, Woodruff RA Jr, Winokur G, Munoz R. *Arch Gen Psychiatry* 1972;26:57–63.
7. Spitzer RL, Endicott J, Robins E. *Research diagnostic criteria (RDC) for a selected group of functional disorders,* 2nd ed. New York: New York State Psychiatric Institute, 1975.
8. American Psychiatric Association. *Diagnostic and statistical manual of mental disorders* 3d ed. (DSM-III). Washington DC: American Psychiatric Association, 1980.
9. Watson GD, Chandarana PC, Merskey H. *Br J Psychiatry* 1981;138:33–36.
10. Lewis Sir T, Pickering GW, Rothschild P. *Heart* 1931;5:359–383.
11. Merskey H. *The analysis of hysteria.* London: Bailliere, Tindall, 1979.
12. Pozniak-Patewicz E. *Headache* 1976;15:261–266.
13. Sternbach RA. *Pain: A psychophysiological analysis.* New York: Academic Press, 1968.
14. Wright JP. *J Hist Ideas* 1980;41:233–247.
15. Reynolds R. *Br Med J* 1869;2:483–485; discussion, 378–279.
16. Charcot JM. Lectures on "*The diseases of the nervous system,*" delivered at La Salpetriere, 1885, Vol III (Savill T, trans). London: The New Sydenham Society, 1889.
17. Gould R, Miller BL, Goldberg MA, Benson DF. *J Nerve Ment Dis* 1986;174:593–598.
18. Slater E. *Br Med J* 1965;1:1395–1396.
19. Merskey H. *Br J Psychiatry* 1986;149:23–28.

20. Wall PD. In: Wall PD, Melzack R, eds. *Textbook of pain*. Edinburgh: Churchill Livingstone, 1984;80–87.
21. McMahon SB, Wall PD. *Pain* 1984;19:235–247.
22. Cook AJ, Woolf CJ, Wall PD, et al. *Nature* 1987;325:151–153.
23. Wall PD, Woolf CJ. *J Physiology* 1984;356:443–458.
24. Woolf CJ, Wall PD. *J Neurosci* 1986;6:1433–1442.
25. Miller H. *Br Med J* 1961;1:919–925, 992–998.
26. Mendelson G. *Med J Aust* 1982;2:132–134.
27. Peck CJ, Fordyce WE, Black RG. *Washington Law Rev* 1978;53:251–278.
28. Pelz M, Merskey H. *Pain* 1982;14:293–301.
29. Chapman SL, Brena SF, Bradford LA. *Pain* 1981;11:255–268.
30. Melzack R, Katz J, Jeans MJ. *Pain* 1985;23:101–112.
31. Dworkin RH, Richlin DM, Handlin DS, Brand L. *Pain* 1985;24:343–353.
32. Blumer D, Heilbronn M. *J Nerv Ment Dis* 1982;170:381–406.
33. Merskey H, Lau CL, Russell ES, Brooke RI, James M, Lappano S, Nielsen J, Tilsworth RH. *Pain* 1987;30:141–157.
34. Marbach JJ, Amit Z, Bodner RJ, Dohrenwend BP, Lennon MC. Paper presented at *Joint Meeting of Canadian Pain Society and American Pain Society*, Toronto, Nov 10–13, 1988.
35. McCain GA, Scudds RA. *Pain* 1988;33:273–287.
36. Merskey H. *J Rheumatol* 1989 (in press).
37. Hudson JI, Hudson MS, Pliner LF, Goldenberg DL, Pope HG. *Am J Psychiatry* 1985;142:441–446.
38. Shepherd M, Cooper B, Brown MC, Kalton G. *Psychiatric illness in general practice*. London: Oxford University Press, 1966.
39. Fordyce WE. *Behavioral methods in chronic pain and illness*. St. Louis: CV Mosby Company, 1976.
40. Anderson KO, Keefe FR, Bradley LA, McDaniel LK, Young LD, Turner RA, Agudelo CA, Semble EL, Pisko EJ. *Pain* 1988;3:25–32.
41. Fordyce WE, Fowler R, Lehmann J, De Lateur BJ. *J Chronic Dis* 1968;21:179–190.
42. Crook J, Tunks E. In: Fields HL, Dubner R, Cervero F, eds. *Advances in Pain Research and Therapy*, vol 9. New York: Raven Press, 1985;871–877.

On arising in the morning, they feel unrefreshed and physically exhausted even though their duration of sleep is no different from that of normal subjects. Morning generalized stiffness and aching, longer than 15 min in duration, are more commonly reported in patients (75.2%) than in normal subjects (57.7%) (3a) On those rare occasions that they may sleep deeply, these patients report awakening in the morning feeling rested with little discomfort and fatigue.

Sleep disturbance is associated with pain severity and pain disability. Pilowsky et al. (5) reported on 100 patients who attended a hospital pain clinic. Thirty percent reported fair to good sleep and 70% described poor sleep. Those with poor sleep reported more pain, spent more time reclining, and described more physical disability with respect to body care, home management, ambulation, and recreation. They complained of more emotional distress and had depressive and anxiety symptoms. They reported more hypochondriacal disease conviction and affective disturbances. There were no differences between the groups in matters related to litigation or compensation claims. While the research does show an association of sleep quality to symptoms, the causal connection cannot be defined. Furthermore, the population was not sufficiently characterized other than having chronic pain for which there was no adequate physical cause or adequate response to conventional treatment.

SLEEP-WAKE PHYSIOLOGY AND FIBROMYALGIA

The Alpha Electroencephalographic Sleep Anomaly

Efforts to characterize the physiology of the sleep of fibromyalgia patients led to the discovery of the alpha (7.5 to 11.0 Hz) electroencephalographic (EEG) non–rapid eye movement (NREM) sleep anomaly (6). This sleep anomaly is found more often in fibromyalgia patients than in age- and sex-matched normal controls (4). We interpreted this anomaly as evidence for an arousal disorder within sleep and as a biological indicator of nonrestorative sleep. Normally the alpha rhythm is recorded over the posterior scalp region during quiet wakefulness. This alpha frequency typically disappears with onset of stage 1 sleep. Stimulations to induce behavioral arousals are accompanied by the appearance of the alpha frequency in the sleep EEG. The alpha frequency during sleep differs from the waking alpha by being prominently displayed over central and prefrontal regions of the scalp.

When first described by Hauri and Hawkins (7), the term "alpha-delta sleep" was used to characterize the anomalous mixture of a faster frequency alpha, superimposed on a slower or delta (0.5 to 2.0 Hz) frequency of slow wave (deep) sleep (7). They reported the alpha-delta sleep pattern in a heterogeneous group of nine psychiatric patients who were not well characterized except that they shared symptoms of "a general feeling of chronic somatic malaise and fatigue." However, the alpha frequency is not confined to slow wave or delta sleep, but may occur during stages 1 and 2, NREM sleep, and rarely in REM sleep. Therefore, we prefer to term this EEG sleep pattern the "alpha EEG NREM sleep anomaly" (6). Since our first report, we have observed this sleep anomaly during NREM sleep in more than 100 fibromyalgia patients studied in our laboratory. Unlike normal subjects or patients with chronic insomnia or dysthymia, who show an average of approximately 25% of NREM sleep occupied by alpha EEG sleep, fibromyalgia patients have an average of 60% of NREM sleep occupied by the alpha EEG sleep anomaly (8,9). This EEG sleep disturbance in fibromyalgia patients has been confirmed by other investigators (1,10–14,33). Furthermore, it has been reported in eight of 26 patients with chronic pain (15).

Specificity of Alpha EEG Sleep for Fibromyalgia

Whereas the alpha EEG sleep anomaly may be a sensitive indictor for fibromyalgia syndrome, it does not appear to be a specific indicator for the disorder. In fact, the anomaly has been found in some healthy people who have no special complaints (16,17). Scheuler et al. (18) reported on this anomaly in 36 of 240 subjects who had no current illness. They observed 20 of 39 healthy people in six families who had the alpha sleep pattern. It occurred predominantly in women (21 versus 11 men), as with fibromyalgia syndrome. They speculated that the alpha sleep pattern might be a genetically determined sleep anomaly. If it is an anomalous sleep trait within the population, then this alpha EEG sleep pattern may predispose certain individuals to the fibromyalgia syndrome under special, adverse circumstances. There is some anecdotal evidence in support of this hypothesis. In our study of noise-induced deprivation of REM sleep, one healthy subject was observed to have the alpha EEG sleep anomaly during the three nights of undisturbed baseline sleep. Of the seven subjects who participated in the experiment, he was the only one to have experienced the appearance of widespread musculoskeletal pain and fatigue during the three nights of REM deprivation (21). His symptoms abated during the subsequent two nights of undisturbed sleep.

Aerobic Fitness, Sleep, and Fibromyalgia

The physiological state of aerobic fitness appears to modulate the contribution of the alpha EEG sleep to the pain and fatigue symptoms. In an experiment with six asymptomatic, sedentary subjects, the alpha EEG sleep anomaly was artificially induced by noise disruption of stage 4 sleep over three consecutive nights. During that time, they described diffuse aching, increased tenderness in localized "fibrositic" regions, and chronic fatigue. Their alpha sleep anomaly was no longer present during the next two nights of undisturbed sleep and their daytime symptoms receded. However, when the same experiment was carried out on three long-distance runners, no tender points were demonstrated and no somatic complaints were described, even though the noise had artifically induced the same alpha EEG NREM sleep anomaly (19). The study suggested that cardiorespiratory fitness may prove beneficial for fibromyalgia patients. McCain (20) showed that patients with fibromyalgia who were trained to become aerobically fit had improvement in their pain measures. Further studies are required to determine the contributions of the alpha EEG sleep anomaly to symptoms in various states of fitness where the alpha EEG sleep anomaly is or is not a trait.

Sleep Physiology in Chronic Insomnia Versus Fibromyalgia

To challenge the specificity of a particular sleep anomaly for fibromyalgia syndrome, we hypothesized that those people who complain of chronic sleep difficulties are likely to show the alpha EEG sleep anomaly. That is, patients with persistent or conditioned difficulty in initiating sleep in the absence of any known medical or psychiatric disorder would show sleep physiology and symptoms similar to those with fibromyalgia syndrome. We compared 30 patients with chronic sleep-onset or conditioned insomnia with 30 age- and sex-matched patients with fibromyalgia (21). The data did not support the hypothesis that the chronic insomniacs would show the alpha EEG NREM sleep anomaly and the symptoms of fibromyalgia syndrome. The insomniacs showed less alpha EEG sleep and pain symtoms than the fibromyalgia patients. Insomniacs described fewer somatic complaints but rated as similar moderate fatigue before and after sleep.

The absence of significant observer-rated alpha EEG frequency in the sleep of our insomnia patients is consistent with the observation of Freedman (22), who analyzed EEG frequency power spectra in sleep-onset insomniacs as compared with normal sleepers. He showed that the insomniacs had less alpha EEG activity than normal sleepers while awake, but no difference in frequencies up to 16 Hz throughout all stages of NREM and REM sleep. However, insomniacs showed high cortical arousal, as indicated by more beta EEG activity (18 to 30 Hz) during light sleep (stage 1) following sleep onset and during dreaming or REM sleep. Insomniacs appear to have a different sleep EEG pattern of physiological arousal as compared with fibromyalgia patients, in whom the alpha EEG sleep arousal pattern persists for much of stages 2, 3, and 4 NREM sleep.

Alpha EEG Sleep and Symptoms of Fibromyalgia

If alpha EEG sleep does play a role in the fibromyalgia syndrome, the sleep anomaly should be related to the symptoms of the disorder. The increased localized point tenderness, self-rating of pain, and fatigue on awakening in the morning compared with the evening presleep measures are consistent with the theory that a nonrestorative sleep physiological disturbance may be contributing to these symptoms (6). Furthermore, by pharmacological manipulations of the sleep EEG frequencies with chlorpromazine or L-tryptophan, we have shown that the alpha and delta frequencies are related to pain, energy, and mood. The mean percentage time per minute or mean percentage power per minute of alpha frequency during sleep correlated with an overnight increase in pain measures and hostility and with a decrease in energy. On the other hand, mean percentage time per minute of delta frequency in sleep was related to overnight decrease in pain. Mean percentage delta power per minute was associated with decreased emotional distress and increased energy (23). The data are consitent with the notion that the alpha frequency during sleep is an indicator of the symptoms of unrefreshing sleep, and that the delta frequency (or slow wave, deep sleep) relates to restorative sleep symtpoms. Furthermore, these studies highlight the importance of sleep physiology in the symptoms of fibromyalgia syndrome.

Because various psychological, environmental, and biological influences can affect sleep, theoretically any sleep-related modulating influence that would promote unrefreshing sleep would affect the fibromyalgia syndrome. In fact, research has shown that various psychologically distressing events, environmental disturbances, primary sleep physiology disorders, and painful joint disease contribute to the constellation of a nonrestorative sleep disorder, diffuse pain, fatigue, and emotional stress. Research addressing these various influences on sleep physiology and symptoms of fibromyalgia will be reviewed.

PSYCHOLOGICAL STRESS AND FIBROMYALGIA

Several studies suggest that psychologically distressing situations are followed by diffuse muscular aching, fatigue, and unrefreshing sleep. In the first report of the alpha EEG sleep anomaly in the fibromyalgia syndrome, all patients described major stressful life situations that occurred at the time of onset of their sleep disturbance, musculoskeletal, and mood symptoms. Typically, they had experienced a frightening but minor automobile or industrial accident or they had become helplessly involved in insoluble domestic difficulties (6). A subsequent study of 11 patients who had diffuse pain and fatigue symptoms following an automobile or industrial accident showed the alpha EEG sleep anomaly but less prominently as compared with patients whose fibromyalgia syndrome was not related to any known traumatic event (9). A recent study of 21 postaccident pain patients versus fibromyalgia patients confirmed the original observations of similar pain and fatigue symptoms associated with the alpha EEG sleep anomaly. There were no differences between those who had an industrial versus an automobile accident. Because the matter of litigation is thought to confound symptoms, 15 patients with ongoing litigation were compared with six patients with resolved litigation. There was no evidence for any confounding effect of litigation on the severity of symptoms and the prominence of the alpha EEG sleep anomaly (21).

The speculation that the emotional stress of combat during war often influenced the appearance of diffuse pain and fatigue in United States soldiers during World War II gave rise to the concept of "psychogenic rheumatism" (76). Similar symptoms reported by soldiers in English hospitals, however, were given a different diagnostic label, "fibrositis" (24). The two terms have created some confusion in the literature (25–27). However, more recently a 2-year follow-up study of Israeli soldiers who suffered emotional distress following war experience showed they were likely to complain of chest and back pain in comparison with soldiers with a similar war experience who were free of combat stress (28). Lavie et al. (29) reported the presence of alpha EEG sleep in four of 11 Israeli war veterans who complained of diffuse pain, headaches, emotional distress, and sleep difficulties. These studies suggest that, like automobile or work-related accidents, stressful combat experience without physical injury may contribute to physiological sleep changes and the emergence of fibromyalgia symptoms. Likewise, the sleep disturbances and symptoms following emotionally traumatic civilian situations (e.g., rape) merit study.

ENVIRONMENTAL NOISE AND FIBROMYALGIA

Our experiment on the artificial induction of the alpha EEG anomaly with noise stimuli during stage 4 NREM sleep of sedentary healthy volunteers showed they experienced symptoms similar to those of fibromyalgia patients (6). Epidemiological studies on the adverse effects of noise provide additional confirmation of the role of noxious environmental influences on the sleep and symptoms of fibromyalgia. People living in the vicinity of London's Heathrow Airport who claimed they were sensitive to the noise of aircraft were likely to complain of sleep difficulties, rheumatic pain, undue tiredness, and emotional distress (30). This sensitivity to noise has been reported in fibromyalgia patients (31). Pathological auditory brainstem responses found in 11 of 36 fibromyalgia patients with dysesthesia suggest the possibility of altered central nervous system functioning in response to perceptual stimuli (32). Further study is required of other noxious environmental influences to which fibromyalgia patients claim sensitivity—for example, to adverse weather and allergens.

PRIMARY SLEEP PATHOLOGIES

If persistently disturbed sleep physiology is significant to the symptoms of fibromyalgia, specific primary sleep physiological disorders known to be associated with repetitive EEG arousals during sleep might be expected in some patients with fibromyalgia syndrome. Two such pathologies have been identified. Patients with obstructive sleep apnea were more likely to fulfill criteria for fibromyalgia syndrome than were patients from a general medical clinic (33). Similarly, some patients with sleep-related periodic involuntary leg movements describe typical fibromyalgia symptoms (34,35). However, both of these sleep disorders are commonly associated with complaints of excessive daytime somnolence.

Whereas no study has been carried out to differentiate the EEG sleep physiology in somnolent versus "fibromyalgic" patients with obstructive sleep apnea, such research has been reported in patients with sleep-related periodic involuntary leg movements (nocturnal myoclonus) (34). The patients with sleep-related periodic leg movements and fibromyalgia symptoms were more likely to be women, have more pain, have morning fatigue, show alpha EEG sleep before the leg movements, and have more sleep-stage changes than those who complained of only daytime sleepiness. Furthermore, those with restless legs during sleep and fibromyalgia symptoms were more likely to be older (average age: 50 years) and have a later onset of their symptoms in comparison with those fibromyalgia patients who had the alpha EEG sleep anomaly and no periodic leg movements (35).

RHEUMATIC DISEASE AND FIBROMYALGIA

Rheumatoid Arthritis and Fibromyalgia

In accordance with the theory that noxious influences affect the alpha EEG arousal disturbance, nonrestorative sleep, fatigue, and pain symptoms, we would predict that chronic painful inflammatory articular disease is accompanied by the same sleep anomaly and symptoms seen in fibromyalgia. In fact, the morning symptoms of increased musculoskeletal stiffness, pain, fatigue, and weakness are characteristic features of acute flares of rheumatoid arthritis. The mechanisms for these symptoms are not well understood. In a study of the sleep physiology and morning symptoms of 15 patients with acute classical rheumatoid arthritis, all were found to have an alpha EEG NREM sleep anomaly. An overnight increase in tenderness in the peripheral joints and in fibromyalgic local regions, as well as increased weakness and diminished energy, were also found. One patient who experienced a remission in symptoms showed an improvement in sleep physiology (36). Similar EEG arousal disturbances in sleep were found in a group of chronic rheumatoid arthritis patients attending an outpatient clinic (37). Experimental sleep physiological studies show that rats with adjuvant arthritis have fragmented sleep with episodes of wakefulness and decreased deep sleep throughout the diurnal sleep-wake cycle (38). These findings are in agreement with the proposition relating noxious influences to sleep disturbance and musculoskeletal symptoms. Therefore, acute rheumatoid flares with nocturnal intrusions of articular pain stimuli during sleep might induce an alpha EEG NREM sleep disturbance and the characteristic nonrestorative sleep morning symptoms of articular and nonarticular pain and stiffness, and fatigue (36). Broadly speaking, fibromyalgia symptoms of nonrestorative sleep, diffuse pain, stiffness, and fatigue, which are found to be common in patients with rheumatoid arthritis, are also likely concomitants of other rheumatic diseases (2).

Osteoarthritis and Fibromyalgia

The presence of disordered sleep physiology has been shown to relate to morning pain and stiffness in some patients with osteoarthritis of the fingers (39). Their symptoms could not be related to articular pathology because radiological changes were similar to a matched group of patients who had no morning complaints. The patients who complained of these morning symptoms were likely to have sleep-related periodic involuntary movements and more disordered EEG sleep. Once again, these observations indicate that the sleep disturbance contributes to morning pain symptoms.

Leigh et al. (40) also found evidence for increased stage 1 sleep disturbance in patients with osteoarthritis of the hip or knee in comparison to controls. However, it is important to determine whether the sleep disturbance relates to a primary sleep disorder (e.g., sleep apnea or nocturnal myoclonus) or is secondary to the discomfort of movement of the affected joints during sleep. In the former case, management of the primary sleep disorder would be expected to be associated with improvement in sleep and nonarticular complaints. In fact, such improvement did occur in several patients with diffuse musculoskeletal pain in whom coincident sleep-related periodic movements during sleep were effectively controlled with nitrazepam (41). On the other hand, if the sleep disturbance results from nocturnal discomfort of the arthritic joint, then the sleep disturbance might be used as an indicator of response to surgical or pharmacological treatment (40).

CENTRAL NERVOUS SYSTEM DYSFUNCTION AND FIBROMYALGIA SYNDROME

Inflammation, Chronic Fatigue Syndrome, and Fibromyalgia

In the absence of demonstrable infectious agents or reproducible structural pathology, an inflammation etiology for fibromyalgia syndrome is no longer acceptable (25). However, many patients experience symptoms similar to fibromyalgia following infectious mononucleosis–like or "flulike" febrile illness. Various viral, parasitic, and mycoplasmic agents have been found in some of the patients, but no specific infectious agent has been proven to be etiological for this so-called postinfectious neuromyasthenia, or chronic fatigue syndrome. Recent attention has focused on the possibility that such patients suffer from a chronic Epstein-Barr viral infection that affects the central nervous system to repoduce the persistent symptoms. However, the specificity of this virus is doubtful because no differences have been found in patients versus asymptomatic normal controls (42). Fibromyalgia patients frequently report symptoms similar to those of patients with chronic fatigue syndrome (43). Our studies have shown that, compared with fibromyalgia patients, such postinfectious chronic fatigue patients have similar disordered sleep physiologies, localized tenderness, and complaints of diffuse pain and fatigue (44,45).

Immune Functions and Fibromyalgia

There is the possibility that altered immunological functions precipitated by a viral illness may play a key role in the sleep disorder and somatic and psychological symptoms. The alpha EEG sleep anomaly has been observed in HIV-seropositive patients (46). Some fibromyalgia patients show altered serology with slightly positive antinuclear antibody and depressed levels of immunoglobulin (Ig) A and C3 or C4 complement fractions (47). Analogous unexplained immune changes have also been reported in fibromyalgia patients who have Raynaud's phenomenon (48). Some fibromyalgia patients have also shown unexplained deposits of IgG at the dermal-epidermal junction of their forearm skin (48,49). Furthermore, animal studies have indicated that certain peptides, such as interleukin-1 (IL-1), alpha-2 interferon, tumor necrosis factor, vasoactive intestinal peptide, and prostaglandin D_2, carry immunological and somnogenic properties (50). Human studies have shown dramatic changes during sleep in certain immune functional measures such as IL-1, IL-2, pokeweed mitogen, and natural killer cell response activities (51). The patterns of these immune functions are changed with sleep deprivation (52).

The contribution of the immune system to altered sleep physiology and symptoms of fibromyalgia remains to be unraveled. A recent report (53) describing the acute onset of sleep disturbance, aching muscles, tender points and stiffness following the intravenous administration of IL-2 in combination with lymphocyte-activated killer cells in patients with cancer is consitent with the theory that certain immunologically active substances may be involved in the altered sleep physiology and symptoms of fibromyalgia. Of interest, serum IL-2 levels have been shown to be elevated in chronic fatigue syndrome patients compared to normal subjects (54). Once more, if prostaglandins are shown to be important for sleep physiology in humans, it is understandable that prostaglandin synthetase inhibitors show no effect on the symptoms of fibromyalgia (55). Such substances (indomethacin, diclofenac) suppress slow-wave sleep in rats (56). Research on the role of cytokine immune modulators and their inhibitors on sleep and symptoms may provide major advances in our understanding of the chronic disability that follows or accompanies infectious and various rheumatic and connective tissue diseases (see Chapter 18, *this volume*).

Serotonin Metabolism and Fibromyalgia

Although studies shown an association between disordered sleep physiology and fibromyalgia, the research does not show how specific neurotransmitters that are known to relate to sleep may be related to the alpha EEG sleep and symptoms. There is considerable evidence to suggest that a biogenic amine metabolic transformation, occurring within the central nervous system, mediates both the sleep disorder and the perception of pain, (26). Research studies in animals and humans have shown that serotonin metabolism in the central nervous system plays a role in the regulation of NREM sleep, pain sensitivity, and affective states (57). An inverse relationship between brain serotonergic activity and pain has been demonstrated in several animal studies (58–63). The analgesic effect of narcotics is potentiated by serotonin precursors (64,65) and reduced by serotonin depletors (66). In humans, a pain syndrome comparable to the constellation of symptoms found in fibromyalgia patients was incidentally produced after the administration of p-chlorophenyalanine, an inhibitor of brain serotonin synthesis (67a). The widespread musculoskeletal pain symptoms disappeared when the drug was stopped and recurred when it was administered again.

Based on the assumption, demonstrated in rats, that positive relationships exist for plasma free tryptophan, brain tryptophan, and brain serotonin, we studied plasma free tryptophan levels in patient with fibromyalgia syndrome. The concentration of plasma free tryptophan was inversely related to the subjective morning pain (26). However, 5 g of L-tryptophan at bedtime had no effect on reducing alpha EEG sleep and pain symptoms in patients (23).

Furthermore, a double-blind, placebo-controlled study of L-5hydroxy-tryptophan and carbidopa given at bedtime showed no therapeutic effect. The research was terminated because the drug provoked nausea and vomiting that interrupted the sleep of the fibromyalgia patients (H. Moldofsky, F. A. Lue, unpublished observations). Nevertheless, low doses of tricyclic medications that influence central nervous system serotonin metabolism (amitriptyline) have been found to be beneficial for these patients' sleep and symptoms (67). Amitriptyline (10 to 30 mg) effectively reduced "alpha-delta" sleep from an average of 90.3 min to 63.2 min with coincident improvement in nonrestorative sleep, fatigue, and malaise in five patients (68). Platelet binding of 3H-imipramine was higher for the untreated fibromyalgia patients than for treated controls. With successful response to treatment, there was normalization of the platelet receptor density (69). These recent findings provide support for the notion that aspects of serotonin metabolism play a role in the sleep and symptoms of fibromyalgia syndrome.

Substance P and Fibromyalgia

Substance P has been considered to be a primary afferent transmitter for pain. Of particular interest is the observation of increased levels of substance P in the cerebralospinal fluid of fibromyalgia patients (70). However, substance P is not specific for pain, but is a neuroactive peptide that is widely distributed throughout the nervous system (75). It is associated with behavioral activation so that it may contribute to arousal disturbances (71), and it enhances immune functions (72).

Endorphin Metabolism and Fibromyalgia

Some authors have speculated on the possible influence of the endogenous opiate system β-endorphins, on the pain of fibromyalgia syndrome (20). The literature on endogenous opioid peptides and pain does not suggest a simple relationship (73). No change in β-endorphin or β-enkephalin levels have been found in chronic pain, but a depressed level of dynorphin-like function has been reported (74). To determine how the endogenous opiate system might be affecting sleep and symptoms, we conducted a pilot study on the effect of naloxone, a specific μ-receptor narcotic antagonist, on sleep physiology and symptoms of fibromyalgia. After the administration of 1 mg naloxone intramuscularly at bedtime, wakefulness and stage 1 sleep increased, and stages 2, 3, and 4 NREM sleep decreased. The next morning, pain measures were dramatically increased over measures taken on the previous baseline nights and days. Additional studies are necessary to determine the contribution of not only endorphins but also various peptides that affect the sleep and symptoms of fibromyalgia.

SUMMARY

The symptoms of widespread aching and stiffness, tender points at specific anatomical sites, chronic fatigue, and nonrestorative sleep comprise a syndrome or specific symptomatic outcome that may be precipitated by various psychological envirommental, or physiological distress conditions. That is, the fibromyalgia syndrome has been shown to occur in some people after an emotionally stressful but physically noninjurious automobile or industrial accident, following war or combat stress, and with disruption of EEG NREM slow-wave sleep by noise. In some cases, it occurs following a flulike febrile illness or occurs in association with primary sleep physiological disorders that disrupt the continuity of sleep—that is, obstructive sleep apnea or periodic involuntary movements (nocturnal myoclonus). Finally, nocturnal discomfort from articular disease may disturb sleep and contribute to coincident fibromyalgia symptoms.

These exogenous and endogenous noxious events produce an arousal disturbance in sleep indicated by the alpha EEG NREM sleep anomaly and possibly alter brain metabolism of substances that are associated with sleep-arousal and pain mechanisms, such as serotonin, endorphins, substance P, and peptides that affect the immune system. While the alpha EEG sleep anomaly is not specific for fibromyalgia, this indicator of disordered sleep physiology is a core biological correlate of the nonrestorative sleep, pain, and fatigue symptoms of fibromyalgia. In some cases, the emotional distress of these symptoms or personality features that heighten psychological sensitivity may serve to perpetuate the arousal disturbance in sleep, nonrestorative sleep, and daytime complaints. The theory may provide a useful model for investigating both the linkages in the chain of psychological and biological events that affect the syndrome and methods of therapeutic intervention.

Acknowledgment. This research was supported by the Medical Research Council of Canada, grant no. MA-7733.

REFERENCES

1. Campbell SM, Clark S, Tindall EA, et al. *Arthritis Rheum* 1983;26:817–824,
2. Wolfe F, Hawley DJ, Cathey MA, et al. *J Rheumatol* 1985;12:1159–1163.
3. Yunus MB, Masi AT. *Arthritis Rheum* 1985;28:138–145.
3a.Wolfe F, Smythe HA, Yunus MB, et al. *Arthritis Rheum* (in press).
4. Anch AM, Saskin P, Moldofsky H. *Sleep Res* 1989;17:327.
5. Pilowsky I, Crettenden I, Townley M. *Pain* 1985;23:27–33.
6. Moldofsky H, Scarisbrick P, England R, et al. *Psychosom Med* 1975;37:341–351.
7. Hauri P, Hawkins DR. *Electroencephalogr Clin Neurophysiol* 1973;34:233–237.
8. Gupta M, Moldofsky H. *Can J Psychiatry* 1986;31:608–616.
9. Saskin P, Moldofsky H, Lue FA. *Psychosom Med* 1986;48:319–323.
10. Sims RW, Gunderman, J, Howard F, et al. *Ann Rheum Dis* 1988;47:40–42.
11. Hamm C, Derman S, Russell IJ. *Arthritis Rheum* 1989;32(suppl):S70.

12. Herisson C, Simon L, Touchon J, et al. *Arthritis Rheum* 1989;32(suppl):570.
13. Shackell BS, Horne JA. *Sleep Res* 1987;16:432.
14. Ware JC, Russell J, Campos E. *Sleep Res* 1986;15:210.
15. Wittig RM, Zorick FJ, Blumer D, et al. *J Nerv Ment Dis* 1982;170:429–431.
16. Dumermuth G, Walz W, Lavizzari GS, et al. *Eur Neurol* 1972;7:275–296.
17. Scheuler W, Stinshoff D, Kubicki S. *Neuropsychobiology* 1983;10:183–189.
18. Scheuler W, Kubicki S, Marquardt J, et al. In: Koella WP, Obal F, Schulz H, et al., eds. *Sleep '86.* Stuttgart: Gustav Fischer Verlag, 1988.
19. Moldofsky H, Scarisbrick P. *Psychosom Med* 1976;38:35–44.
20. McCain GA. *Am J Med* 1986;81:73–77.
21. Saskin P, Moldofsky H, Salem L, et al. *Sleep Res* 1987;16:421.
22. Freedman RR. *EEG Clin Neurophysiol* 1986;63:408–413.
23. Moldofsky H, Lue FA. *Electroencephalogr Clin Neurophysiol* 1980;50:71–80.
24. Boland EW. *Ann Rheum Dis* 1947;6:195–203.
25. Bennett RM. *West J Med* 1981;134:405–413.
26. Moldofsky H, Warsh JJ. *Pain* 1978;5:65–71.
27. Rotes-Querol J. *Clin Rheum Dis* 1979;5:797–805.
28. Solomon Z, Mikolincer M, Kotler M. *J Psychosom Res* 1987;31:463–469.
29. Lavie P, Hefez A, Halperin G, et al. *Am J Psychiatry* 1979;136:175–178.
30. Tarnapolsky A, Watkin G, Hand DJ. *Psychol Med* 1980;10:683–698.
31. Gerster KC, Handj-Kjilani A. *J Rheumatol* 1984;11:678–680.
32. Rosenthal U, Johansson G, Orndahl G. *Scand J Rehab Med* 1987;19:147–152.
33. Molony RR, MacPeek DM, Schiffman PL, et al. *J Rheumatol* 1986;13:797–800.
34. Moldofsky H, Tullis C, Lue FA, et al. *Psychosom Med* 1984;46:145–151.
35. Moldofsky H, Tullis C, Lue FA. *J Rheumatol* 1986;13:614–617.
36. Moldofsky H, Lue FA, Smythe HA. *J Rheumatol* 1983;10:373–379.
37. Mahowald MW, Mahowald ML, Bundlie SR, et al. *Sleep Res* 1987;16:487.
38. Landis CA, Robinson Cr, Levine JD. *Pain* 1988;34:93–99.
39. Moldofsky H, Lue FA, Saskin P. *J Rheumatol* 1987;14:124–128.
40. Leigh TJ, Hindmarch I, Bird HA, et al. *Ann Rheum Dis* 1988;47:40–42.
41. Moldofsky H, Tullis C, Quance G, et al. *Can J Neurol Sci* 1986;13:52–54.
42. Buchwald D, Sullivan JL, Komaroff AL. *JAMA* 1987;257:2303–2307.
43. Buchwald D, Goldenberg DL, Sullivan JL, et al. *Arthritis Rheum* 1987;30:1132–1136.
44. Moldofsky H, Saskin P, Salem L, et al. *Sleep Res* 1987;16:492.
45. Whelton CL, Saskin P, Salit I, et al. *Sleep Res* 1988;17:307.
46. Norman SS, Kiel M, Nay KN, et al. *Sleep Res* 1989;17:353.
47. Salit IE. *Can Med Assoc J* 1985;133:659–663.
48. Dinerman H, Goldenberg DL, Felson DT. *J Rheumatol* 1986;13:368–373.
49. Caro XJ, Wolfe F, Johnston WH, et al. *J Rheumatol* 1986;13:1086–1092.
50. Kureger JM, Karnovsky ML. *Ann NY Acad Sci* 1987;496:510–516.
51. Moldofsky H, Lue FA, Eisen J, et al. *Psychosom Med* 1986;48:309–318.
52. Moldofsky H, Lue FA, Davidson R, et al. *FASEB J* 1989;3:1972–1977.
53. Wallace DJ, Margolin K, Waller P. *Ann Internl Med* 1988;108:909.
54. Cheney PR, Damer SE, Bell DS. *Ann Int Med* 1980;110:321.
55. Ferraccioli G, Chirelli L, Scita F, et al. *J Rheumatol* 1987;14:820–825.
56. Naito K, Osama H, Vena R, et al. *Brain Res* 1988;453:329–336.
57. Chase TN, Murphy DI. *Annu Rev Pharmacol Toxicol* 1983;13:181–197.
58. Harvey JA, Lints CE. *Science* 1965;148:250–252.
59. Harvey JA, Schlosberg AJ, Yunger LM. *Fed Proc* 1975;34:796–801.
60. Messing RB, Fisher LA, Phebus L, et al. *Life Sci* 1986;18:707–714.
61. Riley GJ, Shaw M. *Lancet* 1976;2:249.
62. Samanin R, Valzelli L. *Arch Int Pharmacodyn Ther* 1972;196:138–141.
63. Tenen SS. *Psychopharmacology (Berlin)* 1967;10:204–219.
64. Dewey WL, Harris LS, Howes JF, et al. *Pharmacol Exp Ther* 1970;175:435–442.
65. Major CT, Pleuvry BJ. *Br J Pharmacol* 1971;42:512–521.
66. Tenen SS. *Psychopharmacology (Berlin)* 1968;12:278–285.
67. Carette S, McCain GA, Bell DA. *Arthritis Rheum* 1986;29:655–659.
67a.Sicuteri F. *Headache* 1972;12:69–72.

68. Watson R, Liebmann KO, Jenson J. *Sleep Res* 1985;14:226.
69. Russell IJ, Bowden CL, Michalek J, et al. *Arthritis Rheum* 1987;30:S63.
70. Vaeroy H, Helle R, Forre O, et al. *Pain* 1988;32:21–26.
71. Cooper JR, Bloom FE, Roth RH. *The Biochemical Basis of Neuropharmacology.* New York: Oxford University Press, 1986;362–366.
72. Payan DG, Levine JD, Goetzl EJ. *J Immunol* 1984;132:1601–1604.
73. Woolf CJ, Wall PD. *Nature* 1983;306:739–740.
74. Clement-Jones V, Besser GM. *Br Med Bull* 1983;39:95.
75. Mayer DJ, Frenk H. In: Nemeroff CB, ed. *Neuropeptides and neurological disorders.* Baltimore: Johns Hopkins University Press, 1988;199–280.
76. Moldofsky H. In Hill OW, ed. *Modern trends in psychosomatic medicine.* London: Butterworth's, 1976;187–195.

Advances in Pain Research and Therapy, Vol. 17,
edited by James R. Fricton and Essam Awad.
Raven Press, Ltd., New York © 1990.

14

Segmental Hyperesthesia and Tenderness of the Back in Pain Conditions

Johannes Fossgreen

Department of Rheumatology, Physical Medicine and Rehabilitation, Aarhus Amtssygehus, University Hospital, DK 8000 Aarhus C, Denmark

Clinical observations indicate that visceral diseases are frequently accompanied by referred pain to definite areas of the body surface. The cutaneous areas are often termed "Head zones" in reference to the basic investigations by Henry Head in 1893 (1). Since these early investigations of referred pain, hyperaesthesia (skin sensitivity) and muscle tenderness have also been found to be related to diseases of visceral and somatic structures. The purpose of this chapter is to present some of these findings as they are related to the back.

VISCERAL DISEASES, REFERRED PAIN, AND SEGMENTAL ALTERATIONS

The clinician is familiar with the occurrence of referred pain in connection with internal organ disease, such as pain in the right shoulder region associated with gallstone attacks, pain in the left shoulder and arm in ischemic heart disease, and pain in the lower back with diseases of the internal female genital organs, and with many more visceral diseases (2–4). However, nociceptive and other afferent input from the viscera may not only cause referred pain but also give rise to alterations in the dermatomes, myotomes, and probably sclerotomes that are segmentally linked to the organ in question.

In the dermatomes, hyperesthetic areas may appear and vasomotoric, pilomotoric, and sudomotoric changes can also be observed (3–5). In the myotomes, muscle tenderness and hypertonicity of certain muscles may occur, and in the sclerotomes tenderness of the periosteum can occur (4,6–9). Regarding the spine, segmental restricted mobility corresponding to the segments related to the diseased internal organ may occur, probably as a result of contraction of the deep muscles of the spine resulting in movement restriction of two or more adjacent segments (2,4,10).

SEGMENTAL PAIN SYNDROMES OF THE SPINE

Referred pain, segmental hyperesthesia, and tenderness can also be caused by nociception from spinal ligaments (11), muscles (7,12), intervertebral joints (13–15), and pericapsular tissue of the intervertebral joints (13).

In human experiments, 6% hypertonic saline solution, which is a pain-provoking irritant, was injected (0.1 to 1.0 ml) into spinal muscles and ligaments (5,7,11,16). The injections provoked two types of pain. The first appeared within a few seconds, had a quality described as sharp and stinging, and disappeared after a few minutes. The second was a referred pain with roughly segmental distribution. The referred pain arose about 30 sec after the injection and lasted for several minutes and even hours. With a delay of about 5 min, hyperesthesia and hyperalgesia occurred in the distant areas. When injecting hypertonic saline into lumbar facet joints, a similar reaction has been observed (14,15). Reddening of the skin and muscle spasm could also be observed. McCall et al. (13) investigated the referred pain pattern after intrarticular and pericapsular injection of hypertonic saline solution. In both locations, an aching, cramplike deep pain sensation was reported, but the peak intensity of pain was higher following the pericapsular injections.

Some clinical observations suggest that pain syndromes similar to pain arising from visceral organs may also originate from structures in the spine. Glover (17) described the "hyperesthesia syndrome," which he found extremely common in back pain cases. Whatever the ultimate diagnosis, the syndrome may occur at any spinal level from the occiput to the coccyx. The syndrome comprises one symptom and three signs: (a) clearly defined area of hyperesthesia adjacent to the spine, (b) a localized paravertebral tender spot associated with the area of hyperesthesia, (c) a dull ache in the same area (the only symptom), and (d) limitation of movement of the trunk by pain.

Chest pain is often considered a sign of disease in the internal organs of the chest as well as the abdomen and is a frequent cause of admission to cardiac units. However, there are several references that suggest chest pain could emanate from the thoracic spine as well as the chest wall (16,18–31). This condition is called "thoracic segmental pain syndrome" or "thoracic facet joint syndrome," assuming that the facet joints most likely may be involved (32).

The onset of this syndrome is often acute and related to small, uncontrolled movements of the spine. The pain may be severe and described as a stab in the back. The pain is localized to the affected segment and in typical cases, pain radiation occurs. Painfully restricted movements of the spine in one or more directions can be observed. Movements in other directions are pain free or pain relieving. This is an important diagnostic sign.

Often there is pain aggravation on deep breathing. In the paravertebral muscles corresponding to the involved segments, tightness and tenderness can be found. Furthermore, areas of hyper- or dysesthesia can be demonstrated. Chronic cases of the thoracic facet joint syndrome may be very difficult with regard to differential diagnosis and therapy. All paraclinical tests are normal and the diagnosis must be based on a thorough clinical examination and exclusion of other diseases.

The frequency of the thoracic facet joint syndrome has been sparsely investigated. Ollie (27) found segmental pain distribution in 127 patients among 600 patients with chest pain. In a Danish study (32) of patients admitted to a cardiac unit during a 2-year period, 1,097 patients presented with chest pain. The patients were examined with regard to segmental tenderness of the spine and paravertebral muscles and hyper- or dysesthetic areas. A thoracic segmental pain syndrome was found in 143 patients (13%) and was the third most frequent diagnosis. The syndrome occurred most frequently in the age groups spanning 41 to 80 years, with a peak at 41 to 50 years.

In another study from general practice (33), among 162 patients with chest pain, 37% had pain originating from musculoskeletal structures. A thoracic facet joint syndrome was diagnosed in 23% of the patients.

In conclusion, the thoracic facet joint syndrome, or rather the thoracic segmental pain syndrome, is a relatively frequent cause of chest pain. The basic pathology of this pain syndrome is not clarified, but spinal structures, especially the facet joints, seem to play a role in the pathogenesis.

CHRONIC NONORGANIC UPPER ABDOMINAL PAIN SYNDROME

Upper abdominal pain is a common complaint in the population, and 15 to 20% of European men and women have episodic upper dyspepsia. Among those patients seen in outpatient clinics of a hospital, considerable numbers are discharged without the diagnosis of a well-defined disease (34). The patients who have no demonstrable lesions to explain the abdominal pain are often suspected of being on illicit drugs or being neurotic, and their pain is considered to be "not real."

Patients with chronic nonorganic upper abdominal pain were investigated with regard to their pain threshold and autonomic responses to psychological stressors (34–37), and the presence of symptoms and signs of back pathology were compared blindly with healthy controls (38). The group of patients from the latter study consisted of 16 males and 23 females with a mean age 34 and 35 years, respectively, and a mean duration of symptoms of 11 years for males and 9 years for females. The healthy volunteers were comprised of 10 males and 14 females. The patients and controls completed a questionnaire and were clinically examined randomly with the examiner blind to their status. Standardized clinical examination included tests for segmental skin sensitivity, tenderness of subcutaneous and deep structures, and palpatory segmental movement examination.

The results from the questionnaire showed that 72% of the patients complained of back pain compared with 17% of the controls ($p < .001$). Examination revealed that segmental changes comprising all above-mentioned parameters occurred in 62% of the patients and 21% of the controls ($p < .005$). Disturbed skin sensitivity, mostly hyperesthesia, was found in 31% of the patients and none of the controls ($p < .001$). The segmental pathological findings were mainly localized to the region between the tenth thoracic and first lumbar segments.

In conclusion, a group of patients with chronic nonorganic upper abdominal pain had complaints of back pain more often than healthy controls. Random blinded clinical examinations demonstrated more segmental changes in sensory function (mainly hyperesthesia), more muscle tenderness, and, to some extent, greater restricted movement of spinal segments in patients than controls. The segmental changes were mainly localized to the lower thoracic area. It appears that the sympathetic innervation of the viscera at segments T-10 to L-1 supplies a diverse number of abdominal organs.

The mechanism underlying these symptoms and signs in chronic nonorganic upper abdominal pain is not known. It is hypothesized that the back pain and segmental changes may be referred pain from hitherto unrevealed visceral pathology. The segmental distribution is consistent with the sympathetic innervation of the viscera (2,4). Furthermore, a dysfunction of the spine involving both visceral and somatic components, possibly in the intervertebral foramina causing nerve root irritation, may also be considered. This would imply somatovisceral mechanisms (39–41). Finally, it is possible that the syndrome is brought about by a dysfunction of the sympathetic nervous system itself. Long-lasting sympathetic tone may cause contraction in segmental muscles (8). It has been shown that muscle spindles are influenced by stimulation of the sympathetic system (42,43).

SOME NEUROPHYSIOLOGICAL MECHANISMS

Pain from viscera is diffuse, dull, and aching. It is often accompanied by referred pain to cutaneous and other somatic structures with the same spinal segments that receive input from the internal organs (3,44–46). Pain from deep somatic structures such as muscles, ligaments, joints, and periosteum is essentially similar to visceral pain, with referred pain occurring to distant areas within the same segment (6,39).

Regardless of the primary site of pain, changes such as muscle tenderness and hypertonicity may occur in segmental muscles (47), especially in long-lasting sympathetic hyperactivity (6,8). For example, it has been shown that patients with more than one attack of renal or urethral calculosis had lowered pain thresholds on selective electrical stimulation of the muscles, subcutaneous tissue, and skin at the first lumbar segment on the side of the calculosis (9).

Cervero (47) stated that visceral pain from the upper abdominal viscera is mediated by the activation of few visceral fibers. The spinal cord projections of these fibers converge onto neurons described as viscerosomatic neurons, which are also activated by inputs from the skin and from somatic structures such as muscles, tendons, and ligaments (6,48). These observations support the "convergence-projection theory" of Ruch (49), which explains some of the characteristics of referred visceral sensation.

Some of the viscerosomatic neurons project their axons to supraspinal levels via the spinoreticular and spinothalamic tracts. On the other side, the sensory neurons are subjected to supraspinal control of descending signals that comprise both tonic inhibition and phasic excitation. Thus, nociceptive input to the spinal cord generates extensive divergence in the central nervous system (6,50). The sympathetic nervous system has a widespread distribution throughout the body, innervating not only the visceral organs but also peripheral blood vessels, sweat glands, and hair follicles. Even the muscle spindles are subjected to sympathetic influence (42,43). Branching of sensory axons in the dorsal nerve roots and peripheral nerves has been found (46), but whether the branching can explain certain types of referred pain is a matter for discussion.

CONCLUSION

In conclusion, it appears from clinical and a number of experimental observations that referred pain with segmental hyperesthesia and muscle tenderness of the back may be brought about from three different sources: first, by diseases in the visceral organs; second, by diseases and dysfunctions of structures of the spine; and third, by a chronic abdominal pain syndrome without any demonstrated pathology in the visceral organ.

REFERENCES

1. Head H. *Brain* 1893;16:1–133; 1894;17:339–480.
2. Beal MC. *J Am Osteopath Assoc* 1983;82:822–832.
3. Brodal A. *Neurological anatomy in relation to clinical medicine*, 3rd ed. New York: Oxford University Press, 1981;773–776.

4. Hansen K, Schliack H. *Segmentale Innervation. Ihre Bedeutung für Klinik und Praxis.* Stuttgart: Georg Thieme, 1962.
5. Lewis T, Kellgren JH. *Clin Sci* 1939;1:47–71.
6. Cervero, F. In: Schmidt RF, Schaible HG, Vahle-Hinz C, eds. *Fine afferent nerve fibres in pain.* Weinheim: VCH Verlagsgesellschaft, 1987;321–331.
7. Feinstein B. In: Buerger AA, Tobis JS, eds. *Approaches to the validation of manipulative therapy.* Springfield, IL: Charles C Thomas, 1977;134–174.
8. Korr IM, ed. *The neurobiologic mechanisms in manipulative therapy.* New York: Plenum Press, 1978;229–268.
9. Vecchiet L, Giamberardino MA, Dragani L, Albe-Fessard D. *Pain* 1989;36:289–295.
10. Beal MC. *J Am Osteopath Assoc* 1985;85:786–801.
11. Hockaday JM, Whitty CW. *Brain* 1987;90:481–496.
12. Kellgren JH. *Clin Sci* 1985;3:175–190.
13. McCall IW, Park WM, O'Brien JP. *Spine* 1979;4:441–446.
14. Mooney V, Robertson J. *Clin Orthop* 1976;15:149–156.
15. Park WM. *Clin Rheum Dis* 1980;6:118–120.
16. Gunther L, Kerr WJ. *Arch Intern Med* 1929;43:212–248.
17. Glover JR. In: Buerger AA, Tobis JS, eds. *Approaches to the validation of manipulative therapy.* Springfield, IL: Charles C Thomas, 1977;175–186.
18. Bonica JJ. *The management of pain.* London: Kimpton, 1953;1168.
19. Cyriax J. *Textbook of orthopaedic medicine.* vol I, 4th ed. London: Cassell, 1962;331.
20. Davis D. *Radicular syndromes simulation coronary disease.* Chicago: Year Book, Medical Publ, 1957.
21. Epstein SE, Gerber LH, Borer JS. *JAMA* 1979;241:2793–2797.
22. Grieve GP. In: Grieve GP, ed. *Modern manual therapy of the vertebral column.* Edinburgh: Churchill Livingstone, 1986;377–404.
23. Hohmann D. *Die degnerativen Veränderungen der costotransversal Gelenke.* Stuttgart: Enke, 1968.
24. Judovitch B, Bates W. *Pain syndromes.* Philadelphia: FA Davis, 1950;130.
25. Lewit K. *Manuelle Medizine in der medizinischen Rehabilitation,* 2 Aufl. Müchen: Urban & Schwarzenberg, 1977;455.
26. Menell J. *The science and art of joint manipulation.* London: Churchill, 1952;145,151.
27. Ollie JA. *Can Med Ass J* 1957;37:209.
28. Raney FL JR. *J Bone Joint Surg [AM]* 1966;48:1451–1452.
29. Sampson JJ, Cheitlin MD. *Cardiovasc Dis* 1971;8:507–531.
30. Stoddard A. *Manual of osteopathic practice.* London: Hutchinson, 1969;199.
31. Travell J, Simons DG. *Myofascial pain and dysfunction: The trigger point manual.* Baltimore: Williams & Wilkins, 1983;46.
32. Bechgaard P, Fossgreen J. *Münich Med Wochenschr* 1980;122:759–760.
33. Schmidt H, Hansen JG, Bitsch N, Steinmetz E. *Vgeskr Loeger* 1984;146:2008–2011.
34. Jörgensen LS, Bönlökke L, Wamberg P. *Scand J Gastroenterol* 1985;20:4–50.
35. Jörgensen LS, Bönlökke L, Christensen NJ. *Scand J Gastroenterol* 1986;21:605–613.
36. Sloth H, Jörgensen LS. *Scand J Gastroenterol* 1988;32:1275–1280.
37. Sloth H, Jörgensen LS. *Scand J Gastroenterol* 1989 (in press).
38. Jörgensen LS, Fossgreen J. 1989 (in press).
39. Appenzeller O. In: Korr IM, ed. *The neurobiologic mechanisms in manipulative therapy.* New York: Plenum Press, 1978;179–217.
40. Maigne R. *Arch Phys Med Rehabil* 1980;61:389–395.
41. Risling M, Hildebrand C, Dalsgaard CJ. In: Schmidt RF, Schaible HG, Vahle-Hinz C, eds. *Fine afferent nerve fibres and pain.* Weinheim: VCH Verlagsgesellschaft, 1987;33–44.
42. Hunt CC. *J Physiol (Lond)* 1960;151:332–341.
43. Kieschke J, Mense S, Prabhakar NR. *Progr Brain Res* 1988;74:91–97.
44. Appenzeller O. *The autonomic nervous system,* 3rd ed. Amsterdam: Elsevier Biomedical Press, 1982;314–317.
45. Perl ER. In: Darian-Smith I, ed. *Handbook of physiology, Section 1: The nervous system,* vol III, part 2. Bethesda, MD: American Physiological Society, 1984;915–975.
46. Willis WD. *The pain system.* Basel: S Karger, 1985;63–65.
47. Tattersall JEH, Cervero F. *Progr Brain Res* 1986;67:189–205.

48. Tattersall JEH, Cervero F. In: Schmidt RF, Schaible HG, Vahle-Hinz C, eds. *Fine afferent nerve fibres and brain*. Weinheim: VCH Verlagsgesellschaft, 1987;313–320.
49. Ruch TC. In: Fulton JF, ed. *Howell's textbook of physiology*, Philadelphia: WB Saunders, 1946;385–401.
50. Lumb BM. *Progr Brain Res* 1986;67:279–293.

Advances in Pain Research and Therapy, Vol. 17,
edited by James R. Fricton and Essam Awad.
Raven Press, Ltd., New York © 1990.

15

Histopathological Changes in Fibrositis

Essam A. Awad

*Department of Physical Medicine & Rehabilitation, University of Minnesota
Health Sciences Center, Minneapolis, Minnesota 55455*

My interest in fibrositis, which now includes two disorders, fibromyalgia and myofacial pain, goes back to 32 years ago when I started out as a general practitioner. At that time, I used to inject the so-called fibrositic nodules in the cervical scapular area muscles with a French medication called thiod-acaine. This came in large 20-ml ampules and was a combination of procaine, sulfur, and iodine. The latter two components were thought to be fibrinolytic. Today, after 32 years, I find myself often treating my fibrositis patients with almost the same solution, by procaine or other local anesthetic injections. These often alleviate the symptoms for a few days to a few weeks, just as thiodacaine used to do. In addition I now use some new medications such as amitriptyline, exercise programs, and physical therapy measures such as heat, massage, and ultrasound to manage their symptoms. My frustration as to the understanding of the underlying mechanisms and pathological changes involved in Fibromyalgia and myofascial pain syndromes continues.

In this chapter, an attempt is made to review the literature in the area of pathological features of fibrositis, as it was historically studied. I will also attempt to answer the question as to why there is a fibrositic nodule, and why it is tender. I have selected what I believe is the most pertinent literature covering muscle biopsy studies. At first glance, these reports often seem confusing and inconclusive. However, with more careful analysis they point to several similar findings.

REVIEW OF BIOPSY STUDIES

Perhaps one of the earliest studies was that by Stockman (1) who reported hyperplasia of the connective tissue and the presence of serofibrinous exudate in fibrositic muscles. He attributed this condition to small colonies of microbes and made the assumption that these microbes were destroyed by the tissue. One year later Schade (2) found only normal muscle biopsy specimens from fibrositic tissues.

Collins (3) criticized Stockman's work and said that he could not reach any conclusions as to the cause of the fibrositic nodule. He pointed out, however, that Stockman's most significant finding was a negative one: the absence of leukocytic infiltrations and sterility of the culture prepared from the fibrositic tissues. Glogowski and Wallroff (4) noted increased interstitial substance, variation in size of the muscle fibers, increase in the number of nuclei, and interstitial swelling. They reported the same observations made by Stockman (1) as to the swelling and increased interstitial substance in the fibrositic muscle.

Brendstrup et al. (5) studied biopsies from 12 patients. Muscle samples were taken from symmetrical areas of the paraspinal muscles, where one side demonstrated fibrositic nodules and the other side was normal and served as a control. Palpation was done before the operation (discectomy for herniated nucleus pulposus) with the patient under general anesthesia and the muscles being relaxed by an injection of curare. Thus, the identification of the fibrositic nodule was on the basis of change in consistency and not muscle contraction. In nine of the 12 fibrositic specimens a metachromatic substance was found in the interfibrillar connective tissue indicative of acid mucoplysaccharides; in addition, edema and relative increases in the number of nuclei, mast cells, and lymphocytes were noted. Only two specimens were absolutely normal. Chemical analysis showed an average increase of 8% in the fluid content of the fibrositic muscles and evidence of increase in the volume of the extracellular space. All biopsies from the unaffected side were normal.

Miehlke et al. (6) studies 77 muscle biopsies and described nonspecific dystrophic changes, disruption of the cross-striations, increase in the mast cells, nuclei, and acid mucopolysaccharides, distortion of the mitochondria, and proliferation of the connective tissue. Histochemistry showed a deficit of aldolase compared with lactic acid in 59 biopsies. The findings were interpreted as due to hypoxia.

Christensen and Moesmann (7) described fibrinous exudation and degeneration of some muscle fibers in the fibrositic muscles. The degenerative muscle fibers were replaced by connective tissue or newly formed muscle fibers.

Personal Research

Awad (8) studied muscle biopsies from ten patients 23 to 57 years of age. The duration, severity, and extent of the disorders were reported elsewhere (8). Five patients complained of pain in the neck muscles and the other five had pain in the thigh and leg muscles, resulting in the so-called buckling

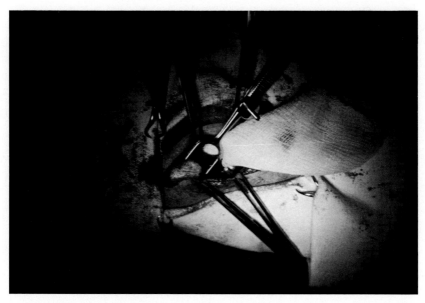

FIG. 1. Muscle biopsy clamped *in situ* before cutting. Gauze is placed under biopsy to demonstrate how it was freed.

knee syndrome (9). In all cases the diagnosis of fibrositis was made by the referring physician. Each patient underwent routine history and physical examinations. A very important step in the examination was deep palpation of the area involved after oiling the skin. Mineral oil was used generously to eliminate the friction between the examiner's fingers and the patient's skin. Certain areas of muscle are usually swollen and extremely tender in the acute stage, and firmer and tougher in cases of long duration. While these changes are clearly defined, they are not obvious without careful search.

Great care was taken to mark the nodule to be biopsied on the skin with an indelible pen. Under sterile conditions a local anesthetic was infiltrated under the skin, followed by incision of the skin and subcutaneous tissues. The muscle fascia was exposed. In the case of the trapezius muscle, this was ill defined. In case of the vastus lateralis in the thigh, incision of the fascia lata, which is membranous, was immediately followed by outward protrusion of some muscle fascicles. This herniation of muscle through the incision was seen in three cases and was an indication of swelling or increased volume of the muscle.

Muscle fasicles approximately 1 cm wide and 2 cm long were freed lengthwise by blunt dissection using the tip of a curved hemostat and clamped *in situ* before cutting the biopsy specimen (Fig. 1). The muscle clamp was a

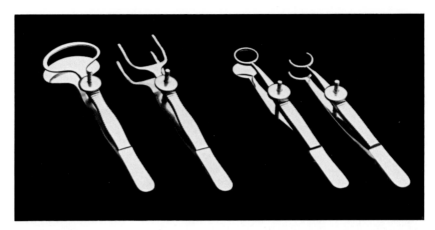

FIG. 2. Awad's biopsy clamps, two sizes, made from chalazion clamps.

modified chalazion clamp in which the plate side was filed and the circular side was opened to form two opposing jaws (Fig. 2). I had originally developed this clamp for the purpose of prevention of contraction artifact, which distorts the muscle architecture and makes it extemely difficult to read the tissue under the microscope. The specimen was fixed in gluteraldehyde while in the clamp (Fig. 3). Another advantage of this clamping

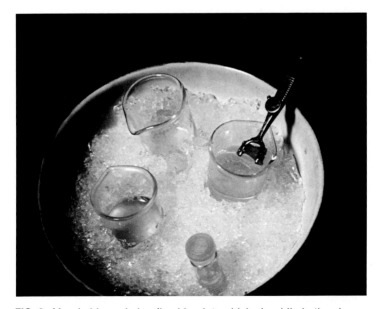

FIG. 3. Muscle biopsy being fixed in gluteraldehyde while in the clamp.

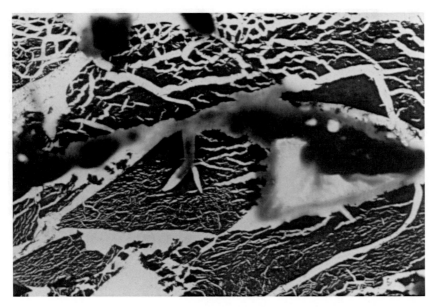

FIG. 4. Cross-section of muscle biopsy from fibrositic nodule showing large accumulations of mucoid amorphous substance between the muscle fascicles. (Toluidine blue, ×86.)

process is that it has resulted in trapping of the fluid content of the muscle within the biopsy sample. This is primarily the ground substance of the connective tissue of the muscle.

On microscopic examination the muscle fibers appeared mostly normal and were medium or large in size. In four cases, a few small fibers were seen, indicating some degree of atrophy. Some occasional degenerating fibers were noted in three cases. In all cases the number of interstitial nuclei seemed to be increased, with a tendency toward pyknosis.

In eight cases, areas of amorphous substance in between the muscle fasicles were noted. After cutting more sections deeper into the tissue blocks, it was realized that the mass of this amorphous substance was larger and spread between the muscle fasicles. This substance was identified as acid mucopolysaccharides because it stained metachromatically with toluidine blue. In some cross-sections this substance was present in multiple clumps within the muscle (Figs. 4 and 5). Some of these masses are equal to or larger in size than the neighboring muscle fasicles. This amorphous substance consitututes a space-occupying lesion, and indeed is a major component of the localized swelling of muscle, or the so-called fibrositic nodule. It is known that acid mucopolysaccharides, now called proteoglycans, have a proteincore and negatively charged repeating units of glucosaminoglycans, which are viscous and have enormous water-binding properties. Under nor-

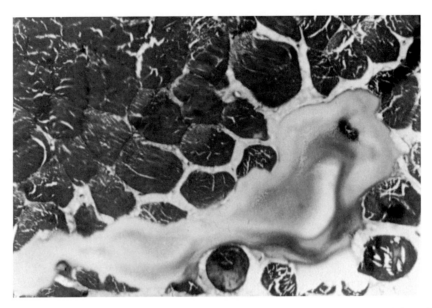

FIG. 5. Cross-section of muscle biopsy from a fibrositic nodule showing accumulation of mucoid amorphous substance between the muscle fibers. (Hematoxylin and eosin, ×400.)

mal conditions the acid mucopolysaccharides are present in small amounts in the muscle extracellular matrix. They merge and interdigitate with the perimysium and tendon components of the muscle. They store bioactive molecules important in function and in the reparative process.

The ultrastructure of most of the muscle fibers appeared normal. Some muscle fibers showed interfibrillar lipid droplets or subsarcolemmal lysosomes. The spaces between some muscle fibers were distended because of the presence of amorphous material, which appeared similar to the basement membrane substance (Fig. 6). This was believed to be mucopolysaccharides of the same nature as the metachromatic substance seen under the light microscope. Several mast cells were observed (Fig. 7). These were variable in shape, contained a large asymmetrical nucleus, and were identified by their characteristic cytoplasmic large, round, membrane-limited, electron-dense granules. The mast cells were noted to be discharging some granules into the intercellular space. These granules are known to contain acid mucopolysaccharides (histamine). In three cases, extravasation of blood was noted between the muscle fibers. Blood platelets were seen in large clusters in what appeared to be a platelet clot. Platelets were recognized by the lack of nuclei, finely granular cytoplasm, large electron-dense granules similar to those of a megakaryocyte, mitochondria, and a smooth endoplasmic reticulum.

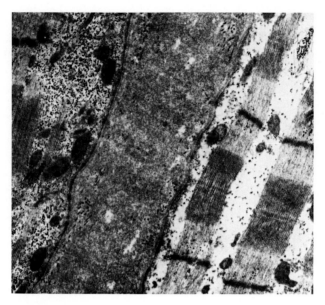

FIG. 6. Electron micrograph showing amorphous substance between portions of two muscle fibers. (×30,000.)

Other Recent Reports

Fassbender and Wegner (10), in biopsy studies, were unable to demonstrate inflammation by light microscopy. However, using electron microscopy they found destruction of myofilaments in the I band region, up to complete lysis of the contractile elements. They reported changes in the endothelial cells of muscle capillaries, which they stated were probably due to relative hypoxia of the muscle fibers. They also reported juvenescence of the connective tissue cells to mesenchymal transformation, with accelerated proliferation and ground substance formation. They clearly stated that the muscular and connective tissue components of soft tissue rheumatism are based on local disturbances of oxygen supply.

Henriksson et al. (11, see also Chapter 16 *this volume*) reported on biopsies from 15 patients with fibromyalgia. Nine had moth-eaten fibers due to focal loss of NADH diaphorase activity in type I fibers. There was variation in size of the muscle fibers and some ragged red fibers. They described abnormal mitochondria and Z line streaming in all five cases studied by electron microscopy.

Kalyan-Raman et al. (12) studied 12 patients with fibromyalgia. The upper trapezius muscle was biopsied. Mild nonspecific changes were seen in nine cases by light microscopy. Five patients showed moth-eaten type I fibers

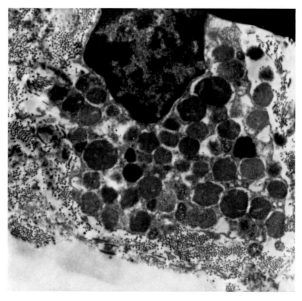

FIG. 7. Electron micrograph showing a portion of a mast cell from the connective tissue of a fibrositic nodule. (×30,000.)

and several showed type II fiber atrophy. Electron microscopy showed extensive segmental necrosis of the myofibrils with glycogen deposition. Ten showed abnormal mitochondria and dilation of the sarcoplasmic reticulum. Papillary projections of the sarcolemma were noted.

Bengtsson et al. (13; see also Chapter 16, *this volume*) studied 55 patients with primary fibromyalgia; 41 of 77 biopsies were taken from the upper trapezius muscle, and 31 from tender points. Findings reported included ragged red fibers and moth-eaten fibers, both of which can be induced by experimental hypoxia. Electron microscopic examination showed swollen capillary organelles and abnormal mitochondria.

DISCUSSION

A critical look at these 12 biopsy studies in fibrositis or fibromyalgia shows the following:

The most common findings was the presence of increased amounts of mucopolysaccharides in between the muscle fascicles (seven reports).

The next most common findings were increased amounts of connective tissue (five reports), and destruction of some myofilaments and abnormal mitochondria (four reports).

Less frequently reported were the presence of swelling, increased nuclei, increased mast cells, and moth-eaten fibers (three reports).

Least frequently noted were changes in the endothelium of the capillaries (two reports) and increased glycogen deposition (one report).

The increased amount of acid mucopolysaccharides in the fibrositic nodules essentially constitutes—in addition to its chemical nature—a space-occupying lesion that produces a mass effect. I believe that this is the reason for feeling the fibrositic nodule and/or the swelling of the muscle on palpation. This mass effect results in stretching of the surrounding muscle fibers, leading to their hyperirritability, and perhaps contributes to the phenomenon described by Dexter and Simons (14) as the "local twitch response." Accumulation of mucopolysaccharides does compromise energy supply and impairs the oxygen flow to the muscle fibers, making performance of work difficult. It is possible that the low pH value or acidity sensitizes the sensory nociceptive nerve endings, causing them to fire spontaneously and to respond to subliminal stimuli, leading to the sensation of pain. It is accepted that connective tissue has a combined structure of protein-polysaccharide, collagen fibers, and water. Its physical and chemical properties are a function of the relative amounts of each component present, including the hydrogen ion concentration, electrolytes, temperature, osmotic pressure, barometric pressure, mechanical stimulation, and immobility (1).

Several questions arise as to whether a change in the acid mucopolysaccharide synthesis occurs in fibrositis. Is there an increase in the production, a decrease in the degradation, or a change in the quality of the ground substance of the connective tissue of the muscle? Is there a gel-sol transformation that interferes with muscles gliding smoothly over neighboring structures? Does the change in acid mucopolysaccharides result in an increased coefficient of friction? Do the acid mucopolysaccharides tend to gel with inactivity and cold or become more soluble during movement, exercise, or with increase in tissue temperature?

Qualitative changes in the connective tissue of muscle could not be relied upon since the distribution of the connective tissue components in any muscle is variable. Whether a biopsy was taken from an area near or far from a tendon or tendinous intersection will have an effect on the amount of connective tissue observed in it. Occasional muscle atrophy or disruption of some myofilaments is nonspecific and may reflect disuse atrophy rather than fibrositis. Abnormal mitochondria must be very carefully interpreted since these fine structures are likely to undergo changes in the immediate postbiopsy period. If the core of the biopsy specimen is not instantaneously exposed to the fixative solution mitochondrial changes do occur.

Further efforts in research should be directed toward the connective tissue elements of the muscle, including its ground substance, if we are to answer the questions raised above.

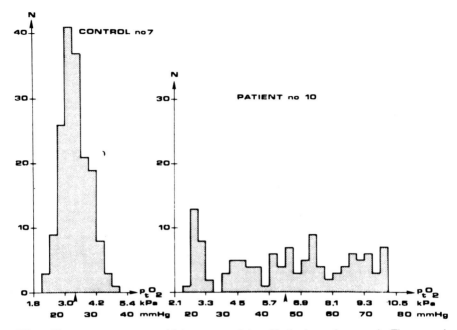

FIG. 1. Tissue oxygen pressure histograms registered in the trapezius muscle. The normal histogram from a control (*left*) is Gaussian in shape. The "scattered" histogram (*right*) is from a patient with fibromyalgia. The histogram distribution types are statistically different with $p < .001$. (From Lund et al., ref. 12, with permission.)

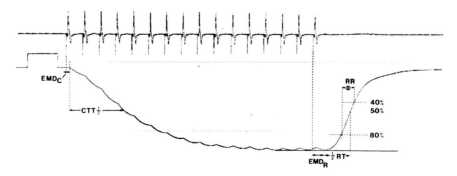

FIG. 2. Muscle relaxation time is determined after a stimulation of 32 impulses at 20 Hz. Relaxation time is expressed as percentage force loss /10 msec (RR) or percentage force loss from the tetanic contraction level 100 msec after the maximum of the last contraction. (From Bäckman et al., ref. 11, with permission.)

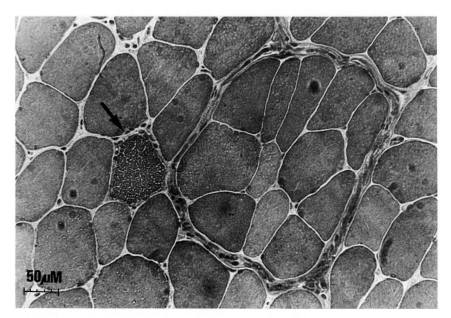

FIG. 3. Section of trapezius muscle from 49-year-old female patient with fibromyalgia. A "ragged red" fiber is seen (*arrow*). (Gomori-trichrome staining.)

with localized work-related myalgia (20). The ragged red fibers, however, were also found in 17% of the biopsies from healthy controls (Fig. 3).

Any factor or factors that can influence microcirculation in the muscle could start a series of events leading to fibromyalgia. Such a factor could be a metabolic disturbance, such as low serotonin values (see Chapter 20, *this volume*), or increased activity in muscle sympathetic nerves. It could also be an altered central motor control leading to an incoordinated contraction/relaxation pattern (21).

In all our studies, fibromyalgia patients who fulfilled the diagnostic criteria of Yunus et al. (3) have been compared with people with no muscular pain or muscle fatigue. No comparison has been made between fibromyalgia patients and patients with other pain syndromes with generalized muscular pain. The conclusion from our studies is that laboratory tests of muscle metabolism should be included in the diagnostic criteria required for fibromyalgia patients, especially when these patients are participating in different research projects.

WHICH MUSCLE SHOULD BE EXAMINED?

The diagnostic tests should be performed in muscles that are frequently painful. It should be observed that diagnostic findings are not found in all

TABLE 2. *Muscles used for different laboratory investigations in patients with fibromyalgia*

Muscle	Laboratory method	Pathology[a]
Trapezius	Muscle histochemistry	+
	Tissue oxygen tension	+
	Electromyography	−
	Determination of ATP and PC	+
Deltoid	Muscle histochemistry	+
Brachioradials	Tissue oxygen tension	+
Adductor pollicis	Relaxation time	+
Biceps	Electromyography	−
Anterior tibial	Determination of ATP and PC	−
	Electromyography	−
Vastus lateralis	Morphological changes in glycerinated muscle fibers (22)	+

[a] +, Pathology found; −, pathology not found.

muscles. An overview of muscles used for our different investigations is given in Table 2. The upper part of trapezius muscle is almost always painful in fibromyalgia and this might be a suitable muscle for diagnostic tests. The anterior tibial muscle has, on the other hand, not proved to be a muscle suitable for diagnostic studies in fibromyalgia.

MUSCULAR VERSUS EXTRAMUSCULAR SYMPTOMS OF THE FIBROMYALGIA SYNDROME

Many fibromyalgia patients have symptoms from other organs and organ systems as well. Vertigo, for example, is frequently found in otoneurological studies of fibromyalgia patients (23). Some patients have both peripheral (paresthesia and numbness) and central nervous symptoms (24). Whether the symptoms from organs other than muscles are caused by the same factor or factors that cause the muscular symptoms is not known. Some of the extramuscular symptoms could be a nonspecific effect of the chronic pain.

The extramuscular symptomatology varies from one fibromyalgia patient to another, but the muscular symptomatology is constant and consistent in virtually all fibromyalgia patients. That is why we propose that the diagnosis of fibromyalgia syndrome in the future should be based on both muscular symptomatology and laboratory tests of muscle function and metabolism.

REFERENCES

1. Quimby L, Block S, Gratwick G. *J Rheumatol* 1988;15:1264–1270.
2. Smythe H, Moldofsky H. *Bull Rheum Dis* 1977;28:928–931.
3. Yunus MB, Masi AT, Calabro JJ, Miller KA, Feigenbaum SL. *Semin Arthritis* 1981;11:151–171.

4. Wolfe F, Smythe HA, Yunus MB, Bennett RM, Bombardier C, Goldenberg DM, Tugwell P, Multicenter Fibromyalgia Criteria Committee. *Arthritis Rheum* 1989;32(suppl 4):S47 (abstr).
5. Torebjörk HE, Ochoa JL, Schady W. *Pain* 1984;18:145–156.
6. Arner S, Meyerson BA. *Pain* 1988;33:11–23.
7. Cherry DA, Gourlay GK, McLachlan M, Cousins MJ. *Pain* 1984;21:143–152.
8. Bengtsson A, Bengtsson M. *Pain* 1988;33:161–167.
9. Cathey MA, Wolfe F, Kleinheksel SM, Miller S, Pitetti K. *Arthritis Care Res* 1988;1–14.
10. Gundmark I, Henriksson C. *Aktivitetsmönster vid primär fibromyalgi.* Linköping, Sweden: Linköping University, Dept of Social Science, 1984.
11. Bäckman E, Bengtsson A, Bengtsson M, Lennmarken C, Henriksson KG. *Acta Neurol Scand* 1982;77:187–191.
12. Lund N, Bengtsson A, Thorborg P. *Scand J Rheumatol* 1986;15:165–173.
13. Bengtsson A, Henriksson KG, Larsson J. *Scand J Rheumatol* 1986;15:1–6.
14. Bengtsson A, Henriksson KG, Larsson J. *Arthritis Rheum* 1986;29:817–821.
15. Kessler M, Lübbers DW. *Pflügers Arch* 1966;291:88.
16. Lassen NA. *J Clin Invest* 1964;43:1805.
17. Nilsson GE, Tenland T, Öberg P. **IEEE** *Trans Biomed Eng* 1980;22:1–00.
18. Harris RC, Hultman E, Nordesjö LO. *Scand J Clin Lab Invest* 1974;33:109–120.
19. Lennmarken C, Bergman T, Larsson J, Larsson L-E. *Clin Physiol* 1885;5:243–255.
20. Bengtsson A, Henriksson KG. *J Rheumatol* (in press).
21. Elert J, Rantapää Dahlqvist SB, Henriksson-Larsénk, Gerdle B. *Scand J Rheum* 1989.
22. Bartels EM, Danneskiøld-Samsøe B. *Lancet* 1986;1:755–757.
23. Ödqvist LM, Thell J, Bengtsson A, Larsby B. In: Clausson C-F, Kirtare MV, eds. *Vertigo, nausea, tinnitus and hearing loss in cardiovascular diseases.* City: Publisher, 1986;429–433.
24. Bengtsson A, Henriksson KG, Jorfeldt L, Kägedahl B, Lennmarken C, Lindtröm F. *Scand J Rheumatol* 1986;15:340–347.

Advances in Pain Research and Therapy, Vol. 17,
edited by James R. Fricton and Essam Awad.
Raven Press, Ltd., New York © 1990.

17

New Diagnostic Tools in Primary Fibromyalgia

Findings from the Copenhagen Research Group on Fibromyalgia

*Rasmus Bach-Andersen, ‡Søren Jacobsen, ‡Bente
Danneskiold-Samsøe, §Else Bartels, **Karl Erik Jensen,
**Carsten Thomsen, **Ole Henriksen, and †Peter Arlien-
Søborg

*Departments of *Rheumatology, **Magnetic Resonance, and †Neurology,
Hvidovre Hospital, University of Copenhagen, Copenhagen, Denmark;
‡Department of Rheumatology, Frederiksberg Hospital, Copenhagen, Denmark,
and §Biophysics Group, Open University, Oxford, England*

Primary fibromyalgia (PF) is a nonarticular rheumatic disorder that is characterized by generalized musculoskeletal pain, stiffness, fatigue, disturbed sleep, and a number of musculoskeletal tender points in the absence of laboratory and x-ray results indicating any other rheumatic disese (1–3). The prevalence of this condition has been estimated to be about 5% of a rheumatic disease population (4,5). The etiology and pathogenesis of fibromyalgia is unknown but hypothesis including sleep disturbances (1), pain modulation disorders (6), and neurotransmitter imbalance (7) have been proposed.

Recently, interesting laboratory abnormalities focusing on muscle function have been revealed. These laboratory abnormalities include alterations in levels of high-energy phosphates in PF muscle (8), abnormal muscle oxygenation (9), and reduced dynamic muscle strength (10). Psychological disturbances such as neurotic changes and depression have been suggested to be present in PF (11); whether this is primary or secondary to PF is still unknown. Current research on fibromyalgia has focused on it's underlying biological characteristics. The purpose of this chapter is to review this current research, present new findings from the Copenhagen Research Group on Fibromyalgia, and discuss these findings in terms of their potential usefulness as new diagnostic tools.

MUSCLE FUNCTION

Exhaustion and fatigue of muscle in PF has directed attention to the functional capacities of these muscles. Previous studies have presented statements that PF patients do not suffer from clinical objective muscle weakness (12,13). Isometric and isokinetic muscle strength of quadriceps muscle as tested with an isokinetic dynamometer in PF was found to be 41 to 51% decreased as compared with matched normal subjects. Other methods of muscle strength measurements have been applied in PF patients; maximal voluntary hand grip strength has been found to be reduced about 40% compared with healthy controls (14), and the maximal workload of calf muscles has been documented to be about 50% of the expected value (15).

Muscle Strength and Disease Activity

The reduction in maximal voluntary strength in PF patients has been shown to be related to the disease impact (16,17). The number of tender points and subjective symptoms correlated to the muscle strength of the patients. It has been suggested that some degree of disability does exist in PF (18). These findings are of great importance in supporting patient reports of difficulties in activities of daily life due to pain and fatigue when applying for disability compensation.

Mechanism for Reduced Muscle Function

A cardinal question in PF research is whether the cause of the illness is muscular, neuromuscular, or central in origin. Also, the impaired muscle function in primary fibromyalgia may be due to central or peripheral mechanisms.

In favor of peripheral mechanisms are studies that have shown metabolic and morphological changes in muscles of PF patients. The muscle content of high-energy metabolites has been found to be decreased (8). Histopathological findings include "rubber band" morphology (19) and ragged red fibers (20). Electromyographic examinations have not revealed convincing evidence for neuromuscular transmission defects (21).

In favor of a partial central mechanism is the ability to obtain a near-normal muscle strength by electrical nerve stimulation (14). Some of the central mechanisms for reduced muscle function may be the lack of motivation or pain effects with negative feedback on motor unit recruitment. Primary fibromyalgia has been suggested to be a disorder of pain modulation (6) and as such, this would be consistent with reduced muscle function due to pain. It has therefore been suggested that maximal voluntary muscle strength, evaluated by isokinetic measurements be used as a parameter for measuring the disease impact on the patients (17).

Other findings direct interest toward a central mechanism of muscle fatigue. Recently, the similarity between primary fibromyalgia and benign myalgic encephalomyelitis has been described (22), and abnormal auditory brainstem responses in about one third of the patients (23) would also be consistent with central nervous system dysfunction. It is therefore of great interest that focal cerebral pathology of unknown origin has been determined in some patients with primary fibromyalgia using magnetic resonance imaging (24).

^{31}P Nuclear Magnetic Resonance Spectroscopy

Since the first ^{31}P nuclear magnetic resonance spectrum from intact muscle was obtained in 1974 the interest in this noninvasive method has grown rapidly. ^{31}P NMR spectroscopy provides data on the bioenergetics of muscles at rest as well as during exercise. In our experimental setting, we have studied the calf muscles with a simple surface coil. The amount of muscle examined depends on the size of the coil—in our studies approximately 60 to 70 mm^3 of muscle tissue. The high-energy phosphorus metabolites phosphocreatine (PC) and adenosine triphosphate (ATP) together with inorganic phosphorus (Pi) can be detected in our ^{31}P NMR spectra. The calf muscles can be stressed by voluntary contraction, during aerobic as well as anaerobic conditions, performed in a specially built ergometer (15,25).

Our study of the calf muscle in normal subjects during exercise confirms that all PC can be depleted. In our examinations of patients with PF, the main result was an inability to deplete the muscle PC level below 30% of the resting value (15). This observation suggests some kind of as yet unknown disorder of skeletal muscle metabolism in PF patients.

Abnormal ^{31}P NMR spectra have been reported in patients with weakness, fatigability, and muscle pain (26). Recently abnormal Pi/PC ratios have been obtained from PF patients at rest (27), suggesting mitochondrial defects. We have not found this in our PF patients (15).

The recovery of the Pi/PC concentration ratio after aerobic as well as anaerobic work was normal in the PF patients, which also indicates that the enzyme systems are normal in the muscle mitochondria. Furthermore, this is in contrast to the finding of abnormal oxygenation of muscle surface, suggesting changes in microcirculation (96), which have been supported by the observation of lower exercising blood flow in PF patients than in controls (28).

ELECTRICAL CHARGES OF SINGLE MUSCLE FIBERS

By measuring Donnan potentials using microelectrodes, it is now possible to estimate the fixed electrical charges in the A and I bands of the striated muscle fibers. Glycerinated fibers from the quadriceps muscle of both PF patients and controls were examined. The electrical charges on contractile proteins in the A and I bands of the muscle fibers did not differ in the two groups, which indicates that the contractile filaments in the muscle fibers are normal (29).

MORPHOLOGY IN SINGLE MUSCLE FIBERS

In conventional histology of muscle fibers from PF patients, no changes have been observed to date by our group. However, by microscopic examination of fibers from glycerinated standard biopsies of the quadriceps muscle, a characteristic pattern could be observed (29). A pattern of "rubber bands" was observed along the length of the PF fibers. These "rubber bands" are readily seen as constrictions of the fiber, and sometimes threads were found connecting one fiber with another. No such morphological patterns have been observed either in healthy muscles or in muscle from other rheumatic patients, including rheumatoid arthritis patients (S. Jacobsen, E. M. Bartels, B. Schiøtt-Christensen, B. Danneskiold-Samsøe, unpublished observations, 1989) and polymyositis patients (29a). Staining results point toward the "rubber bands" being reticular fibers, which are always present in a muscle but not as constrictions around the cells. Why these "rubber bands" have not been stripped off with the membranes during the glycerol treatment is not known, but they may be the cause of PF or perhaps are only a secondary phenomenon to the real cause of the disease.

Since these first observations, further investigations have been made to estimate the sensitivity and specificity of the "rubber band" morphology method.

Validity of "Rubber Band" Patterns as a Diagnostic Tool

Muscle biopsies from 118 patients consecutively referred to us suffering from muscle pain and fatigue were investigated for "rubber band" morphology (30). The biopsies were examined by a physician and a technician, both specially trained in microscopical methods. Neither the physician nor the technician had any knowledge of the patients from whom the biopsies were taken while examining the biopsies.

Eighty-one of the 118 patients fulfilled the clinical criteria for fibromyalgia syndrome; 37 of the 118 patients had regional muscle tension and pain. A majority 78% of the patients who fulfilled the clinical criteria for PF showed "rubber band" morphology, with a varying number of bands per fiber. Sixty-five percent of the patients who did not fulfill the clinical criteria for PF showed no "rubber band" morphology, and their biopsy specimens appeared normal. Sensitivity of "rubber-band" morphology to clinical diagnosis was 78%, and specificity was 65%. These results indicate a close relationship between the "rubber band" morphology and the fibromyalgia syndrome.

Furthermore, muscle biopsies from 14 patients with rheumatoid arthritis, seven patients with polymyositis, seven patients with myotonia congenita, and 15 healthy persons were investigated. No "rubber band" morphology was found in muscle biopsies from these subjects.

In conclusion, the described morphological examination of glycerinated single fiber is suggested as a new specific diagnostic test for PF when coupled with other objective methods [e.g., isokinetic strength measurements (10), relaxation rate (14), and content of energy-holding compounds in PF muscle (8)].

OTHER FINDINGS OF INTEREST

Effects of Sleep Disturbances

Poor sleep is another of the cardinal symptoms of PF (1,31), which has been suggested to be a perpetuating factor in PF. The concentration of procollagen type III aminoterminal propeptide (P-III-NP) in PF serum was compared to that in healthy controls.

During the production and secretion of collagen, the procollagen has an NH_2-terminal and COOH-terminal polypeptide attached at each end of the molecule. In the extracellular space these polypeptides are split off. By measuring the NH_2-terminal polypeptide—the P-III-NP—an expression of type III collagen production can be obtained.

Primary fibromyalgia patients as a group had a lower serum level of P-III-NP than the controls. When dividing PF patients into those with no sleep disturbances and those with sleep disturbances, the latter group turned out to be those with the lowest serum concentration of P-III-NP (32). It has also been found that PF patients with low serum concentration of P-III-NP have more symptoms, more tender points, lower muscle strength, and more distrubed sleep than PF patients with normal P-III-NP values (33).

Cranial Magnetic Resonance Imaging

Cranial magnetic resonance imaging in seven patients with fibromyalgia has revealed clearly pathological white matter lesions in five of these patients. The lesions were diffusely distributed and had a size of 3×3 to 5×5 mm (24). These findings are presently being further investigated. There may be a connection between these CNS lesions and the findings of CNS dysfunction in fibromyalgia patients with dysesthesia (23,34).

Autoimmune Screening

Studies have described an increased occurrence of antinuclear autoantibodies (ANAs) in PF. Even though presence of ANA is connected to inflammatory rheumatic disease, no evidence has been found that PF should be of such a nature, supported by the fact that prednisone treatment has no effect in PF.

In 20 patients with PF and 19 matched healthy controls, sera were examined for various antibodies: anti–parietal cell antibodies, anti–adrenal cortex antibodies, antimicrosomal antibodies, antithyroglobulin antibodies, granulocyte-sepcific ANA, antineutrophil cytoplasmic antibodies, anti–smooth muscle antibodies, anti–striated muscle antibodies, antisarcolemma antibodies, rheumatoid factor (immunoglobulins M and A), ANAs (HEP-2 cells), anti-DNA antibodies, and anti-ENA antibodies (35).

It was remarkable that 40 and 55% of the PF patients had antibodies against striated muscle and smooth muscle, respectively, whereas none of the controls had any. Occurrence of striated muscle antibodies in PF patients may be due to an increased exposure of intracellular muscle antigens to the immune system. Liberation of these muscle antigens could take place as a result of sporadic muscle fiber degeneration, which has been described earlier in some PF patients (36). Smooth muscle antibodies are known to occur in some infections (e.g., acute hepatitis and Epstein-Barr virus infections). Acute ongoing infections were ruled out in our patients, but it has been proposed that chronic viral infection may be associated with PF (22) and could therefore account for the presence of smooth muscle antibodies.

CONCLUSION

We conclude from our studies that:

1. The dynamic muscle strength is decreased; this may be connected to the abnormal bioenergetics of energy-rich phosphocreatine in working PF muscle.
2. The fixed electrical charge in the A and I bands is normal, suggesting normal conditions in the contractile apparatus.
3. The morphology of single muscle fibers is characterized by "rubber bands" in some patients with PF.
4. Lack of recovery and restitution after a night's sleep may have an influence on collagen synthesis.
5. Antibodies against striated muscle antigen and smooth muscle antigen are present in some patients. This is interpreted for the striated muscle antibodies to be a result of an increased exposure of intracellular muscle antigens to the immune system and for the smooth muscle antibodies in line with other chronic viral infection, such as hepatitis and Epstein-

Barr virus infections, as a chronic viral infection either of primary or secondary relevance to the still obscure pathogenesis of the fibromyalgia syndrome.

The present and most used criteria for PF (3) have been extremely important for the PF research, but it has now been suggested that they be revised (37) to include tender points as the major cornerstone in the diagnosis of fibromyalgia. We think it is of great importance to test the presented objective findings and laboratory tests in fibromyaliga relative to these new criteria in order to narrow the scope of patients and thereby produce new and better diagnostic tools for the fibromyalgia syndrome.

REFERENCES

1. Smythe H, Moldofsky H. *Bull Rheum Dis* 1978;28:928–931.
2. Yunus MB. *J Rheumatol* 1983;10:841–844.
3. Yunus MB, Masi AT, Calabro JJ, Miller KA, Feigenbaum SL. *Semin Arthritis Rheum* 1981;11:151–171.
4. The American Rheumatism Association Committee on Rheumatologic Practice. *Arthritis Rheum* 1977;20:1278–1281.
5. Wolfe F, Cathey MA. *J Rheumatol* 1983;10:965–968.
6. Smythe HA. *Clin Rheum Dis* 1979;5:823–832.
7. Wallace DJ. *Mount Sinai J Med* 1984;51:124–131.
8. Bengtsson A, Henriksson KG, Larsson J. *Arthritis Rheum* 1986;29:817–821.
9. Lund N, Bengtsson A, Thorborg P. *Scand J Rheumatol* 1986;15:165–173.
10. Jacobsen S, Danneskiold-Samsøe B. *Scand J Rheumatol* 1987;160:61 – 65.
11. Ahles TA, Yunus MB, Riley SD, Bradley JM, Masi AT. *Arthritis Rheum* 1984;27:1101–1106.
12. Kaplan H. *Medical Times* 1977;105:49–51.
13. Yunus MB. *Compr Therapy* 1984;10:21–28.
14. Bäckman E, Bengtsson A, Bengtsson M, Henriksson KG. *Acta Neurol Scand* 1988;77:187–191.
15. Jacobsen S, Jensen KE, Thomsen C, Danneskiold-Sansøe B, Andersen RB, Henriksen O. Paper presented at 1st International Symposium in Myofascial Pain and Fibromyalgia.
16. Jacobsen S, Danneskiold-Samsøe B, Andersen RB. *Scand J Rheumatol [Suppl.]* 1988;72:37 (abstr).
17. Jacobsen S, Danneskiold-Samsøe B, Andersen RB. Paper presented at 1st International Symposium in Myofascial Pain and Fibromyalgia.
18. Hawley DJ, Wolfe F, Cathey MA. *J Rheumatol* 1988;15:1551–1556.
19. Bartels EM, Danneskiold-Samsøe B. *Lancet* 1986;1:755–757.
20. Bengtsson A, Henriksson KG, Larsson J. *Scand J Rheumatol* 1986;15;1–6.
21. Bengtsson A, Henriksson KG, Jorfeldt L, Kägedal B, Lennmarken C, Lindstrøm F. *Scand J Rheumatol* 1986;15:340–347.
22. Goldenberg DL. *Semin Arthritis Rheum* 1988;18:111–120.
23. Rosenhall U, Johansson G, Ørndahl G. *Scand J Rehabil Med* 1987;19:147–152.
24. Jacobsen S, Jensen KE, Thomsen C, Danneskiold-Samsøe B, Andersen RB, Henriksen O. Paper presented at 1st International Symposium in Myofascial Pain and Fibromyalgia.
25. Jensen KE, Jacobsen S, Thomsen C, Andersen RB, Henriksen O. *Radiology* 1988;169(suppl. P):238 (abstr).
26. Radda GK, Bore PJ, Rajagopalan B. *Br Med Bull* 1983;40:155–159.
27. Mathur AK, Gatter RA, Bank WJ, Schumacher HR. *Arthritis Rheum* 1988;31(4):S23 (abstr).
28. Bonafede P, Nelson D, Clark S, Goldberg L, Bennett RM. *Arthritis Rheum* 1987;30(4):S14 (abstr).
29. Bartels EM, Danneskiold-Samsøe B. *Scand J Rheumatol [Suppl.]* 1986;59:19 (abstr).

29a.Bartels EM, Jacobson S, Rasmussen L, Danneskiold-Samsøe B. *J Rheumatol* 1989 (in press).
30. Jacobsen S, Danneskiold-Samsøe B, Bartels E, Andersen RB. Paper presented at 1st International Symposium in Myofascial Pain and Fibromyalgia.
31. Jacobsen S, Danneskiold-Samsøe B, Andersen RB. Paper presented at 1st International Symposium in Myofascial Pain and Fibromyalgia.
32. Jensen LT, Jacobsen S, Hørslev-Petersen K. *Br J Med* 1988;27:496 (letter).
33. Jacobsen S, Jensen LT, Danneskiold-Samsøe B, Andersen RB. Paper presented at 1st International Symposium in Myofascial Pain and Fibromyalgia.
34. Rosenhall U, Johansson G, Ørndahl G. *Scand J Rehabil Med* 1987;19:139–145.
35. Jacobsen S, Høier-Madsen M, Danneskiold-Samsøe B, Andersen RB, Wiik A. Paper presented at 1st International Symposium in Myofascial Pain and Fibromyalgia.
36. Henriksson KG, Bengtsson A, Larsson J, Thornell LE. *Scand J Rheumatol [Suppl.]* 1987;69:12 (abstr).
37. Wolfe F, Smythe HA, Yunus MB, et al. *Arthritis Rheum* 1989;32(suppl. 4):S47 (abstr).

Advances in Pain Research and Therapy, Vol. 17,
edited by James R. Fricton and Essam Awad.
Raven Press, Ltd., New York © 1990.

18

Fibromyalgia, Cytokines, Fatigue Syndromes, and Immune Regulation

*Daniel J. Wallace, **James B. Peter, **Ralph L. Bowman,
**Susan B. Wormsley, and *Stuart Silverman

*Department of Medicine/Division of Rheumatology, Cedars-Sinai Medical
Center, UCLA School of Medicine, Los Angeles, California 90024; and
**Specialty Laboratories, Inc, Santa Monica, California 90904

The cause of primary fibromyalgia (fibrositis) syndrome (PFS) is unknown. It has been estimated that between 3 and 6 million Americans have PFS (1,2), and nearly that many have secondary fibromyalgia, according to at least 46 documented sources (3). Primary and secondary fibromyalgia have similar clinical presentations and common treatment approaches (4). Fibromyalgia has a devastating socioeconomic impact resulting in billions of dollars in lost productivity annually in the United States (5). Recent efforts to explore the etiology of PFS have included the examination of immune parameters. This report summarizes prior studies, reports on our work in this area, compares the results of PFS investigations with those in the closely related chronic fatigue syndrome and myalgic encephalomyelitis, discusses newer developments evolving around neuropeptides and their relationship to PFS, and outlines opportunities for further studies.

PFS, IMMUNE PARAMETERS, AND CYTOKINES

Slightly increased frequencies of Raynaud's phenomenon, alopecia, and sicca syndrome have been reported in PFS (6–8). Nearly all patients with a positive antinuclear antibody (ANA) or rheumatoid factor and PFS fall into this grouping, but some studies have excluded patients with positive serologies. In 1984, Caro (9) reported that 76% of 25 patients with PFS had immunoglobulin (Ig) G deposition at the dermal-epidermal junction, but the largest independent recent study found this in only 4 of 36 patients (11%) (6). It has been well documented that fibrositis is associated with neurogenic inflammation (10) or cold-induced vasospasm (11) or what has been called enhanced vascular permeability (9), characterized by vasodilation and dermatographia (mediated axon reflex response). It is therefore probable that most investigators who described livedo reticularis or Raynaud's phenomenon in PFS are simply using different terms to denote neurogenic inflammation and local autonomic changes. There is no evidence that circulating immune complexes, ANA, C4 complement, anti-DNA antibody, sedimentation rate, muscle enzymes, or any other serological measure is abnormal in PFS (6,12,13), and despite an early report no human leukocyte antigen (HLA) phenotype is associated with PFS (14,15).

The administration of certain cytokines modulates symptoms associated with fibrositis. For example, interleukin-2 (IL-2) promotes stiffness and aching (16), interferon alpha (IFN-α) can cause fatigue and disorientation (17), and interleukin-1 (IL-1) and tumor necrosis factor (TNF) are somnogenic (18). In 1988, our group reported that patients with terminal cancer developed a transient fibrositis after receiving IL-2 therapy (16). We then designed a study to test the hypothesis that PFS might be associated with alterations in immune regulation and that abnormal cytokine levels might explain some of the symptoms of PFS.

Patient Selection and Methods

Sixteen patients who fulfilled Yunus et al.'s (19) proposed criteria for PFS were studied. All had generalized aches and pain or prominent stiffness, involving three or more specific antomical sites, for at least 3 months and absence of any secondary causes with normal laboratory testing for complete blood count (CBC), erythrocyte sedimentation rate (ESR), rheumatoid factor, antinuclear antibody (ANA) and muscle enzymes. The patients also had at least five tender points and three or more of the minor criteria symptoms. Their mean age was 50.1 (range 31 to 74). Eleven were caucasian, one hispanic, and four black. All had been under treatment for PFS for at least 2 years and thus had the chronicity said to be typical of PFS (20). None of the patients were being treated with steroids or immunsuppressive agents. All participants filled out a questionnaire from which a Fatigue Severity Scale was derived (21).

At their first study visit, patients had the following tests performed using published techniques: lymphocyte mitogenic stimulation, including phytohemagglutinin (PHA), concanavalin A (Con A), and pokeweed mitogen (PWM) stimulation indices (22,23); lymphocyte enumeration, including total white blood cell count, and total lymphocyte count; flow cytometric quantitation (24) of the CD2, CD4, CD5, CD20, NKH-1, CD8, Leu 7, and CD8/Leu 7BR subsets of lymphocytes; and CD4/CD8 ratios of heparinized (10 U/ml) peripheral blood. Inteferon alpha was assayed in serum by a low-level, two-site immunoradiometric technique that allows reproducible mea-

TABLE 1. *Patient characteristics (N = 15)*

Index features	Symptoms and percentage	
Mean Age: 50.1 years	Greater than or equal to	
Female sex: 93%	5 tender points	100
Caucasian: 69%	Worse with stress	100
Black: 25%	Fatigue	100
Hispanic: 6%	Worse with exercise	94
	Worse with weather	94
Mean Westergran	Anxiety	88
ESR: 11.6 mm/hr	Nonrestorative sleep	81
	Subjective edema	44
	Irritable colon	38
	Chronic headache	31
	Numbness	31

surement down to 5 U/ml Interferon gamma (IFN-γ) (25), interleukin-1 beta (IL-1β), IL-2, and interleukin-2 receptor (IL-2R) were measured in serum as described previously (26–29). Tumor necrosis factor alpha (TNF-α) was measured by radioimmunoassay (30).

In 15 of the 16 patients, lymphocyte subset analysis and cytokine levels were repeated on three to five serial visits over a 6-month period. The control group consisted of 55 apparently healthy individuals who attended a community health fair. This included 28 men and 30 women with a mean age of 35.6 years (range 20 to 65). Comparisons between the study and control groups were made using the unpaired *t*-test. The alpha level was set at 0.05 for all statistical comparisons (31).

Humoral immunity was evaluated by mesuring IgG subsets 1, 2, 3, and 4. Circulating immune complexes were assessed by four methods: Raji cell, polyethylene glycol, C1q binding, and conglutinin binding (32). Epstein-Barr virus (EBV) antibodies assayed by the indirect fluorescent antibody (IFA) technique included IgG and IgM antibodies to viral capsid antigen and IgG antibodies to early antigen and to nuclear antigen. For determination of EBV antibodies, sera from the 15 PFS patients and 15 non-PFS patients matched for age and gender were read blindly by two individuals.

Results

The similarity of symptoms, signs, and clinical and laboratory features of our patient population to those reported in a study on diagnostic criteria (19) suggests that our cohort is representative of what has been called PFS (Table 1). In addition, this group's Fatigue Severity Scale was 5.6 out of 7, in comparison with 4.5 for inflammatory arthritis patients and less than 2 for controls (13). Lymphocyte subset analysis revealed that the average CD4/CD8 ratio was elevated ($p < .025$) for PFS patients when compared to 55

TABLE 2. *Lymphocyte and subset levels: PFS versus control comparisons*

	PFS group (N = 15)	Control range (N = 55)
Lymphs: %	36 ± 11	35 ± 8
per mm^3	2050 ± 805	1996 ± 555
CD2 (%)	84 ± 6	81 ± 10
CD20 (%)	6 ± 3	8 ± 4
CD4 (%)	56 ± 11[a]	42 ± 8
CD8 (%)	18 ± 7	22 ± 8
CD4/CD8 ratio	3.8 ± 2.0[b]	2.2 ± 1.0
CD5 (%)	78 ± 7	73 ± 8
Kappa (%)	5 ± 2	5 ± 2
Lambda (%)	4 ± 2	4 ± 1
Leu7 (%)	6 ± 4	7 ± 5
CD8/Leu7 Br (%)	3 ± 2	4 ± 4
NKH-1 (%)	7 ± 3	7 ± 5

[a] $p < .001$.
[b] $p < .025$.

controls (Table 2). Fifteen patients had CD4/CD8 ratios determined three to five times over a 6-month period. Nine of the patients had at least one of their determinations elevated above the normal range. Four of the nine patients had CD4/CD8 ratios that were elevated on all visits during the 6-month study (Fig. 1). The elevated CD4/CD8 ratios were due primarily to increased

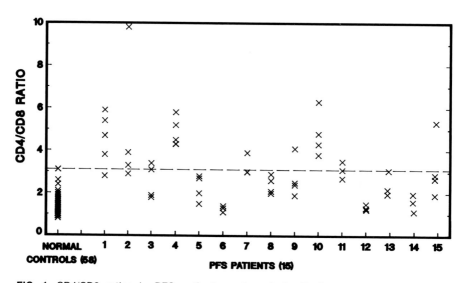

· **FIG. 1.** CD4/CD8 ratios in PFS patients and controls. Each × represents a single determination.

TABLE 3. *Other laboratory assays: PFS versus control comparisons*

	PFS group (N = 15)	Control range (N = 55)
Cytokines		
IL-1 (pg/ml)	<20	<20
IL-2 (units/ml)	<5	<5
IL-2R (units/ml)	297 ± 90	273 ± 102
IFN-α (units/ml)	<10	<10
IFN-γ (units/ml)	<5	<5
TNF (pg/ml)	407 ± 89	417 ± 88
Mitogen stimulation		
PHA (index)	142 ± 101	114 ± 29
Con A (index)	71 ± 72	78 ± 21
PWM (index)	25 ± 25	28 ± 12
IgG subclasses		
IgGl (mg/dl)	644 ± 191	400–950
IgG2 (mg/dl)	301 ± 110	70–450
IgG3 (mg/dl)	44 ± 33	20–90
IgG4 (mg/dl)	56 ± 61	3–90
Circulating immune complexes[a]		
Raji cell (μg AHG Eq/ml)	<12	<12
C1q binding (%)	<13	<13
Polyethylene glycol (μg IgG/ml)	<30	<30
Conglutinin (μg AHG Eq/ml)	<5	<5

[a] AHG, aggregated human gamma globulin.

mean percentages of CD4-positive lymphocytes (helper) ($p < .001$), although five out of 15 and six out 15 also had decreased percentages and absolute numbers of CD8-positive lymphocytes, respectively. All other lymphocyte markers were within normal ranges.

Cytokines IL:-1β, IL-2, TNF-α, IFN-α, and IL-2 receptor levels were obtained on three to four occasions in 15 of the patients. Eight out of 15 patients had elevated IL-2 levels on at least one of the five study visits. Similarly, six out of 15 had elevated INF-α levels and three out 15 had elevated IL-1β levels. However, neither the percentage of patients with cytokines in the detectable range nor the mean levels were significant when compared with the control group (Table 3).

IgG1, IgG2, IgG3, and IgG4 subclass levels were all within the normal range for the patient group. All 15 patients for whom mitogen stimulation indices were obtained had normal results. Titer of antibodies to EBV capsid antigen (IgG and IgM), early antigen, and nuclear antigen were essentially identical in the 15 patients, compared to 15 age- and gender-matched controls (data not shown). We also evaluated circulating immune complex levels in all 15 patients by four assays (Raji cell, C1q binding, polyethylene glycol, and conglutinin binding). All 60 determinations were within normal limits.

PFS, CHRONIC FATIGUE SYNDROME, AND MYALGIC
ENCEPHALOMYELITIS: COMPARATIVE IMMUNOLOGY

For many years, patients with a clinical picture similar too what rheumatologists now call PFS presented themselves to physicians in other specialities (33). From the 1930s to the late 1950s, a syndrome known variously as epidemic neuromyasthenia, myalgic encephalomyelitis (ME), or Icelandic disease frequently appeared in the literature (reviewed in ref. 34). Even though 30 years have elapsed since the last known case in the United States had been reported, this disorder is still quite common in the United Kingdom and has been the subject of recent investigations (35–38).

In the United States, reports of a chronic mononucleosis syndrome, postviral fatigue syndrome, and chronic Epstein-Barr viral (CEBV) disorder have appeared throughout this decade (39–44). In 1988, 15 authors of the most important papers in this area agreed that the commonalities of the patients they described warranted a new, all-encompassing disease classification, the chronic fatigue syndrome (CFS) (45). In 1987, Goldenberg et al. (rheumatology), Komaroff (internal medicine), and their colleagues published the results of a collaborative effort that could not find any substantial clinical or serological differences between the CEBV (now CFS) and PFS patients followed at different clinics of the same institution (46). Some obvious differences between PFS, CFS, and ME still exist. First, only the latter two entities are associated with sore throat, rash, fever, and adenopathy. However, Buchwald et al. (46) showed that the incidence of these symptoms in their PFS group of 50 patients was not significantly different from what has been reported in CFS. Our group is also able to confirm these findings (data not shown). Second, ME and CFS are almost always postinfectious (even though the inciting agent is rarely if ever isolated), whereas many other causes of fibromyalgia have been described (e.g., trauma, hypothyroidism, poor posture, rheumatoid arthritis, viral infection). Nevertheless, these inducing factors are excluded by definition in PFS and patients with these features are denoted as suffering from "secondary fibromyalgia." Also, PFS implies the ascendency of musculoskeletal complaints above all other features. These are present in most but not all patients with ME and CFS.

Immunological investigators have examined various aspects of ME and CFS. For example, viral infection in a group of patients with postviral fatigue syndrome has been suggested by elevated levels of IgM and IgG antibodies to enteroviruses (47). Others have described phenotypic and functional deficiency of natural killer cells as well as IgG subclass deficiencies in patients with chronic fatigue syndrome (47–50). Recently, a controlled immunological study of 50 patients appeared. The number of patients with musculoskeletal symptoms was not stated. Mitogenic stimulation indices were increased in the postinfected group, half had circulating immune complexes, and CD4/CD8 ratios were unchanged overall (51). Unfortunately, all of the

TABLE 4. *Comparison of clinical manifestations of PFS, CF, and ME (%)*

	PFS[a]	CFS[b]	ME[c]
Female sex	94	70	67
Myalgia	100	80	80
Arthralgia	100	75	80
Fatigue	100	100	100
Poor sleep	81	70	Most
Psychological problems	80	65	75
Chronicity	90	90	90
Complaints of fever	28	75	Most
Complaints of swollen glands	33	80	23
Headache	31	90	57
Elevated sedimentation rate	0	4	—

[a] Data from current study and Yunus et al. (19).
[b] Data from Straus (52).
[c] Data from Shelokov (35), Wessely (38), and Dillon et al. (37).

studies listed in Table 4 are either poorly controlled, small in scale, or uncontrolled.

Our observations suggest that, except for a nonspecific persistent tendency toward increased CD4/CD8 ratios in a subset of those with the disease, patients with well-established, chronic PFS do not differ from control groups in cytokine levels, IgG subclasses, EBV titers, lymphocyte subsets, measurements of mitogenic stimulation, or circulating immune complexes. Clearly, if PFS has an immunological basis, more sophisticated studies are in order. For example, cytokines still could play a role in PFS (e.g., resulting in a pain modulation syndrome) and one might consider measuring *in vitro* cytokine production in this group of patients. Interferon alpha production by peripheral blood mononuclear cells was found to be excessive in a group of patients with postviral fatigue syndrome (53). It is, of course, possible that cytokines in the serum could go undetected because of a short half-life of cytokines bound to soluble cytokine-bound receptors. A summary of these comparisons is shown in Table 5. The chief differentiating feature is the presence of circulating immune complexes in two controlled CFS studies and its absence in two controlled PFS studies. Perhaps an early postviral state is associated with circulating immune complexes. All of our PFS patients were studied after 2 years of symptoms.

PFS, NEUROPEPTIDES, CYTOKINES, AND IMMUNE REGULATION

Pain is modulated by neuropeptides, including substance P and β-endorphin. Over the last few years, a neuropeptide-immune linkage has been firmly established. β-Endorphin has been shown to increase IL-2 production, decrease T rosette formation and lymphocyte proliferation, increase autologous mixed lymphocyte reaction, and decrease the inhibitory effects of pros-

TABLE 5. *Immunological assessments in PFS, CFS, and ME*

Measure	PFS[a]	CFS	ME
Mitogen stimulation	Normal	Normal or ↑ (43,44) ↓ Natural killer activity (54)	— —
Lymphocyte enumeration	Usually normal ⅓ have ↑ T_4/T_8 ratio	Normal (40,44) Slight ↑ T_4 (p = .08) (43) ↓ T_4/T_8 ratio (51)	—
Cytokines	Normal	↑ IFN-α (44) Normal IFN (43) Slight ↑ IFN production (*in vitro*) (53) Normal IFN-γ production (56) ↑ IL-2 (57) Normal IL-1 production (58)	Normal (55)
Circulating immune complexes	Normal (see also ref. 59)	↑ in 60–67% (44,51)	—
IgG subclasses	Normal (no subclass ↓)	↓ various IgG subclasses (47–50)	—

[a] Data from current study except as noted.

taglandin (PG) E_2 released by adherent cells in stimulated cell fractions. It can also enhance leukocyte macrophage inhibitory factor production (60–62). Substance P can stimulate T cells, induce phagocytosis of macrophages by polymorphs, and initiate wheal and flare reactions via vasodilation. It also induces the production of charge-containing cytokines (63–65). It is made by 10 to 20% of the sensory neurons in the dorsal root ganglion (unmyelinated C fibers) and transported antegrade and retrograde. Increased peripheral utilization results in neurogenic inflammation. The neuroimmune link has been solidified by evidence that lymphocytes contain opiate-like receptors and cytokines IL-1 and IL-2 have brain receptors (66,67). Furthermore, 20 to 30% of substance P binds to human peripheral blood lymphocytes (equally to T helper and suppressor populations and to B cells to a lesser extent). In 1988, Lotz et al. (68) found that substance P and the related neuropeptide substance K can stimulate the production of IL-1, IL-6, and TNF. They also reported that certain monocyte functions such as arachidonic acid metabolism, chemotaxis, and oxidative burst are in part regulated by substance P. Although PFS patients were observed to have normal serum β-endorphin and substance P levels (69,70), a Norwegian group recently presented a controlled study that demonstrated elevated cerebrospinal fluid substance P values (71). It is probable that neuropeptide serum levels are of little value, or that their receptor sites and tissue deposition are more important. For example, a patient with chronic unilateral pain was found to have increased deposits of neuropeptides in the appropriate dorsal horn lamini (72).

SUMMARY AND FUTURE DIRECTIONS

We have shown that CFS, ME, and PFS are overlapping disorders that are manifestated by alterations in pain modulation and fatigue. The administration of cytokines can produce many manifestations of these disorders, although serum cytokine levels are not abnormal when compared to those of a control group. Even though neuropeptides (which mediate pain) interact with lymphocytes, no abnormalities in immune regulation are apparent in PFS. The administration of substance P can induce neurogenic inflammation and pain, both of which are observed in PFS. Most current approaches to fibromyalgia involve the administration of agents that support the analgesic effects of serotonin derivatives, induce restorative sleep, relax muscles, and improve conditioning so that unfit muscle will not be susceptible to microtrauma. The authors of this review propose that an additional approach might involve a trial of agents that are known antagonists to certain neuropeptides, such as somatostatin or calcinonin (67,73). For example, calcitonin has been reported to have analgesic properties in patients with metastatic cancer, osteoporosis, and reflex sympathetic properties in patients with metastatic cancer, osteoporosis, and reflex sympathetic dystrophy (74,75; S. Silverman, unpublished observations). Fibromyalgia represents a heterogenoeous population of patients with symptoms of varible similarity. Our observations should improve current efforts to define more rigorously the immunological features that are characteristic of some patients with PFS. These evolving distinctions will assist physicians in understanding the clinical features of this often misunderstood, common, devastating group of disorders.

REFERENCES

1. Wallace DJ. *J Rheumatol* 1985;12:913–915.
2. Goldenberg DL. *JAMA* 1987;57:2782–2787.
3. Hench PK. *Clin Rheum Dis* 1989;15:19–29.
4. Wolfe F, Cathey MA. *J Rheumatol* 1983;10:965–968.
5. Cathey MA, Wolfe, F, Kleinheksel SM, Hawley DJ. *Am J Med* 1986;81:78–84.
6. Dinerman H, Goldenberg D, Felson DT. *J Rheumatol* 1986;13:368–373.
7. Caro XJ, Wolfe F, Johnston WH, Smith AL. *J Rheumatol* 1986;13:1086–1092.
8. Bennett RM. *JAMA* 1987;257:2802–2803.
9. Caro XJ. *Arthritis Rheum* 1984;27:1174–1179.
10. Littlejohn GO, Weinstein C, Helme RD. *J Rheumatol* 1987;14:1022–1025.
11. Ingram S, Nelson D, Porter J, Campbell S, Bennett R. *Arthritis Rheum* 1987;30:S13.
12. Caro XJ. *Am J Med* 1986;81:43–49.
13. Bengtsson A, Henriksson KG, Jorfeldt L, Kagedal B, Lennmarken C, Lindstrom F. *Scand J Rheumatol* 1986;15:340–347.
14. Burda CD, Cox FR, Osborne P. *Clin Exp Rheumatol* 1986;4:355–357.

15. Russell IJ, Wolfe F, Burda C. Paper presented to the Study Group Session on Nonarticular Rheumatism, 50th Annual ARA Meeting, 1986.
16. Wallace DJ, Margolin K, Waller P. *Ann Intern Med* 1988;108:909.
17. McDonald EM, Mann AH, Thomas HC. *Lancet* 1987;2:1175–1178.
18. Krueger JM, Walter J, Dinarello CA, Wolff SM, Chedid L. *Am J Physiol* 1984;246:994–999.
19. Yunus M, Masi AT, Calabro JJ, Miller KA, Feigenbaum SL. *Arthritis Rheum* 1981;11:151–171.
20. Felson DT, Goldenberg DL. *Arthritis Rheum* 1986;29:1522–1526.
21. Krupp L, LaRocca NG, Muir-Nash J, Steinberg AD. *Neurology* 1988;38(suppl 1):99–100.
22. Maluish A, Strong DM. In: Rose NR, Friedman H, Fahey JL, eds. *Manual of clinical laboratory immunology*. Washington, DC: American Society for Microbiology, 1986;274–281.
23. Dean JH, Connor R, Herberman RB, Silva J, McCoy JL, Oldham RK. *Int J Cancer* 1977;20:359–370.
24. Zatz MM, Mathieson BJ, Kanelopoulos-Langevin C, Sharrow SO. *J Immunol* 1981;126:608–613.
25. Protzman WP, Minnicozzi M, Jacobs SL, Surprenant DI, Schwartz J, Oden EM. *J Clin Microbiol* 1985;22:596–599.
26. Hirsch RL, Panitch HS, Johnson KP. *J Clin Immunol* 1985;5:386–389.
27. Lisi PJ, Chu C-W, Koch GA, Endres S, Lonnemann G, Dinarello *Lymphokine Res* 1987;6:229–244.
28. Cornaby A, Simpson MA, Vann Rice R, Dempsey RA, Madras PN, Monoca AP. *Transplant Proc* ;1988;20:108–110.
29. Pui C-H, Ip SH, Kung P. *Blood* 1987;70:624–628.
30. Girardin E, Grau GE, Dayer J-M, Roux-Lombard P, Lambert P-H. *N Eng JMed* 1988;319:397–400.
31. Conover W, ed. *Practical non-parametic statistics*. New York: John Wiley and Sons, 1980.
32. Theofilopoulos AN, Aguado MT. In: Rose NR, Friedman H, Fahey JL, eds. *Manual of clinical laboratory immunology*, Washington, DC: American Society for Microbiology, 1986;197–203.
33. Goldenberg DL. *Semin Arthritis Rheum* 1988;18:111–120.
34. Wallace DJ. *Mt Sinai J Med* 1984;51:124–131.
35. Shelokov A. In: *Infectious diseases*. Philadelphia: Harper & Row, 1983;1421–1424.
36. Keighley BD, Bell EJ. *J R Coll Gen Pract* 1983;33:339–342.
37. Dillon MJ, Marshall WC, Dudgeon JA. *Br J Med* 1974;1:301–305.
38. Wessely S. *J R Soc Med* 1989;82:215–216.
39. Jones JF, Straus SE. *Annu Rev Med* 1987;38:195–209.
40. DuBois RE, Seeley JK, Brus I. *South Med J* 1984;77:1376–1382.
41. Holmes GP, Kaplan JE, Stewart JA, Hunt B, Pinsky PF, Schonberger LB. *JAMA* 1987;257:2297–2302.
42. Buchwald D, Sullivan JL, Komaroff AL. *JAMA* 197;257:2303–2307.
43. Straus SE, Tosato G, Armstrong G. *Ann Intern Med* 1985;102:7–16.
44. Jones JF, Ray CG, Minnich LL, Hicks MJ, Kibler R, Lucas DO. *Ann Intern Med* 1985;102:1–7.
45. Holmes GP, Kaplan JE, Gantz NM. *Ann Intern Med* 1988;108:387–389.
46. Buchwald D, Goldenberg DL, Sullivan JL, Komaroff AL. *Arthritis Rheum* 1987;30:1132–1136.
47. Rousef GE, Mann GF, Smith DG, Bell EJ, Murugesan V, McCartney RA, Mowbray JF. *Lancet* 1988;1:146–149.
48. Komaroff AL, Gelaer AM, Wormsley SB. *Lancet* 1988;1:1288–1289.
49. Linde A, Hammarstrom L, Smith CIE. *Lancet* 1988;1:885–886.
50. Read R, Spickett G, Harvey J, Edwards AJ, Larson HE. *Lancet* 1988;1:241.
51. Behan PO, Wilhelmina M, Behan H, Bell EJ. *J Infect* 1985;10:211–222.
52. Straus SE. *J Infect Dis* 1988;157:405–412.
53. Lever AML, Lewis DM, Bannister BA, Fry M, Berry N. *Lancet* 1988;2:101.
54. Caligiuri M, Murray C, Buchwald D, Levine H. *J Immunol* 1987;139:3306–3313.
55. Lloyd A, Hanna DA, Wakefield D. *Lancet* 1988;1:471.

56. Morte S, Castilla A, Civiera MP, Serrano M, Prieto J. *Lancet* 1988;2:623.
57. Cheney PR, Dorman SE, Bell DS. *Ann Intern Med* 1989;110:321.
58. Morte S, Castilla A, Civiera MP, Serrano M, Prieto J. *J Infect Dis* 1989;159:362.
59. Caro XJ. *Clin Rheum Dis* 1989;15:169–186.
60. Kusnecov AW, Husband AJ, King MG, Pang G, Smith R. *Brain Behav Immunol* 1987;1:88–97.
61. Froelich CJ. *J Neuroimmunol* 1987;17:1–10.
62. Gilmore W, Weiner LP. *J Neuroimmunol* 1988;18:125–138.
63. Lofstrom B, Pernow B, Wahren J. *Acta Physiol Scand* 1965;63:311.
64. Payan DG, Levine JD, Goetzl EG. *J Immunol* 1984;132:1601–1604.
65. Werner H, Paegelow I, Meyer-Rienecker H, Bienert M. *Ann NY Acad Sci* 1987;496:312–315.
66. Wiedermann CJ. *Immunol Lett* 1987;16:371–378.
67. Farrar WL, Hill JM, Harel-Bellan A, Vincour M. *Immunol Rev* 1987;100:361–378.
68. Lotz M, Carson D, Vaughn J. *Science* 1988;241:1218–1221.
69. Yunus MB, Denko CW, Masi AT. *J Rheumatol* 1986;13:183–186.
70. Raynolds WJ, Chiu B, Inman RD. *J Rheumatol* 1988;15:1802–1803.
71. Vaeroy H, Helle R, Forre O, Kass E, Terneius L. *Pain* 1988;32:21–26.
72. Williams S, Wells L, Hunt S. *Lancet* 1988;1:1047–1048.
73. Brain SD, William TJ. *Nature* 1988;335:73–75.
74. Gobelet C, Meier JL, Schaffner W, Bischof-Delaloye A, Gerster JC, Burckhardt P. *Clin Rheumatol* 1986;5:382–388.
75. Szanto J, Jozsef S, Rado J, Juhos E, Hindy I, Eckhardt S. *Oncology* 1986;43:69–72.

Advances in Pain Research and Therapy, Vol. 17,
edited by James R. Fricton and Essam Awad.
Raven Press, Ltd., New York © 1990.

19

Management of the Fibromyalgia Syndrome

Glenn A. McCain

Department of Medicine, University Hospital,
London, Ontario, N6A 5A5 Canada

Fibromyalgia is a chronic painful syndrome that presents difficulties for successful long-term management. We now know that the natural history of fibromyalgia appears to be one of continuous and unremitting pain. For example, one current report has shown that only 5% of individuals with fibromyalgia sustained remission of all symptoms during a 3-year follow-up period (1). Over 60% of the patients studied continued to report significant fatigue and nonrestorative sleep despite the fact that 83% received medication for their complaints during the study period. A list of therapeutic regimens purported to be of benefit in fibromyalgia is given in Table 1. Even though some of these therapies have been studied with acceptable scientific rigor, no wholly acceptable approach to treatment has been forthcoming. This is exemplified by two recent studies in which patients were asked about the effectiveness of their previous treatment regimens. Cathey et al. (15) surveyed 81 patients about medications used during the previous year of their illness. They noted that the average patient used 4.7 drugs during the year and was taking 3.8 medications at year's end. Of the 50% of patients who reported using cyclobenzaprine or amitriptyline only one third had improved sufficiently to report moderate or great improvement. Interestingly, analgesics were often noted to be more effective than either of these medications.

Similarly, various nonmedicinal therapies, including relaxation training and chiropractic treatment, were rated no better. Goldenberg et al. (16) recently reported similar results after follow-up of 87 patients treated over a 3-year period in their Rheumatic Diseases Clinic. Their results indicate that up to 50% of patients fail to respond to numerous pharmacological and nonpharmacological therapies. Taken together, these studies confirm the clinical observation that patients with fibromyalgia are indeed difficult treat-

TABLE 1. *Proposed medicinal treatments for fibromyalgia syndrome*

Treatment		Current status
Class	Agent	
Tricyclic antidepressant	Amitriptyline	Effective (2,3)
	Cyclobenzaprine	Effective (4–6)
	Dothiepin	Possibly effective (7)
	Imipramine	Not effective (8)
Major tranquilizer	Chlorpromazine	Possibly effective (9)
Serotonin precursor	L-Tryptophan	Not effective (10)
Benzodiazepine	Alprazolam	Effective (11)
	Temazopam	Not determined
NSAID[a]	Naproxen	Not effective (3)
Corticosteroid	Prednisone	Not effective (12)
Other	Regional sympathetic blockade	Possibly effective (13)
	S-adenosylmethionine (SAMe)	Possibly effective (14)

[a] Nonsteroidal antiinflammatory drug.

ment problems such that the average patient will require multiple treatment modalities over the natural history of the disease, often with limited success.

There are many reasons for the difficulties encountered in developing effective modalities of treatment in fibromyalgia. One compelling reason is that the syndrome is not associated with known alterations in the anatomy or physiology of the structures from which pain emanates. Furthermore, laboratory tests are characteristically normal. Treatment approaches have therefore been based on necessarily arbitrary footings, often with precarious pathological and/or physiological rationales. Thus, those treatments that have been shown to be successful in randomized clinical trials often show weak effects. As often as not they say more about what might be at fault in fibromyalgia than about what can be done to treat it successfully.

Another factor hampering rapid progress is the difficulty in development of responsive outcome measures for interventional studies. At present the only objective measure of this painful condition is the demonstration of fi-brositic tender points. The measurement of pain threshold over fibrositic tender points has only recently conformed to acceptable standards of valid-ity, reproducibility, and rater reliability. Unfortunately, improvements in other outcome measures have not always been correlated with, or accom-panied by, clinically significant improvements in pain tolerances and pain thresholds over these tender points (2). Consequently, less powerful means of evaluating efficacy prevail. Recently Hawley et al. (17) demonstrated the usefulness of the Health American Questionnaire (HAQ), a standard mea-sure of functional status used widely for determination of disability in rheu-matoid arthritis. There is at present a need to incorporate such functional outcome measures in clinical trials. Functional outcome measures of this type may allow future investigators to study the effects of various interventions in more predictable fashion.

This chapter, while taking into account these difficulties, will concentrate on recent evidence for efficacy of both medicinal and nonmedicinal treatments purported to be effective in the treatment of fibromyalgia. Where appropriate these studies will be described in detail so that the reader may be aware of the particular study design, the outcome measures used, and, most importantly, the magnitude of the effect of the intervention studied.

MEDICINAL TREATMENTS—INTERVENTIONAL STUDIES USING DRUG THERAPY

Tricyclic Antidepressants

Acceptably designed clinical trials have now been completed showing efficacy for both amitriptyline and clyclobenzaprine in fibromyalgia. These two related compounds are used in much smaller doses (10 to 50 mg of amitriptyline and 10 to 30 mg of cyclobenzaprine/day) than those recommended for the treatment of major depression, suggesting an alternative mechanism of action for these drugs in controlling the pain of fibromyalgia. The rationale for the use of these agents was prompted by a series of seminal investigations by Moldofsky et al. (9,10). In these experiments it was noted that sleep electroencephalographic (EEG) recordings of fibromyalgia patients exhibited a periodic fast alpha wave (8 to 10 cps) intrusion into the normally slow delta wave (1 to 3 cps) pattern of stage 4 sleep. Alpha wave activity, which is more characteristic of an "awake" EEG pattern, was thought to represent an endogenous arousal system leading to an altered density and duration of stage 4 sleep. The clinical correlate of this observation was nonrestorative sleep, so commonly complained of by patients with fibromyalgia. This hypothesis was strengthened when it was reported that normal volunteers, when deprived of delta slow-wave sleep by hand arousal, developed not only symptoms of fibromyalgia but also exquisite fibrositic tender points (10).

Further sleep studies were undertaken to incriminate altered biogenic amine metabolism when it was noted that plasma free tryptophan, a precursor of serotonin, was low in those most severely affected by pain in fibromyalgia. Chlorpromazine 100 mg at bedtime improved slow-wave sleep as well as the fatigue and pain experienced by fibromyalgia patients. Five grams of tryptophan per day, however, failed to cause significant improvement despite reproducible changes in sleep stages on EEG recordings (10). Since these experiments were reported there has been considerable circumstantial evidence for the role of serotonin in the control of pain in fibromyalgia. For example, administration of *p*-chlorophenylalanine (pCPA), which inhibits central nervous system production of serotonin, results in a painful syndrome very similar to fibromyalgia (18). L-5-Hydroxytryptophan in combination with a peripheral decarboxylase inhibitor has been reported to ameliorate pain in a patient with postanoxic encephalopathy and myoclonus (19). In addition, animal studies have shown that pain sensitivity is related to the level of brain serotonin, with lower pain thresholds present after serotonin depletion (20,21).

Serotonin is known to function as a neurotransmitter in various areas in the brain, including a spinal inhibitory pathway connecting neurons in brainstem periaqueductal gray and the substantia gelatinosa of the spinal cord. Activity of these neurons inhibits transmission of painful stimuli in spinothalamic tracts, probably by their tonic inhibitory influence over opioid-dependent neurotransmission in internuncial neurons of laminae I, II, and V of the dorsal horn (for detailed review see ref. 22). This serotonin-dependent pathway has been implicated as a possible physiological correlate of pain inhibition said to originate in higher levels of the central nervous system as postulated in the gate control theory of pain transmission put forward by Melzak and Wall (23,24). The existence of this pathway may explain the potentiation of the analgesic effects of narcotic analgesics by serotonin precursors and, alternatively, its diminution by serotonin antagonists (25). Serotonin depletion, therefore, might perpetuate the chronic pain of fibromyalgia so that drugs such as amitriptyline and cyclobenzaprine, which competitively prevent the reuptake of serotonin in selected neuronal pathways, might be expected to lead to improvements in the pain of fibromyalgia. Depression, also thought to be related to a lack of serotonin in specific parts of the brain and often found concomitantly in patients with fibromyalgia, might be similarly improved.

Russell et al. have reported on experiments evaluating serotonin defficiency in fibromyalgia (11). These studies took advantage of the fact that peripheral blood platelets have high-avidity receptors for serotonin on their membrane surfaces. Radiolabeled imipramine may serve as a marker for serotonin reuptake sites on platelet membranes since it competes with serotonin for available receptors *in vitro*. Imipramine, unlike serotonin, is not susceptible to enzymatic degradation, so that measurement of radioactive imipramine uptake *in vitro* is thought to correlate with levels of brain serotonin (26–28). Russell et al.'s data show significantly higher receptor density for serotonin on peripheral blood platelets in fibromyalgia patients compared with pain-free controls (11). More importantly, improvements in clinical outcome measures after treatment with alprazolam and ibuprofen were associated with normalization of platelet receptor densities.

Some clinical evidence for the role of serotonin in other painful sites is worthy of mention in this context. Ward (29) recently noted that administration of fenfluramine, a relatively selective releaser of serotonin, led to decreased pain-reporting behavior in a subset of patients with low back pain.

This subset was comprised only of those patients who subsequently responded to treatment with antidepressants. Amitriptyline and cyclobenzaprine, therefore, might be expected to work because of their ability to prevent serotonin reuptake in critical parts of the central nervous system and spinal cord. This in turn would lead to a mustering of the patient's endogenous pain control mechanisms and return to homeostasis. Other clues to the mechanism of action of tricyclic antidepressants are emerging. Littlejohn et al. (30) recently postulated increased peripheral neurogenic hypersensitivity in fibromyalgia. Tricyclic antidepressants, therefore, might exert some benefit through their known anticholinergic effects, reducing hypersensitivity in peripheral sensory afferents to that their mode of action may be more pleiomorphic than discussed here.

Clinical Trials

Amitriptyline

There are at least two well-controlled studies of the effects of amitriptyline in patients with fibromyalgia. Carette et al. (2) reported on 59 patients who completed a 9-week double-blind trial comparing 50 mg of amitriptyline with placebo. Twenty-seven patients were randomized to the amitriptyline group and 32 to placebo. At the onset of the study patients were matched equally for age, sex, duration of morning stiffness, present pain intensity scores using a visual and analogue pain scale, and tenderness scores over reproducible fibrositic tender points. Pain thresholds over tender points were subjected to tests of intrarater and interrater reliability, and in this study five paired fibrositic tender points were deemed acceptable. Pain thresholds over fibrositic tender points were summed and expressed as Total Myalgic Score (TMS). Outcome measures were obtained at 5 and 9 weeks of treatment and consisted of (a) duration of morning stiffness, (b) self-report inventories of sleep quality, (c) patient and physician global assessment scores, (d) pain visual analogue scores, and (e) total myalgic scores.

Statistically and clinically significant improvement in quality of sleep and physician and patient global assessment scores were evident at 5 and 9 weeks of treatment in patients taking amitriptyline. Seventy-seven percent of patients experienced overall improvement at 5 weeks and 70% at 9 weeks in the amitriptyline group, compared with 43 and 50%, respectively, in the placebo-treatment group. Furthermore, the magnitude of improvement was greater in the amitriptyline group, with 55% of the patients assessing their disease as moderately to markedly improved, compared with 22% receiving placebo. While changes observed in total myalgic scores in the amitriptyline group were statistically significant, they were not deemed to be clinically important by the authors, amounting to only an average of 0.5 kg improvement for individual fibrositic tender points. However, the total mylagic score improved in 26 of 35 patients who reported an overall improvement, while scores remained unchanged or worsened in 15 of 24 patients reporting that their disease was unchanged or worse. There was no significant difference in the duration of morning stiffness between the two groups. Common side effects were drowsiness, agitation, gastrointestinal upset, or the onset of intercurrent illness (varicella, herpes zoster, pneumonia). Seven patients in the amitriptyline group and four patients in the placebo-treated group withdrew from the study. The authors concluded that amitriptyline was superior to placebo with respect to improvement in sleep quality and patient-physician global assessment scores.

These results were replicated in a study by Goldenberg et al. (3). Patients in this study were randomized to four treatment groups as follows: group 1 patients received naproxen 500 mg twice daily plus 25 mg of amitriptyline at bedtime; group 2 patients received naproxen and placebo; group 3 patients received placebo and amitriptyline; group 4 patients received double placebo. Outcome measures were performed at 2, 4, and 6 weeks and included patient global assessment, pain and sleep determination using a visual analogue score, physician global assessment, and pain threshold measurements over fibrositic tender points. A dropout rate similar to that noted in the Carette et al. study was observed, with major side effects of drowsiness and dry mouth accounted for by amitriptyline. The results indicated that group 1 patients fared the best, with statistically significant improvement in global assessments and pain scores. While group 2 patients, taking naproxen only, had improvements only in their pain scores, group 3 patients had significant improvement in both patient global assessment and fibrositic tender point scores. These latter improvements could not be explained by concomitant naproxen use. Combined naproxen and amitriptyline was therefore considered to be an effective regimen in ameliorating the manifestations of fibromyalgia. Importantly, naproxen alone was no better than placebo in this study, so that combined use of amitriptyline and naproxen was not recommended by the authors.

Amitriptyline, therefore, appears to be an effective agent for improving subjective sleep quality, visual analogue pain scores, and objective measurements of tenderness over fibrositic tender points. Furthermore, amitriptyline seems to be effective in improving both physician and patient global assessment scores. These studies open the way for trials of other tricyclic antidepressants in fibromyalgia.

Cyclobenzaprine

Cyclobenzaprine has also been tested in two recent collaborative trials (4–6). Bennett et al. (4,5) reported a study composed of 120 patients. Forty-four percent of the patients studied had fibromyalgia alone, whereas 56% of the patients also had concomitant rheumatoid arthritis, osteoarthritis, or a history of trauma precipitating the syndrome. Patients took cyclobenzaprine 10 to 40 mg at bedtime for 12 weeks in a double-blind crossover design. Patients assessed the efficacy of their treatment program using a take-home diary in which the following measures were recorded on a weekly basis: (a) pain, using a visual analogue scale; (b) quality of sleep, using a visual analogue scale; (c) duration of morning stiffness; and (d) duration of fatigue. Patients were evaluated by physician investigators at baseline and at weeks 1, 2, 4, 8, and 12. The following features were assessed: the degree of global musculoskeletal pain, tightness of shoulder girdle muscles as assessed by palpation, and number and degree of tenderness at 16 representative fibrositic tender points. Physician global assessment was evaluated at the end of the study on a 5-point Likert scale.

The dropout rate due to adverse reactions was not significant in the two treatment groups, and cyclobenzaprine was well tolerated over the 12-week observation period. Major side effects from cylcobenzaprine included dry mouth, drowsiness, and constipation, but these were also observed in the placebo group. Patient's self-evaluation diaries showed a uniform superiority of cyclobenzaprine for the symptoms of pain severity and sleep disturbance. Cyclobenzaprine did not show statistically significant improvements in fatigue and morning stiffness, however. Physician assessments showed improvements in muscle tightness in the shoulder girdle musculature, the number of tender points, and the tender point scores in the cyclobenzaprine-treated group for weeks 2 through 12. At the end of the study period, physician global assessment of patient therapeutic response was significantly greater in patients who had just completed 12 weeks of cyclobenzaprine therapy. A dropout analysis showed that 52% of the patients taking placebo withdrew because of a lack of beneficial response, compared with 16% of patients taking cyclobenzaprine. The results of this study indicated that patients with fibrositis experienced a greater overall improvement when treated with cyclobenzaprine as compared to placebo.

Quimby et al. (6) reported identical results using a similar study design. These studies indicate that cyclobenzaprine may have important salutary effects on the symptoms of patients with fibromyalgia.

Other Drugs

Several other medications have been shown to have little or no effect on the symptoms and signs of fibromyalgia. Imipramine, for example, was found to be ineffective in one report (8). This study was uncontrolled however, so that no assessment of type II error was possible. Imipramine, while theoretically promising, must therefore await the results of a properly designed study.

Similarly, phenothiazines have not been well studied but have been shown to be of limited usefulness because of the unacceptable incidence of side effects (9). They do, however, lead to a predictable improvement in sleep disturbance. Dothiepine has been reported to be superior to placebo in one study when given as a single dose of 75 mg at bedtime (7). Bengtsson et al. (13) have also reported on the beneficial effects of of regional sympathetic blockade in fibromyalgia. Alprazolam in combination with ibuprofen has been mentioned earlier in the context of serotonin deficiency (11). Antiinflammatory medications have shown disappointing results in clinical trials. Prednisone 20 mg/day (12) and naproxen 500 mg/day (3) were no more effective than placebo in properly controlled randomized trials. The novel compound S-adenosylmethionine (SAMe), which has both antidepressant and antiinflammatory properties, has been found to be more effective than placebo in one report (14). This study suffered from less stringent outcome measures and comprised only 17 patients, so that the role of this interesting compound requires further study.

Summary

In summary, several medications appear to demonstrate effectiveness in ameliorating the symptoms of fibromyalgia. The best studied of these are amitriptyline and cyclobenzaprine. Well-designed clinical trials have not been reported in sufficient detail for other tricyclic antidepressants. Nonsteroidal antiinflammatory drugs, while often used for this condition, have not been studied in detail, but preliminary evidence is disappointing. Of note is the fact that prednisone is of no value. Several agents, including the novel compound SAMe, are presently being studied but their role in fibromyalgia must await properly constructed clinical trials.

NONMEDICINAL THERAPIES

It is apparent from the foregoing discussion that drug therapy alone is often insufficient intervention for patients with fibromyalgia. Medicinal therapies are therefore often relegated to an adjunctive role, and it is often necessary to include a number of nonmedicinal modalities of treatment for patients with this disorder. A list of proposed nonmedical treatments is outlined in Table 2. Note that only the minority of such treatments have been studied using acceptable scientific criteria. At present, these modalities of therapy are used with little rationale, often in haphazard sequence, and rarely in consort with medicinal therapies. To date preliminary evidence exists for only two forms of such treatment, cardiovascular fitness training (31) and electromyographic (EMG) biofeedback training (32).

TABLE 2. *Proposed nonmedical treatments for fibromyalgia syndrome*

Treatment	Current status
Cardiovascular fitness training	Effective (31)
Electromyographic biofeedback training	Effective (32)
Transcutaneous electrical nerve stimulation	Not determined
Interferential current stimulation	Not determined
Acupuncture analgesia	Not determined
Local injection of tender points	Not determined
Postisometric relaxation	Not determined
Ice/heat range-of-motion exercise	Not determined
Laser therapy	Not determined
Massage	Not determined
Hypnosis	Not determined
Cognitive behavioral therapy	Not determined

Cardiovascular Fitness Training

A recent study (31) reported the effects of cardiovascular fitness training (CFT) on the manifestations of primary fibromyalgia. Forty-two patients fulfilling Smythe's original criteria were randomized to a 20-week program of either (a) CFT or (b) a flexibility exercise program (FLEX). Enhanced cardiovascular fitness was attained in 83% of those randomized to CFT and in none of the FLEX group. Significant improvement in pain threshold measurements over fibrositic tender points was noted in the CFT group when compared with FLEX-treated patients. Both physician and patient global assessment scores were also improved in the CFT group. No significant differences were found, however, between the groups in present pain intensity scores as measured by visual analogue scale, percentage total body area involved, or hours per night or nights per week of disturbed sleep. Psychological profiles were no different in the two groups before and after treatment. The authors concluded that CFT improved some objective and subjective measurements of pain in primary fibromyalgia.

Cardiovascular fitness training might be expected to confer benefit by a variety of mechanisms. First, it is well known that exercise leads to a predictable increase in serum levels of β-endorphin–like immunoreactivity, adrenocorticotrophic hormone (ACTH), prolactin, and growth hormone (33–36). These alterations are associated with a state of decreased pain sensitivity known as post-run hypoalgesia. Naloxone, an opioid receptor and antagonist, can abolish post-run hypoalgesia under certain conditions, indicating that strenuous exercise activates the body's endogenous opioid system (37). The beneficial effects of exercise noted in this study may have been due, then, to a harnessing of the body's own analgesic systems mediated primarily through opioid peptides. This notion is supported by a study of Janal et al. (38) in which 12 long-distance runners were evaluated on superficial, thermal, and deep ischemic pain tests before and after a 16-mile run. To determine which of these tests was mediated by endogenous opioids, naloxone or placebo was given before the run in a double-blind crossover design. Only the tourniquet ischemic test proved to be naloxone sensitive, indicating that deep pain, which incidentally is often described by fibromyalgic patients, was mediated through endogenous opioids. Tests of superficial types of pain (thermal) were not naloxone sensitive. It is conceivable, therefore, that CFT might exert some of its effects through activation of the endogenous opioid system.

Second, CFT at levels in excess of 60% of maximal oxygen capacity leads to predictable serum increases in both ACTH and cortisol (37). Because exercise is a complicated stimulus and induces a stress response, it would be expected that cortisol level would be high. This is indeed the case. Cortisol response to exercise occurs despite increased removal and follows the increase the ACTH (37). Therefore, exercise may act akin to stress-induced analgesia in animal models so that elevations of ACTH might be associated with post-run analgesic effect. It has not been proven that fibrositics have low levels of ACTH or that, if these are low, they would revert to normal after exercise. Some preliminary data are available on this point. We recently reported on hormonal changes in patients with fibromyalgia (39). In this study 20 patients with primary fibromyalgia were age and sex matched with rheumatoid arthritis patients who had similar nonrestorative sleep patterns. No differences were noted in diurnal variation of prolactin or growth hormone. However, a significantly smaller difference between peak (0800 hr) and trough (2000 hr) values (percentage variation) for serum cortisol and ACTH was noted for primary fibromyalgic patients compared with rheumatoid arthritis controls. This was noted in 70% of the fibromyalgic patients and in none of the rheumatoid arthritis controls. Abnormal dexamethasone suppression was present in 30% of the primary fibromyalgia patients and in only 5% of the rheumatoid arthritis patients. Four of seven patients with nonsuppressibility of serum cortisol also had abnormal percentage variation of serum ACTH. Overall, 30% of the fibromyalgia and 7% of the rheumatoid arthritis patients showed abnormal variation in ACTH. Further analysis stratified fibromyalgia patients into two groups with symptoms of greater or less than 2 years' duration. The former group showed (a) an even smaller percentage variation between trough and peak serum cortisols and (b) a higher incidence of abnormal dexamethasone suppression tests (54 versus 35%). It is tempting to speculate that exercise may have normalized the pituitary-adrenocortical axis such that the usual mechanisms of pain control were manifest.

EMG Biofeedback Training

Only one controlled study of the effects of biofeedback training (BFT) in primary fibromyalgia has been reported (32). This study consisted of an open trial of 15 patients who underwent 15 sessions of EMG biofeedback over a 5-week observation period. Nine patients had improvement in the number of fibrositic tender points, present pain intensity as measured by visual analogue scores, and morning stiffness. These improvements persisted up to 6 months after BFT had ceased. A follow-up study, randomizing 12 more patients to a similar regimen of EMG BFT or sham biofeedback, showed a significant improvement in visual analogue pain scores, morning stiffness and number of fibrositic tender points in the true EMG BFT group. Again, these differences were significant, both at 5 weeks and 6 months after treatment. While this study has some methodological difficulties, like the small number of patients and possible bias toward patients with psychological problems, it is worthy of attention. A recent report by the same authors indicated that EMG BFT reduces plasma ACTH and β-endorphin during treatment, indicating an opioid and/or neuroendocrine basis for some of the observed beneficial effects in primary fibromyalgia (40).

Implications for Treatment of Pain Using Nonmedicinal Treatment Modalities

It is clear from the foregoing analysis that it is possible to modulate the painful experience of patients with fibromyalgia through nonpharmacological means. Rational use of nonmedicinal therapy might be best predicted on an understanding of the mechanisms of pain production unique to this syndrome. Recent evidence suggests that the painful experience in fibromyalgia differs significantly from that in other painful states such as rheumatoid arthritis. Fibromyalgia patients generally characterize their pain as qualitatively more significant using a larger number of words on the McGill Pain Questionnaire, and indicate dispersal over a larger number of body surfaces. Quantitative estimates of their pain by self-report, however, are usually no different in magnitude than those of matched rheumatoid arthritis patients (41). All studies do seem to agree that measurement of pain threshold and pain tolerance, by whatever means, directly over fibrositic tender points is lower in fibromyalgia patients. However, studies disagree when pain threshold and pain tolerance are measured over nonfibrositic tender points (i.e., over "control" areas).

Campbell et al. (42), for example, reported that nonfibromyalgia patients attending a general medical outpatient clinic did not differ significantly from fibromyalgia patients in pain threshold measurements over four anatomical areas generally not considered to be fibrositic tender points. Alternatively, Scudds et al. (43), using a number of different pain-inducing stimuli, showed fibromyalgia patients to have significant decreases in pain threshold and pain tolerance levels when compared with healthy normal volunteers, but no differences in this respect when compared with age- and sex-matched clinic patients with rheumatoid arthritis. This was true only for dolorimeter readings; no differences were present when a pressure algometer or trains of electrical pulses were used to induce pain. Block et al. (44) agreed that fibromyalgia patients have lower pain tolerances over nonfibrositic tender points but argued that this is a general characteristic of patients with nonarticular rheumatism (patients with generalized muscular aching but no fibrositic tender points on examination). We have recently shown in a controlled double-blinded crossover trial of placebo versus amitriptyline that pain threshold measurements over nonfibrositic tender points do not improve after amitriptyline treatment or return to pretreatment levels during washout and placebo (45). These data taken together suggest some alteration in pain control mechanisms in primary fibromyalgia and implicate dysregulation of one or several descending inhibitory pain control pathways that modulate the painful experience.

There is growing evidence that simple ablation or pharmacological interference with peripheral sensory afferents does not result in prolonged pain relief. Local injection or dry needling of fibrositic tender points, therefore, may not be expected to provide long-lasting relief in PFS. If these techniques do provide long-term benefit it is likely that spinal gating mechanisms are altered or that central inhibitory pathways are activated. Future research in this area should be directed toward elucidation of these mechanisms. "Counterirritant" procedures such as ice, heat, ultrasound, interferential current stimulation, cold (helium-neon) laser, or transcutaneous electrical nerve stimulation might be expected to work through the gating mechanism proposed by Melzak and Wall (23,24). Nonpainful stimuli of these types delivered via large-fiber nonnociceptors may inhibit the pain transmission system at the spinal level. This may also involve activation of both opioid and nonopioid endogenous pain control mechanisms. This does not preclude concomitant activation of neuroendocrine-mediated systems of pain control. That the action of these particular modalities is complex is afforded by a double-blind study of the effects of cold (helium-neon) laser treatment of patients with chronic pain (46). During successful treatment urinary levels of 5-hydroxyindoleacetic acid were elevated, suggesting that this modality may activate endogenous pain pathways subserved by serotonin.

Cognitive behavioral therapy, hypnosis, and relaxation training may also act via more centrally originating pain-inhibitory pathways. It is more likely, however, that any successful modality will act by altering the pain transmission system at several levels. For other types of pain, acupuncture analgesia serves to illustrate this point. There is good evidence that acupuncture analgesia is mediated via the nervous system. For example, injection of local anesthetic around the peripheral nerve supplying an acupoint abolishes analgesia (47). Consensus of opinion indicates that analgesic signals are carried along large myelinated fibers (A fibers), closing the gate to further pain transmission at the spinal level. Since naloxone reverses acupuncture analgesia (48), it has been suggested that peripheral stimulation also activates enkephalin-containing neurons in the spinal cord, resulting in interference with pain transmission. However, since hypophysectomy in animals diminishes analgesia due to acupuncture (49), it might be possible that the pituitary plays a central role, perhaps through the release of β-enkephalin. This concept is corroborated by the observation that both β-endorphin and ACTH are released from the pituitary in response to acupuncture (50). To complicate matters, serotonin has also been implicated; reserpine, which depletes stores of brain serotonin, increases the analgesic effects of acupuncture when given 24 hr prior to treatment (51). Acupuncture analgesia, therefore, is mediated by a number of pain control pathways and systems and illustrates the concept that future successful treatments for primary fibromyalgia must rely on strategies based on a clear understanding of pain transmission systems and their various interactions.

Conclusions

What portends for future studies of nonmedicinal modalities of therapy for patients with fibromyalgia? Clearly the painful experience, as well as those physiological mechanisms that subserve it, are both intricate and interconnected. As scientists, we have so far been able to prove that only a few of these modalities actually work. Our present state of knowledge suggests that we can influence pain transmission by a number of potential mechanisms:

1. Eradication of transmission along nociceptive neurons.
2. Perturbation of spinal gating mechanisms.
3. Enhancement of the activity of descending pain-inhibitory systems through peripheral sensory afferents.
4. Enhancing central inhibitory neurons at the cognitive level.
5. Reducing unbridled discharges in the sympathetic nervous system as a result of the painful experience.
6. A combination of any of the above.

Summary

To date few nonmedicinal treatments for primary fibromyalgia have been studied using acceptable scientific standards. This has led to rather arbitrary use of disparate treatment modalities, often in haphazard sequence. Because primary fibromyalgia syndrome is a chronic painful condition, the rationale for treatment should be based on present concepts of pain perception supported by studies in the basic sciences. Recent clinical studies in the treatment of primary fibromyalgia syndrome conforming to the scientific method are discussed in light of what is presently known about pain transmission and perception.

REFERENCES

1. Felson DT, Goldenberg DL. *Arthritis Rheum* 1986;29:1522–1526.
2. Carette S, McCain GA, Bell DA, Fam A. *Arthritis Rheum* 1986;29:655–659.
3. Goldenberg DL, Felson DT, Dinerman H. *Arthritis Rheum* 1986;29:1371–1377.
4. Bennett RM, Gatter RA, Campbell SM, Andrews RP, Clark RA, Scarlo JA. *Arthritis Rheum* 1988;31:1535–1542.
5. Campbell SM, Gatter RA, Clarke S, Bennett RM. *Arthritism Rheum* 1984;27:S76 (abstr).
6. Quimby LG, Gratwick GM Whitney CA, Block SR. *J Rheumatol* 1989 (in press).
7. Caruso I, Sarzi Puttini PC, et al. *J Int Med Res* 1987;15:154–159.
8. Wysenbeek AJ, Nor F, Lurie Y, Weinburger A. *Ann Rheum Dis* 1985;44:752–753.
9. Moldofsky H, Scarisbrick P, England E. *Psychosom Med* 1975;37:341–351.
10. Moldofsky H, Scarisbrick P. *Psychosom Med* 1976;38:35–44.
11. Russell IJ, Bowden CL, Michalek J, et al. *Arthritis Rheum* 1987;30:S63.
12. Clark S, Tindall E, Bennett RA. *J Rheumatol* 1985;12:980–983.
13. Bengtsson A, Bengtsson M, Lofstrom SJB. *Pain* 1987;31(suppl 4):S295.
14. Tavoni A, Vitali C, Bombardieri S, et al. *Am J Med* 1987; 83(suppl 5A):107–110.
15. Cathey MS, Wolfe F, Kleinheksel SM, et al. *Am J Med* 1986;81:78–84.
16. Goldenberg DL. *Rheum Dis Clin North Am* 1989;15:61–71.
17. Hawley DJ, Wolfe F, Cathey MA. *J Rheumatol* 1988;15:1551–1556.
18. Sicuteri F. *Headache* 1972;12:69–72.
19. Van Woert MH, Sethy VH. *Neurology* 1975;25:135–140.
20. Harvey JA, Schlosberg AJ, Yunger LM. *Fed Proc* 1975;34:796–801.
21. Messing RB, Fisher LA, Phebus L, et al. *Life Sci* 1976;18:707–714.
22. Cassem NH. In: Rubenstein E, Federman DD, eds. *Scientific American Medicine*. New York: Scientific American Inc, 1988;1–14.
23. Melzack R. *The puzzle of pain*. New York: Basic/Harper Torchbooks, 1973.
24. Melzak R, Wall PD. *Science* 1965;150:971.
25. Samanin R, Valzelli L. *Arch Int Pharmacodyn* 1972;196:138–141.
26. Briley MS, Langer RZ, Raisman R, et al. *Science* 1980;209:303–305.
27. Paul SM, Rehavi M, Skolnick P, Ballenger JC, Goodwin FK. *Arch Gen Psychiatry* 1981;38:1315–1317.
28. Suranyi-Cadotte BE, Wood PL, Nair NP, Schwartz G. *Eur J Pharmacol* 1982;85:357–358.
29. Ward NG. *Spine* 1986;11:661–665.
30. Littlejohn GO, Weinstein C, Helme RD. *J Rheumatol* 1987;14:1022–1025.
31. McCain GA, Bell DA, Mai FM, Halliday P. *Arthritis Rheum* 1988;31:1135–1141.
32. Furaccioli G, Chirelli L, Scita F, et al. *J Rheumatol* 1987;14:820–825.
33. Farrell PA. *Med Sci Sports Exerc* 1985;17:1, 89–93.
34. Grossman A. *Clin Cardiol* 1984;71:255–260.
35. Grossman A, Sutton JR. *Med Sci Sports Exerc* 1985; 17:74–81.
36. Harber VI, Sutton JR. *Sports Med* 1984;1:154–171.
37. Howlett TA. *Clin Endocrinol* 1987;26:723–742.
38. Janal MN, Colt EWD, Clark WC, Glusman M. *Pain* 1984;19:13–25.
39. McCain GA, Tilbe KS *J Rheumatol* 1989 (in press).
40. Molina E, Cecchettin M, Fontana S. *Fed Proc* 1987;46:1357.
41. Leavitt HF, Katz RS, Golden HE, Glickman PB, Layfer LF. *Arthritis Rheum* 1986;29:775–781.
42. Campbell SM, Clark S, Tindall EA, et al. *Arthritis Rheum* 1983;26:817–824.
43. Scudds RA, Rollman GB, Harth M, McCain GA. *J Rheumatol* 1987;14:563–569.
44. Block SR, Quimby LG, Gratwick GM. *Arthritis Rheum* 1987;30:4(B40).
45. Scudds RA, McCain GA, Rollman GB, Harth M. *J Rheumatol* 1989 (in press).
46. Walker J. *J Neurol Transm* 1977;40:305–308.

47. Lowe WC. *Introduction to acupuncture anesthesia.* London: Kimpton, 1973.
48. Peng CH, Yang MM, Kok SH, Woo YK. *Comp Med East West* 1978;6:57–60.
49. Pomeranz B, Cheng RS, Law P. *Exp Neurol* 1977;54:172–178.
50. Pomeranz B. *Persistent pain: modern methods of treatment.* London: Academic Press, 1981.

Advances in Pain Research and Therapy, Vol. 17,
edited by James R. Fricton and Essam Awad.
Raven Press, Ltd., New York © 1990.

20

Treatment of Patients with Fibromyalgia Syndrome

Consideration of the Whys and Wherefores

I. Jon Russell

Department of Medicine, The University of Texas Health Science Center, San Antonio, Texas 78284

Fibromyalgia syndrome (FS) is a relatively common clinical disorder characterized by musculoskeletal pain, so widely distributed about the body that patients often say they "hurt all over." The typical physical finding is tenderness to digital palpation at specifiic soft tissues sites. Considerable progress has been made in achieving consensus regarding diagnostic criteria, so investigative attention should now be increasingly directed toward developing rational therapy.

Several distinct issues need to be considered in the course of making therapeutic decisions. They are generic to the management of all medical illnesses, but will herein be applied to FS. It goes without saying that the diagnosis must be correct in order to learn anything constructive from experimental treatment protocols. A better understanding of the responsible pathogenesis is likely to suggest novel approaches to treatment that might not be considered without such insight. Documentation of a therapeutic response to any proposed intervention is dependent upon the use of one or more valid outcome measures. Since most medical treatments incur some risk of adverse effects, the range of modalities to be seriously considered must depend on the perceived severity of the disorder. Finally, each patient presents a unique background of problems and concerns, so treatment regimens that are found to be helpful in the average patient must be tailored to each individual needing care.

The approach used in the following paragraphs is to first raise an issue in the form of a question and then briefly discuss its current status. The purpose is not to be encyclopedic or comprehensive, but to illustrate the concept as it might apply to "designer therapy" for FS.

DIAGNOSIS

Is the diagnosis correct and complete?

It cannot yet be stated that clinicians are in full agreement on uniform criteria for the diagnosis of FS, but that goal may be achieved in the very near future. A representative composite of rheumatology practitioners and active investigators in the field participated in a study (1) designed to establish such criteria. It was generally agreed that patients with FS should have experienced widespread musculoskeletal pain for at least 3 months, in order to exclude the myalgias and arthralgias associated with a variety of self-limiting febrile conditions. When a requirement for subjective tenderness at 11 of 18 specified tender points about the body was added, the criteria provided a very acceptable sensitivity of 88.6% and specificity of 81.1%.

There was no real difference in the way these criteria applied to primary FS patients or to those whose FS was concomitant with another medical condition, so it was suggested that the historical distinction of "secondary FS" be abandoned.

It is still important, of course, to identify other clinical conditions that would merit separate specific treatment. After a thorough history and physical examination, seeking evidence for arthritis, myopathic weakness, chronic infectious diseases, and endocrine dysfunction, the relatively simple laboratory screening profile shown in Table 1 may be appropriate. Based on available evidence, however, it cannot be anticipated that treatment of any associated medical illness will dramatically improve the concomitant symptoms of FS.

TABLE 1. *Diagnostic studies useful in seeking concomitant medical illnesses*

Illness	Tests[a]
Rheumatic disease	
Systemic lupus erythematosus	ANA + ESR
Rheumatoid arthritis	RF + ESR
Polymyositis	CPK
Chronic infections	
Tuberculosis	PPD + ESR
Chronic syphilis	VDRL
Subacute bacterial endocarditis	Culture + ESR
Endocrine disorders	
Hypothyroidism	T_4 + TSH

[a] ANA, antinuclear antibodies; ESR, erythrocyte sedimentation rate; RF, rheumatoid factor; CPK, creatine phosphokinase; PPD, purified protein derivative; VDRL, Venereal Disease Research Laboratories; T_4, thyroxine; TSH, thyroid-stimulating hormone.

PATHOGENESIS

What is the pathogenesis of the disorder?

The etiology of FS is not known, but a variety of abnormalities found in this patient population has led to several different theories regarding its pathogenesis (2–11). Among them, the serotonin deficiency hypothesis (9,11) is appealing because it could potentially explain many of the observed findings in this disorder. In a series of publications, Moldofsky et al. (9,10,12) described the cliinical logic behind their suggestion that serotonin might be involved. Serotonin was known to be a neurotransmitter with a role in the regulation of deep restorative sleep and in the interpretation of painful stimuli (13).

Tryptophan is an essential amino acid and the metabolic precursor or serotonin. Free plasma tryptophan can be actively transferred across the blood-brain barrier into the central nervous system (14). There it is taken up by serotonergic nuclei like the brainstem's raphe nucleus. Stimulation of that nucleus results in the release of serotonin at multiple brain sites (15). Moldofsky and Warsh (12) found relatively normal *free plasma* tryptophan in patients with FS, but demonstrated an inverse relationship between its concentration and the severity of the patient's symptoms. Recogniziing the potential of their findings, Moldofsky's group administered tryptophan to FS patients. As was hoped, there was some improvement in the sleep, but, surprisingly, the musculoskeletal symptoms were worse.

Following Moldofsky's lead, our group in San Antonio measured *total serum* tryptophan [free + protein adherent] in samples from 20 FS patients and matched controls (16). The results indicated a significantly lower level of tryptophan in the patients than in the controls, but the more surprising observation was that six other amino acids were also significantly low. It should be noted that another study examining the levels of *total plasma* amino acids failed to show a difference between FS patients and controls (M. Yunus, personal communication, 1989). The reasons for the apparent discrepancies remain to be explained.

A relative deficiency of several amino acids could potentially explain why Moldofsky and Warsh's tryptophan supplementation experiment (12) produced the results it did. The tryptophan may have corrected the serotonin deficiency, but at the same time precipitated a crisis in protein synthesis. It is known (17) from other amino acid deficiency states that supplementation of only one of several deficient amino acids can cause the deficiency of the others to become hypercritical.

It is curious that seven amino acids would be low in FS patients. If these findings can be confirmed, it will be necessary to determine why this is so. Is there inadequate digestion of proteins, impaired absorption from the gut, disordered urinary excretion, or some even less obvious explanation? A potentially informative dietary experiment with FS patients would be to replace all seven of the deficient amino acids, rather than just tryptophan, and see if the response is better than it was with just tryptophan (12).

Serotonin is the metabolic product of tryptophan's oxidative decarboxylation. To evaluate its status in nine FS patients and their matched controls (18), our group measured the serum concentration of serotonin. The mean value for the patients was found to be significantly lower than that of the controls. It is known that platelets store great quantities of serotonin, which can later be released during clot formation. Since serum was used for that experiment, some of the measured serotonin could have come from platelets activated by the clotting process *in vitro*. Thus, it will be important to determine whether the low serum serotonin measured was due to low circulating plasma levels *in vivo* among the patients or resulted from differences in the way platelet degranulation occurred in the two groups.

Another interesting finding tends to support the impression that plasma serotonin may be low in FS. Peripheral blood platelets have on their surface membranes a serotonin reuptake receptor, which seems to quantitatively parallel the similar receptor in the central nervous system (19). Imipramine and a number of other psychoactive drugs are known to bind to the serotonin reuptake receptor, where they compete with binding by serotonin (20). Peripheral blood platelets from 22 FS patients revealed a significantly higher mean density of those receptors than did those from matched normal controls (18). That might be expected to occur by servo mechanism if the ambient serotonin concentration were too low.

An abnormality in the function of natural killer (NK) cells in FS patients may also be due indirectly to a deficiency of serotonin (21,22). While there were normal numbers of phenotypically positive NK cells in the peripheral blood of FS patients, they did not lyse tumor cell targets as effectively as did NK cells from normal individuals (23). That implies a failure to maintain normal numbers of *activated* NK cells. The explanation may hinge on the fact that serotonin regulates the release of "NK cell cytotoxicity effector factor" from monocytes (21). A decrease in the ambient serotonin concentration in FS patients would apparently down-regulate the NK cell activation and give the observed low level of NK function in FS.

There has been much interest in the study by Vaeroy (24), who reported threefold higher levels of substance P in the cerebrospinal fluid (CSF) of FS patients than in the CSF of normal controls. It was previously known (25) that substance P exerts a dampening effect on the discharges of sensory nerves in the presence of normal or high levels of serotonin. When serotonin levels are lower than normal, substance P fails to exercise that control. A lower than normal level of serotonin could not only alter the central nervous system threshold for incoming painful signals, but may actually cause those signals to be amplified.

Finally, some of the pharmaceutical interventions that have been found to be effective in the treatment of FS (26–29) are known to influence serotonin metabolism or function. Amitriptyline and cyclobenzaprine have similar tricyclic structures. It has been suggested that they increase the available serotonin in the interneural junction by inhibiting its reuptake by the afferent neuron. They may also inhibit the oxidative metabolism of serotonin to 5-hydroxyindoleacetic acid.

Alprazolam also appears to be useful in this disorder (30). Of mechanistic interest was the finding that FS patients taking alprazolam and ibuprofen normalized the density of serotonin reuptake receptors on their peripheral platelets (18). Since platelets are the major repository of serotonin in the peripheral blood, there may be some significance (reviewed in ref. 31) to the observation that alprazolam inhibits the action of platelet-activating factor on platelets (32).

This kind of information will be particularly useful if it eventually leads investigators to consider new therapeutic approaches. The goal would be to use the pathogenic data to design therapy directed at the underlying mechanism of FS to provide a cure, or at least better symptomatic relief than is now possible.

OUTCOME MEASURES

Is there a valid measure of outcome?

When a patient returns to the physician after having tried a therapeutic intervention, it is important that the clinician have some means of determining whether the patient benefited. In a condition such as diabetes or hypertension, a simple check of the blood glucose or resting blood pressure, respectively, may suffice, but in FS the problem is pain. Pain is an individual sensation that is currently impossible to quantify. On the other hand, its severity must be assessed among FS patients in order to document therapeutic responses. Two approaches that have been used in FS with some success are "self-report" and "response to painful stimuli."

Several self-report questionnaire instruments have been developed to help patients describe the magnitude and character of their pain. Perhaps the most useful is the simple 10-cm horizontal line known as the visual analog scale (VAS) (34). The left end of the VAS is labeled "no pain" while its right extremity is labeled "severe pain." The patient simply marks the point on that scale that best describes the severity of pain experienced over the past 7 days. Comparing the pre- and postintervention value provides a valid assessment of response.

The diagnostic criteria for FS (13) require that the examining clinician press on tender points about the musculoskeletal system to determine whether patients have undue tenderness at those sites. About 4 kg of pressure

TABLE 2. *Palpation tenderness severity scale and tender point index*[a]

Severity scale	Patient response to pressure (4 kg/cm^2)
0	Only pressure reported
1 +	Tenderness reported verbally, but la belle indifference, no physical response
2 +	Tenderness reported plus an objective physical response (wince, withdrawal)
3 +	Tenderness reported with emphasis, plus an exaggerated, dramatic physical response (wince, jerk, withdrawal)
4 +	Untouchable area; the anticipated pain is so severe that the patient avoids the expected palpation.

Adapted to table form from Russell et al., ref. 11.
[a] Sum of severities at 16 sites.

(about the amount of pressure required to blanch blood from the examiner's thumb nail) is applied to the tender or control point while observing the patient's response.

A simple 5-point severity scale, based on tenderness to palpation, has been developed (11) and tested extensively (1,30). As shown in Table 2, patients can subjectively report pressure only (= 0) or pain (= 1). The clinician should observe the patient's face and the body part being examined for evidence of a semiinvoluntary physical response resulting from pain induced by the applied pressure. There may be a wince, grimace, or withdrawal (= 2) or dramatic exaggerated withdrawal (= 3) to indicate ''objectification'' of the pain response. If the patient refuses to be examined at a specific site because of anticipated severe pain, the site is given a severity score of 4.

The sum of the severities at all of the examined sites is called the Tender Point Index (TPI). That value, which can be easily obtained in 2 min with the patient, has been shown to decrease with improvement in symptoms and to increase when the pain is more severe. It also provides a semiobjective parameter to follow at low cost to the patient.

Another semiobjective measure comparable to the TPI is the Dolorimeter Pain Index (DPI). A spring-loaded or other strain gauge instrument is pressed against a tender point until the patient reports a change in the resultant sensation from pressure to pain (35). That so-called pain threshold is usually above 4 kg for normal, pain-free controls and less than 4 kg for FS patients. The average of these values at a designated number of sites (DPI) varies inversely with the severity of pain and the TPI (30). The DPI is somewhat easier to standardize than the TPI but has the disadvantage of requiring the purchase of the device and the addition of decimal numbers, whereas the TPI uses the clinician's fingers and involves adding small whole numbers.

Which ever method is used to quantitate the patient's tenderness, it is recommended that a value be recorded at each clinical visit, so the pattern of responses to therapy can be systematically assessed in a relatively objective manner. Coupling this with the patient's self-report will allow a more structured approach to trial of therapeutic interventions for individual patients.

DISEASE SEVERITY

How severe is FS in the average patient?

Approaching this question presents a whole new spectrum of problems to the investigator. The answer cannot realistically be viewed in a vacuum but is best evaluated in relation to other well-recognized disorders. Rheumatoid arthritis has been selected as the comparison disease by several authors because it involves the musculoskeletal system, is known to be painful, and has a well-characterized disabling potential (36).

When well-validated assessment instruments were applied to 101 FS patients (37) in a manner identical to that used in studying 303 rheumatoid arthritis (38), the resultant data indicated little or no difference in the severity of perceived pain, in the effect of these diseases on quality of life, or in their overall severity. Similarly, Cathey et al. (39) found only a slight difference in the work capacity of patients with these disorders. These finding suggest that FS may be comparable in severity to rheumatoid arthritis, at least from the view of the respective patients.

One of the implications of that finding pertains to treatment. Rheumatoid arthritis is recognized to be an aggressive, destructive disease with sufficient disabling potential to merit use of potentially toxic drugs (36). The trend with FS, on the other hand, has been to limit interventions to psychological support, exercise, and benign medications, because it was thought not to warrant any risk from therapy.

Considering the findings described above, one could argue that such an approach is unduly conservative. Perhaps FS patients and their physicians would be justified in considering therapies not now being evaluated because they are expensive or because they carry some risk of side effects. In addition, research seeking innovative approaches to therapy of FS should be backed by financial resources comparable to that now being invested in the study of rheumatoid arthritis.

INDIVIDUALIZATION

What factors should be considered when the physician is called to personalize therapy for a specific patient?

As with any clinical disorder, the severity of FS varies with each affected individual. One patient may only occasionally experience discomfort after physical exertion or during inclement weather. On the other end of that spectrum is the patient who said "Every day, the pain feels like I played volley ball in the hot sun all day at the beach." Adding a generalized sunburn to the muscle soreness of unaccustomed activity makes a painful syndrome that cannot be ignored for a minute. Every move is an agony and brief sleep comes only with exhaustion.

Then, too, each patient has a unique attitude toward medical care. The priorities and goals the patient brings to the doctor-patient relationship must be taken into consideration. Most patients desire relief from pain. Some expect the physician to do whatever it takes to achieve that objective. Others may be willing to accept some residual discomfort rather than having to take daily medication. Just a confident diagnosis is sufficient for some FS patients, because it spells an end to the constant search for understanding, after a multitude of fruitless diagnostic procedures.

Patients should be informed honestly regarding what can and cannot be expected from therapy of this disorder. They should known that therapy for FS is aimed at a reduction in the severity of symptoms and an educated adaptation to the pattern of remissions following exacerbations. They should be told that there is currently no cure for FS, but that the physician will keep the patient up to date with new developments as they become available.

It is helpful to initiate a "management partnership," which means that "We will *work together* to resolve this problem as well as possible for you." That approach gives patients a realistic view of the current status of treatment. It also gives them a combination of responsibility and control over their health outcome, which has been shown to be valuable (40), but lacking in FS patients (41).

It may be useful to determine the frequency with which a FS patient was seen by any health care professional in the prior 12 months, and then schedule to see that patient with about that same frequency during the subsequent 12 months. That gives the patient confidence in the physician's attention and in his/her commitment to the care partnership.

The physician's expectations must also be realistic. A family practice resident once lamented "her illness and I paired off like two gladiators—but alas the patient rooted for her illness" (W. Katon, personal communication), implying that her patient wanted to be sick. On the other hand, if modern-day physicians were to give iron rather than insulin to their type I diabetics, they should not blame the patients if patients fail to improve. In the same way, clinicians must realize that therapy for FS is still largely experimental. As a result, patients may not be entirely responsible for less than optimal outcomes.

Finally, as T. F. Main stated, "The sufferer who frustrates a keen therapist by failing to improve is always in danger of meeting *primitive human behavior* disguised as treatment" (42). Doctors need to maintain a generous, caring attitude toward their FS patients and avoid reacting with anger or defense when patients don't magically get well. In so doing, they will avoid contributing to the problem.

SUMMARY

In summary, it can be stated that the understanding of FS is improving. Not only can the diagnosis be made with confidence and the severity at any point in time be assessed, but a better view of its pathogenesis may be within reach. Treatment must be appropriate to the severity of the symptoms and tailored to the needs of each patient. Realistic expectations on the part of patients and physicians will help to maintain perspective.

REFERENCES

1. Wolfe F, Smythe HA, Yunus MB, Bennett RM, Bombardier C, Goldenberg DL, Tugwell P, Campbell SM, Abeles M, Clark P, Fam AG, Farber SJ, Fiechtner JJ, Franklin CM, Gatter RA, Hamaty D, Lessard J, Lichtbroun AS, Masi AT, McCain GA, Reynolds WJ, Romano TJ, Russell IJ, Sheon RP. *Arthritis Rheum* 1989; 32(suppl 4):S47 (abstr), 1990 (in press).
2. Bengtsson A, Henriksson KG, Larsson J. *Arthritis Rheum* 1986;29:817.
3. Caro XJ. *Arthritis Rheum* 1984;27:1174.
4. Caro XJ. *Am J Med* 1986;81:43–49.
5. Danneskiold-Samsøe B, Christiansen E, Lund B, Andersen RB. *Scand J Rehab Med* 1982;15:17.
6. Gerster JC,, Hadj-Djilani A. *J Rheumatol* 1984;11:678.
7. Hudson JI, Hudson MS, Pliner LF, Goldenberg DL, Pope HG. *Am J Psychol* 1985;142:441.
8. Kalyan-Raman UP, Kalyan-Raman K, Yunus MB, Masi AT. *J Rheumatol* 1984;11:808.
9. Moldofsky H. *Adv Neurol* 1982;33:51–57.
10. Moldofsky H, Scarisbrick BS. *Psychosom Med* 1976;38:35.
11. Russell IJ, Vipraio G, Morgan WW, Bowden CL. *Am J Med* 1986;81(suppl 3A):50–56.
12. Moldofsky H, Warsh JJ. *Pain* 1978;5:65–71.
13. Harvey JA, Schlosberg AJ, Yunger LM. *Fed Proc* 1975;34:1796–1801.
14. Gessa GL, Biggio G, Fadda F. Corsini GU, Tagliamonte A. *J Neurochem* 1974;22:869–870.
15. Mouret J, Coindet J. *Brain Res* 1980;186:273–287.
16. Russell IJ, Vipraio GA, Michalek JE, Fletcher EM, Wall KA. *J Rheumatol* 1989;16(suppl 19):158–163.
17. Anonymous. *Nutr Rev* 1968;26:115–118.
18. Russell IJ, Bowden CL, Michalek J, Fletcher E, Hester GA. *Arthritis Rheum* 1988;30(suppl):S63.
19. Briley MS, Raisman R, Langer SZ. *Eur J Pharmacol* 1979;58:347–348.
20. Paul SM, Rehavi M, Rice KC, Ittah Y, ,Skolnick P. *Life Sci* 1981;28:2753–2760.
21. Helstrand K, Hermodsson S. *J Immunol* 1987;139:869–875.
22. Sternberg EM, Trial J, Parker CW. *J Immunol* 1986;137:276–282.
23. Russell IJ, Vipraio GA, Tovar Z, Michalek J, Fletcher E. *Arthritis Rheum* 1988;31(suppl):S24.
24. Vaeroy H, Helle R, Forre O, Kass E, Terenius L. *Pain* 1988;32:;21–26.
25. Murphy RM, Zemlan FP. *Psychopharmacology (Berlin)* 1987;93:118–121.
26. Bennett RM, Gatter RA, Campbell SM, et al. *Arthritis Rheum* 1988;31:1535–1542.
27. Carette S, McCain GA, Bell DA, et al. *Arthritis Rheum* 1986;29:655–659.
28. Goldenberg DL, Felson DT, Dinerman H. *Arthritis Rheum* 1986;29:1371–1377.
29. Quimby L. Paper presented at the Third Dunlop Symposium, London, Ontario, 1988.

30. Russell IJ, Fletcher EM, Hester GA, Michalek JE, Vipraio GA. *Arthritis Rheum* 1989;32(suppl):S69.
31. Russell IJ. *Rheum Dis Clin North Am* 1989;15:149–168.
32. Chesney CM, Pifer DD, Cagen LM. *Biochem Biophys Res Commun* 1987;144:359–366.
33. Leavitt F, Katz RS, Golden HE, Glickman PB, Layfer LF. *Arthritis Rheum* 1986;29:775–781.
34. Scott J, Huskinsson EC. *Pain* 1976;2:175–184.
35. Simms RW, Goldenberg DL, Felson DT, Mason JH. *Arthritis Rheum* 1988;31:182.
36. Pincus T, Callahan LF, Sale WG, Brooks AL, Payne LE, Vaughn WK. *Arthritis Rheum* 1984;27:864–872.
37. Russell IJ, Fletcher EM, Tsui J, Michalek JE. *Arthritis Rheum* 1989;32:S70.
38. Bombardier C, Ware J, Russell IJ, Larson M, Chalmers A, Read JL. *Am J Med* 1986;81:565.
39. Cathey MA, Wolfe F, Kleinheksel SM. *Arthritis Care Res* 1988;1:85.
40. Strickland BR. *J Consult Clin Psychol* 1978;46:1192–1211.
41. Bishop GA, Russell IJ, Fletcher EM, Caro XJ, Wolfe F. *Arthritis Rheum* 1989 (submitted).
42. Main TF. *Br J Med Psychol* 1957;30:129–145.

Advances in Pain Research and Therapy, Vol. 17,
edited by James R. Fricton and Essam Awad.
Raven Press, Ltd., New York © 1990.

21

Management of Muscular Pain Associated with Articular Dysfunction

K. Lewit

Central Railway Health Institute, Prague, Czechoslovakia

THE CONCEPT OF DYSFUNCTION

The subject of this chapter is pain due to dysfunction, most frequently referred to as "nonspecific pain" (1). This type of pain occurs in over 90% of patients affected by myofascial pain syndromes as well as in dysfunctional joints, which after appropriate treatment allow normal function again. In myofascial pain, a muscle with a trigger point contains fibers that do not properly decontract when the muscle relaxes; this can be relieved almost instantly by spray and stretch or postisometric relaxation (PIR) (2,3). In joint dysfunction, there may be joint restriction, or binding without structural pathology that also is quickly resolved with appropriate treatment. Both of these changes are usually accompanied by painful changes in the connective tissues that also recede immediately if the articular or muscle problem is adequately dealt with.

What does the term "nonspecific pain" imply? It means that no specific pathological or structural lesions can be identified by autopsy or biopsy. As has been pointed out, the changes seen can be relieved immediately after appropriate treatment. This certainly suggests that there are no structural pathological changes, because if these were present, the patient would require much longer to recover or would require surgery. However, clinical thinking has been under the tutelage of the pathologist for so long, that respectable clinicians dealing with the motor system refuse to call the child by its proper name: disturbances of function or simply dysfunction. This is by no means a subterfuge, since true pathology has not yet been found, but is, rather, a fundamental issue. Just as a machine does not work because a ball bearing or a cylinder has burst, it also won't function if the distributor or carburetor is not correctly adjusted. In this case, the structure is basically intact and a mere adjustment will make it function immediately.

This is the basis of what we call "functional pathology" (4) and is the key to the high percentage of patients affected by pain from the motor system. This is also the most important point of distinction from structural pathology, requiring a fundamentally different approach to the patient's problem, a distinction comparable to "hardware" and "software." It also implies, unfortunately, that software is by no means less complicated than hardware, but that a different approach is required.

THE EXPRESSION OF PAIN

One of the immediate consequences of this difference in approach is that we have to rely more on clinical rather than laboratory or instrumental methods in diagnosis, treatment, and even research, because the most frequent symptom of impaired locomotor function is pain. The structure in the motor system that reacts most to stimuli and is the effector of the nervous system is the muscle (5). As a result, it is also the structure that most regularly and intensively expresses pain. This is done by creating trigger points both in its contractile elements and its attachment points (6). Even if a joint is involved, we find trigger points in the corresponding muscles and/or there may be an analgesic posture (as in acute disc lesions) maintained by painful muscle spasm. Even visceral disease expresses pain via the motor system by creating trigger points in muscles (7). This is discussed in more detail in Chapter 14 by Fossgreen (*this volume*).

DISTINCTIONS BETWEEN JOINT AND MUSCLE DYSFUNCTION

Because of the need for a different approach in therapy for nonspecific pain, it is necessary to distinguish between pain due to a muscular trigger point and that due to a restricted (blocked) dysfunctional joint. As will be pointed out, this is not a simple task, and our current knowledge may be aptly called a picture of our present state of ignorance.

Naively, we have been taught that the muscle is concerned with active motion and the joint with passive mobility. However, as Korr (8) has pointed out, "while thinking of muscles as the motors of the body . . . it is important to remember that the same contractile forces are also used to oppose motion." This is demonstrated clearly with the straight leg raising test, in which no joint limits mobility. Moreover, we recently have used "muscle energy techniques" (9) in moving a restricted joint to demonstrate the importance of the muscular factor. In fact, it is not difficult to show that in studying joint movement restriction a muscular factor is usually present. Why then bother about joints and use manipulation? And if manipulation is useful clinically, why does it work and when is it the most effective approach?

There is evidence that both muscular and articular factors are important in nonspecific pain, and one of the two may predominate in any specific

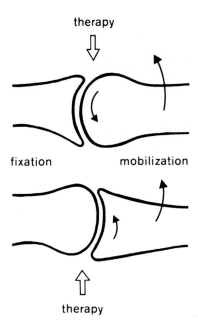

FIG. 1. Joint play is often affected in musculoskeletal dysfunction. This movement is characterized by passive translatory, gapping, and in some cases rotation movement.

case. However, evidence for articular involvement admittedly is purely clinical (10). This includes:

1. There are joints that are neither moved nor opposed by muscles and can still be limited. These include the acromioclavicular, the sacroiliac, and the tibiofibular joints. Interestingly, they can be quickly mobilized with a minimum of force and without using muscle energy techniques.

2. As a rule, joint play is affected first in nonspecific pain. Joint play, according to Mennell (11), is a type of movement that can be induced passively. It is mainly translatory motion between joint surfaces (Fig. 1) (12), but can also include gapping and in some cases rotation. Therefore, this movement cannot be produced by the patient's muscles nor is it likely to be opposed by muscles.

3. In thrusting a joint, we produce a gapping effect in the joint, which is audible, and joint mobility can be restored. This has been explained by a sudden stretch of muscles and tendons at the extreme range of movement. However, by distraction of a joint, we can also produce a gapping effect in a neutral position (Fig. 2). In this case, freeing the joint can then occur without stretching muscles or tendons.

4. In order to demonstrate the role of articulation in nonspecific pain the following experiment was undertaken. Ten patients with nonspecific neck pain but no cervical pathology had the cervical spine examined prior to surgery (mainly abdominal surgery) and reexamined under general aesthesia

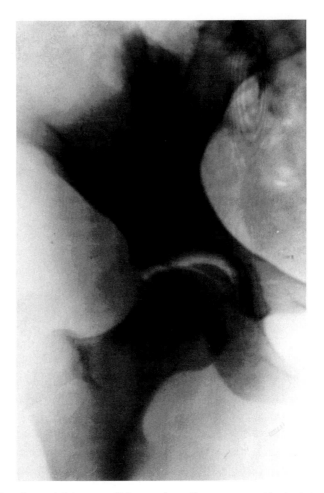

FIG. 2. In thrusting a joint, an audible gapping effect occurs with the joint in neutral position to free the joint and improve mobility.

with myorelaxants. In all cases, movement restriction remained unchanged and was even more easily recognizable during the complete relaxation found with narcosis (13). This suggests that articular factors can play a significant role in this type of pain.

The more difficult question in functional disorders, however, is whether we can separate the muscular and articular factors clinically. In painful conditions, we usually find clear trigger points. In other cases, we often find movement restriction, which may be clinically relevant, with little or no local pain. In such cases, there may be no trigger points in the vicinity of the joint. This is more evident in an extremity joint than in the spinal column. For example, in epicondylar pain there may be restriction due to muscular activity. Restriction of pronation and flexion of the wrist and fingers is evident with extension of the elbow. After relaxation of the supinators, finger and wrist extensors, and biceps, joint play in the elbow may be normal. However, the reverse may also happen: joint play may be impaired, but pronation, flexion of the wrist, and extension of the elbow may be normal.

THE DIFFICULTY IN DIFFERENTIATION

In the majority of cases, we find a combination of both the muscular and articular factors, and we may deal with each. Frequently, when one has been successfully relieved, the other will also improve (14). This is no coincidence since it is a disturbance of function that is involved. Function, however, is not limited to any single structure but implies correlation and interplay between many structures, forming characteristic chains (15). A single structure is but a link in a chain and if its function is impaired, the entire chain is affected. However, one link may be more relevant than others and, by giving treatment to one, we may affect the entire chain. At this stage of ignorance, it is clinical acumen and experience that help us to diagnose—or guess— the relevant link; that is, the most valuable method to date is "trial and error."

There are, however, a few more reasons why a distinction between the muscular, the articular, and even other important factors may be difficult. The first is redundancy of afferents. When McCough et al. (16) severed all involved muscles, they were able to elicit proprioceptive reflexes in the cervical area from the joints only, thus proving the importance of joints as proprioceptive organs. Since then, innumerable patients with artificial hips have their joint afferents removed without any loss of proprioception. Nociception, being even more ubiquitous, will make no exception to this law of redundancy. If function is impaired, all structures involved in dysfunction will indicate this.

There are also other common features involved in nonspecific pain mechanisms, the most important being tension. Dysfunction in the motor system will always create tension: a restricted joint when moved in the restricted direction; a muscular trigger point containing muscle fibers that are shortened and create tension. Increased tension can also occur in the subcutaneous and other connective tissues, particularly the fascia. Obviously, both static and dynamic overloading creates tension, and wherever increased tension arises in the motor system, pain is likely to occur. Tension, as an expression of possible overstrain, may be harmful, eventually resulting in pain, the warning sign of impending danger.

This is closely related to a common barrier phenomenon (17) that was first

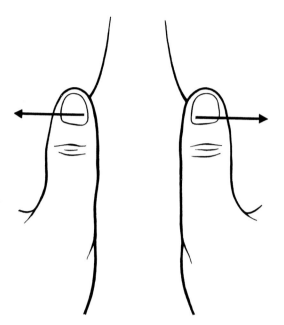

FIG. 3. The common barrier phenomena is exemplified by applying a stretch to a skin area. A barrier is initially met and after a latency period of a few seconds a release takes place.

described in joints. On moving a joint from neutral to end position, there is initially little resistance until we reach a barrier where we gradually meet resistance. This barrier is soft and elastic and can be easily extended under normal conditions. It is the same when we stretch a muscle since we can not do so without moving a joint. Interestingly, the same phenomenon occurs if we stretch the skin or move one layer of soft tissue against another. No resistance occurs at first, until we come to a barrier that can be extended. With myofascial pain this barrier can change: If the range of no resistance is restricted, the barrier becomes abrupt and there is little or no springing. This applies to all tissues or structures involved: the joint, the muscle, and the connective tissues. Even more interestingly, there is a common denominator or mechanism, whether we treat soft tissues, muscular trigger points, or restricted joints. The simplest model, in this case, is soft tissue: we may apply stretch to an area of increased tension on the skin, engage the barrier (take up the slack) and wait, without increasing the force. After a latency of a few seconds, we feel that the resistance gives and a release takes place; this may go on for 10 sec or longer until a new barrier is reached (Fig. 3). The same applies to a skin or connective tissue fold or even to a shortened (tight) muscle (Fig. 4) or scar.

When treating a muscle harboring a trigger point, the patient first gives resistance after the muscle is stretched, then he or she is told to "let go"; after a latency of a few seconds, release takes place and the muscle lengthens by decontraction for 10 sec and even longer. This also happens if we apply

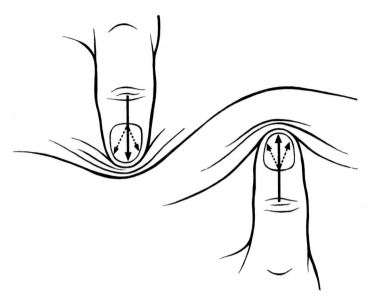

FIG. 4. The common barrier phenomena also applies to a connective tissue fold.

muscle energy techniques to mobilize a restricted joint. In each of these instances, it is essential that the operator senses release taking place so as not to cut it short. Again, whenever we sense release, the tension has been relieved and the pain is usually alleviated.

THE ROLE OF PALPATION AND SOME IMPLICATIONS

Whether it is tension, the barrier phenomenon, or release, we gather knowledge about it through palpation (18). What does palpation imply? Not only does the palpating hand sense diverse qualities such as temperature and moisture; the palpating finger can also move and change its pressure to distinguish one tissue layer from another in order to examine the shape of a structure, its resilience, and its mobility in relation to other structures. By this motion, interaction is created with the patient eliciting changes such as the local twitch response (i.e., snapping a trigger point with resultant contraction of muscle fibers) (3). The reaction of the patient is sensed by the operator and modifies his further examination. A most sophisticated feedback relationship is thus established that can be used for therapy, as we have seen when eliciting the release phenomenon. Palpation can be the most sophisticated form of clinical examination, creating an ideal feedback mechanism between two highly complicated self-regulating systems.

Palpation also gives us a clue to the puzzle of noninflammatory, "non-

Advances in Pain Research and Therapy, Vol. 17,
edited by James R. Fricton and Essam Awad.
Raven Press, Ltd., New York © 1990.

22

Management of Myofascial Pain Syndrome

James R. Fricton

*Department of Diagnostic and Surgical Sciences, University of Minnesota
School of Dentistry, Minneapolis, Minnesota 55455*

Myofascial pain syndromes (MPSs) can range from simple cases with transient single muscle syndromes to complex cases involving multiple muscles and many interrelating contributing factors. Many authors have found success in treatment of MPS using techniques such as exercise, trigger point injections, spray and stretch, transcutaneous electrical nerve stimulation (TENS), and addressing perpetuating factors (1–8). However, the difficulty in management of MPS lies in the critical need to match the level of complexity of the management program with the complexity of the patient. Failure to address the entire problem, including all involved muscles and contributing factors, may lead to failure to resolve the pain and perpetuation of a chronic pain syndrome.

Although there are no controlled studies examining progression of chronic pain syndromes, results from clinical studies reveal that most patients with MPS have seen many clinicians, and received numerous medications and multiple other singular treatment for years without receiving more than temporary improvement. In one study of 164 MPS patients, the mean duration of pain was 5.8 years for males and 6.9 years for females, with a mean of 4.5 past clinicians seen for the pain (9). In another study of 102 consecutive temporomandibular joint (TMJ) and craniofacial pain patients that included 59.8% MPS patients, the mean duration of pain was 6.0 years, with 28.8 previous treatment sessions, 5.1 previous doctors, and 6.4 previous medications (10). These and other studies of chronic pain (11) suggest that regardless of the pathogenesiss of MPS, a major characteristic of these patients is continued pain and the failure of traditional approaches to resolve the problem.

The question arises whether this situation is a result of innate patient characteristics such as poor compliance and psychosocial stressors that would cause any treatment approach to fail, or a result of limited or inappropriate treatment approaches that do not address the whole problem, or that MPS is a chronic untreatable condition. Although the answer may well lie between these extremes and varies with each individual situation, it is the responsibility of each clinician confronted with a patient with MPS to recognize and address the whole problem and maximize the potential for a successful outcome. Treating only those patients with a complexity that matches the treatment strategy available to the clinician can improve success. Simple cases with minimal behavioral and psychosocial involvement can typically be managed by a single clinician. Complex patients should be managed within an interdisciplinary setting that uses a team of clinicians to address different aspects of the problem in a concerted fashion. The purpose of this chapter is to first describe the principles associated with treatment of MPS, including basic concepts of counterstimulation and rehabilitation of muscles and control of contributing factors, and then describe an interdisciplinary team approach to implement this treatment for complex patients.

BASIC CONCEPTS

Once a secure diagnosis of MPS is established, and a full understanding of the person and any contributing factors is achieved, education of the patient and management of the problem can proceed. Evaluation of myofascial pain includes locating the trigger points and muscles involved as well as recognition of all contributing factors. Management of the syndrome naturally follows, including both treating the muscular trigger points and reducing all contributing factors to prevent the trigger points from redeveloping. Treating the muscle includes inactivating the trigger point through repetitive counterstimulation coupled with active and passive muscle stretching and postural rehabilitation (7). The goal is to restore the muscle to normal length, posture, and full joint range of motion. Preventing the redevelopment of a trigger point includes maintaining this exercise program and controlling all contributing factors that initiate the development of trigger points, perpetuate the persistence of trigger points, and result from the chronic pain. In many patients, simply controlling the contributing factors without counterstimulation will improve the condition.

There are many methods suggested for providing repetitive counterstimulation to inactivate trigger points (6,7). Massage, acupressure, and ultrasound provide noninvasive mechanical disruption to inactivate the trigger point. Moist heat applications, ice packs, fluorimethane, and diathermy provide skin and muscle temperature change as a form of counterstimulation. Transcutaneous electrical nerve stimulation, electroacupuncture, and direct current stimulation provide electric currents to stimulate the muscles and trigger points. Acupuncture and trigger point injections of local anesthetic, corticosteroids, saline, or alcohol cause direct mechanical or chemical alteration of trigger points.

TABLE 1. *Treatment planning for myofascial pain syndrome of the head and neck: management of MPS with acute onset with rapid resolution*

Clinical characteristics	Treatment (3 months)
Onset is less than 2 months ago	Fluorimethane spray and stretch (office)
No previous treatment	Home stretching and postural exercises
Defined behavioral factors	
Few trigger points	Control of contributing factors
No other symptoms	Reduce muscle tension habits
Prognosis is excellent	Improve postural habits
	Evaluate for other perpetuating factors

Although counterstimulation can provide short-term relief, the means for achieving long-term pain management is through maintaining a regular muscle stretching and strengthening exercise program as well as long-term control of contributing factors. A home program of muscle stretching exercises will reduce the activity of any remaining trigger points while postural exercises will reduce the susceptibility to reactivation of trigger points by physical strain.

Management of MPSs is a long-term process that is as much under the control of the patient as the clinician. Long-term rehabilitation depends on patient education, and self-responsibility and development of long-term doctor-patient relationships. The difficulty in long-term management often lies not in treating the trigger points, but rather in the complex task of identifying and changing contributing factors, since they can be integrally related to the patient's attitudes, life style, and social and physical environment. Treatment planning should be directed by the complexity of the patient, as noted in Tables 1 through 3.

Interdisciplinary teams have been used to integrate various health professionals in a supportive environment to accomplish both long-term treatment of illness and modification of the contributing factors. Many approaches, such as habit reversal techniques, biofeedback, and stress management have been used to achieve this.

COUNTERSTIMULATION

The two most common techniques of counterstimulation include the spray-and-stretch technique and trigger point injections.

Spray-and-Stretch Technique

With the spray-and-stretch technique, a mild application of a vapocoolant spray, such as Fluorimethane, with simultaneous passive stretching of the

TABLE 2. *Treatment planning for myofascial pain syndrome of the head and neck: management of MPS with recent onset with good response*

Clinical characteristics	Treatment (6 months)
Onset is 1–6 months age Minimal previous treatments Some psychosocial or behavioral factors Various trigger points bilaterally No other symptoms Prognosis is good	Fluorimethane spray and stretch (office and home) Home exercises: jaw, head, neck, and body stretching and posture Stabilization splint Nonsteroidal antiinflammatory drug for 2 weeks (optional)
	Control of contributing factors
	Reduce tension-producing habits Reduce postural habits Behavioral therapy for habit change, relaxation, and pacing skills training if indicated If no continuing success, use physical therapy, trigger point injections, or acupuncture and reevaluate for perpetuating factors

TABLE 3. *Treatment planning for a chronic pain syndrome involving myofascial pain*

Clinical characteristics	Treatment (1 year)
Onset of more than 6 months ago Many previous unsuccessful therapies and medications Many psychological, behavioral, and social factors Many muscles with trigger points Other symptoms may include diminished sensation, dizziness, tinnitus, flushing, joint pathology, migraine Prognosis is guarded for long-term reduction of pain and improvement in function, and is dependent on patient compliance	Physical therapy: mobilization with heat, ultrasound, or other modality Home stretching and postural exercises: jaw, head, neck, and body Stabilization splint Eliminate medications, except short-term antidepressant if there is reactive depression with sleep difficulties; L-tryptophan for sleep disturbance only
	Control of contributing factors
	Reduce bruxism and clenching Improve postural habits Behavioral therapy for dietary and habit change, relaxation, and pacing skills training Consider biofeedback, stress management training, or hypnosis if indicated and desired Education and change of social contributing factors If depression or chemical dependency is present, manage first If no long-term success, consider trigger point injections, reevaluate contributing factors, reevaluate home program, enroll in inpatient chronic pain program

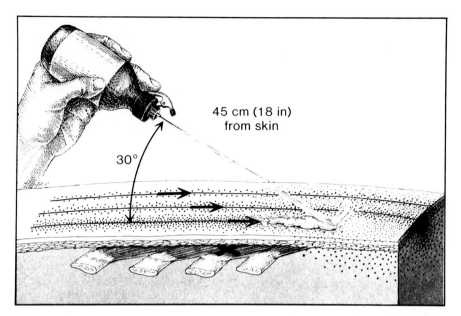

45 cm (18 in) from skin

30°

FIG. 1. Treatment of myofascial pain syndrome using the spray-and-stretch technique involves directing a stream of vapocoolant spray such as fluorimethane on the skin overlying the trigger point and applying it in slow even sweeps toward the zone of reference. The muscle needs to be placed in passive stretch during three or four series of sweeps over the muscle. Warming the muscle between the series of sweeps helps prevent overcooling. (From Travell and Simons, ref. 7, with permission.)

muscle can provide immediate reduction of pain, although lasting relief requires a full managment program. This technique has been described in detail by Travell and Simons (6) and recently studied by Jaeger and Reeves (12). They studied the effect of fluorimethane spray with passive stretch on trigger point sensitivity and referred pain using a pressure algometer and visual analog scales. They found that both the trigger point sensitivity and the referred pain intensity were reduced, suggesting that they are related and can be alleviated with this technique.

The technique involves directing a fine stream of fluorimethane spray from the finely calibrated nozzle toward the skin directly overlying the muscle with the trigger point. A few sweeps of the spray are first passed over the trigger point and zone of reference before adding sufficient manual stretch to the muscle to elicit pain and discomfort. The muscle is put on a progressively increasing passive stretch while the jet stream of spray is directed at an acute angle 30 to 50 cm (1 to 1.5 feet) away (Fig. 1). It is applied in one direction from the trigger point toward its reference zone in slow, even sweeps over adjacent parallel areas at a rate of about 10 cm/sec. This sequence can be repeated up to four times if the clinician warms the muscle with his/her hand or warm moist packs to prevent overcooling after each sequence. Frosting the skin and excessive sweeps should be avoided because it may lower the underlying skeletal muscle temperature, which tends to aggravate trigger points. The range of passive and active motion can be tested before and after spraying as an indication of responsiveness to therapy. Failure to reduce properly identified trigger points with spray and stretch may be due to: (a) inability to secure full muscle length because of bone or joint abnormalities, muscle contracture, or the patient avoiding voluntary relaxation; (b) incorrect spray technique; or (c) failure to reduce perpetuating factors. If spray and stretch fails with repeated trials, direct needling with trigger point injections may be effective.

Trigger Point Injections

Trigger point injections have been shown to reduce pain, increase range of motion, increase exercise tolerance, and increase circulation of muscles (3,4,13–16). The pain relief may last anywhere from the duration of the anesthetic to many months, depending on the chronicity and severity of trigger points, and the success in reducing perpetuating factors. Since a critical factor in needling appears to be the mechanical disruption of the trigger point by the needle and not the injection of the anesthetic, precision in needling of the exact trigger point and the intensity of pain during needling appear to be the major factors in trigger point inactivation (16). However, other mechanisms have also been implicated. In a study of the mechanism of trigger point injections, Fine and colleagues (17) used a double-blind cross-over study to determine if analgesia is reversed with naloxone and, thus, mediated by activation of an endogenous opioid system. The results suggested that naloxone does reverse the short-term analgesic effect of injections compared to placebo and at least, in part, involves this system, but it cannot explain the long-term analgesia usually seen.

Trigger point injections with local anesthetic agents are generally more comfortable than dry needling or injecting other substances, although acupuncture may be helpful for patients with multiple chronic trigger points in multiple muscles. The effect of needling can be complemented with the use of local anesthetics in concentrations less than those required for a nerve conduction block. This can markedly lengthen the relative refractory period of peripheral nerves and limit the maximum frequency of impulse conduction. Local anesthetics can be chosen for their duration, safety, and versatility. Three percent chlorpromazine (short acting) and 5% procaine (medium acting) without vasoconstrictors are suggested. Some clinicians suggest that adding corticosteroids to the local anesthetic will be more effective for inflamed fascial structures such as ligaments and joint capsules.

A number of studies have been completed examining the efficacy and parameters of these injections. Hameroff and associates (3) compared injection of bupivacaine, etidocaine, and saline and found the local anesthetics to be superior to saline. Jaeger and Skootsky (4) compared four conditions (dry needling, injection of saline or procaine, and a placebo skin injection) in a double-blind study of efficacy in changing referred pain and trigger point sensitivity in patients with MPS. They found that reduction in trigger point tenderness was dependent on penetration of the trigger point with a needle and reduction of referred pain was greater with injection of either saline or procaine than dry needling or placebo. Lewit studied the short- and long-term effects of dry needling of MPS trigger points and found immediate improvement in 86.8% of patients and permanent improvement in 29.8% (16). He noted that improvement depended on intensity of the injection and the precision in needling the site of maximal tenderness.

Preparation for the injection technique consists of proper patient selection, education, and consent and, then, positioning of the patient in a comfortable, relaxed position, locating the exact trigger point with palpation, and marking it. Proper aseptic skin preparation is needed. Insertion of the needle requires great care and patience to penetrate the skin quickly for maximum comfort and then insert the needle into the muscle until the precise trigger point in the band of muscle is located with the tip of the needle. The prior use of 5 sec of fluorimethane spray to refrigerate the skin may also be helpful. Movement of the needle in and out of the muscle band, but not the skin, is usually required to locate the trigger point. The "local twitch response," or contraction of the band containing the trigger point, as well as intensification of the dull pain over the muscle or in the zone of reference, will indicate when the trigger point has been "needled." Aspiration and slowly injecting the local anesthetic can follow. Repeating the probing or "peppering" of that area of the muscle band with the needle without removing it will locate any satellite trigger points that may also be causing pain (Figs. 2).

Pain relief should be seen within a few minutes if the pain in the zone of reference is related to the trigger point. After pain relief is achieved, immediate full-range manual stretching of the muscle is accomplished for 1 to 2 min to restore the muscle to normal resting length and determine if other trigger points are present. If present, reducing them can be accomplished with use of spray and stretch over the area or another injection. Shortening activation or a reactive spasm may occasionally occur from unaccustomed gross shortening of an antagonist muscle that contains a trigger point during stretching of the muscle. Stretching both agonist and antagonist muscles with spray and stretch may help prevent this. A mild increase in pain can be observed for 2 to 5 hr after injection, but this subsides within a day or two or with aspirin. Failure to achieve relief longer than the duration of the local anesthetic would indicate failure in locating and "needling" the exact trigger point responsible for the symptoms.

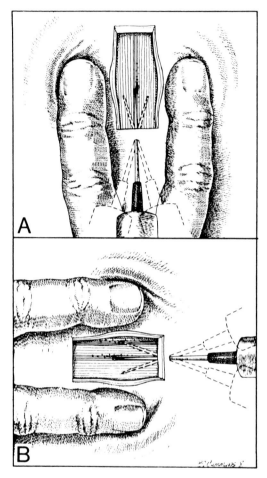

FIG. 2. The technique used with trigger point injections involves repeated probing or "peppering" of the taut band at the trigger point site after injection of a local anesthetic such as 3% chlorpromazine or 5% procaine in the muscle. A local twitch response and intensification of the pain in the zone of reference will indicate when the trigger point has been "needled." Schematic top view of two approaches to the flat injection of a trigger point area in a taut based (*closely spaced black lines*). **A**: Injection away from fingers, which have pinned down the trigger point so it cannot slide away from the needle. *Dotted outline* indicates additional probing to explore for a cluster of trigger points. The fingers are pressing downward and part to maintain pressure for hemostasis. **B**: Injection toward the fingers, with similar finger pressure. Additional trigger points are often found in the immediate vicinity by probing with the needle. (From Travell and Simons, ref. 7, with permission.)

A series of injections may be required in various trigger points to provide long-term relief. Protective splinting can occur with various trigger points in multiple muscles. When one trigger point is obliterated, another asymptomatic trigger point in a complimentary muscle may become symptomatic and refer pain to the same or a new area. The original muscle was shortened as a result of the development of trigger areas, thus protecting the complimentary muscle from being fully stretched and also exhibiting pain. When the original trigger point is reduced, this protective splinting is also reduced because the original muscle is stretched to its normal length. Since inactivation of multiple trigger points in severe cases is a step-by-step process, it is necessary to give multiple injections over a period of weeks to months, at a frequency of about one injection per one or two weeks.

Contraindications to the use of trigger point injections include:

1. Severe acute cases of muscle injury, trauma, or pain.
2. Allergies to the specific anesthetics used.
3. Patient with bleeding difficulties or diathesis, or on anticoagulants.
4. Patient with cellulitis of the area.

Intramuscular infiltration of myofascial trigger points with a diluted local anesthetic containing no vasoconstrictor is a harmless procedure providing proper aseptic technique, aspirating technique, and consideration of anatomy are utilized.

MUSCLE REHABILITATION

The most useful techniques for muscle rehabilitation include muscle stretching, posture, and strengthening exercises. A home program of active and passive muscle stretching exercises will reduce the activity of any remaining trigger points while strengthening exercises will increase muscle conditioning and reduce the muscle's susceptibility to reactivation of trigger points by physical strain. Postural exercises will reduce continuous mechanical strain placed on the involved muscles.

Evaluating the present range of motion of muscles is the first step in prescribing a set of exercises to follow. Range of motion should be determined for the joint involved at initial evaluation. For example, a limited mandibular opening in a patient with MPS will indicate if there are any trigger points within the elevator muscles: temporalis, masseter, and medial pterygoid. If mandibular opening is measured as the interincisal distance, a normal range of opening is generally between 42 and 60 mm, or approximately three knuckles' width (nondominant hand). A mandibular opening with trigger points in the masseter will be approximately between 30 mm and 40 mm, or two knuckles' width (18). If contracture of masticatory muscles is present, the mandibular opening can be as limited as 10 to 20 mm. Other causes of di-

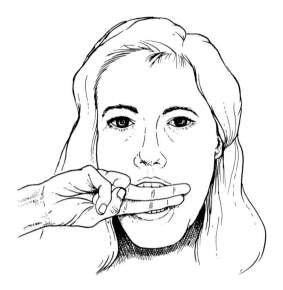

FIG. 3. Jaw stretching exercise. This exercise can be peformed gradually and gently three times daily for 1 min each time with optional simultaneous application of heat or ice. Jaw should be stretched slightly beyond the point of tightness and pain. Patient should avoid overstretching with acutely strained jaws or with acute closed locking from a TMJ internal derangement. (From Fricton J, Kroening R, Hathaway K. *TMJ and craniofacial pain: diagnosis and management.* St. Louis: IEA Publishers, 1988, with permission).

minished mandibular opening include structural disorders of the TMJ, such as ankylosis, internal derangements, and gross osteoarthritis.

Inactivation of the trigger points with passive and active stretching of the muscles will increase the opening to the normal range as well as decrease the pain. Passive stretching of the masticatory muscles during counterstimulation of the trigger point can be accomplished through placing a properly trimmed and sterile cork, tongue blades, or other object between the incisors while the spray and stretch technique is accomplished. Active stretching at home and in the office can be accomplished through exercise, as demonstrated in Fig. 3. It must be emphasized that rapid, jerky stretching of the muscle should be avoided to reduce potential injury to the muscle.

Although the spine has specific characteristics and, thus, differences in treatment from the TMJ, the same general principles can be followed with MPS in the cervical, thoracic, or lumbar region. For example, the range of motion for the neck can be determined by the degree of neck flexion, rotation, and lateral flexion. The normal range of motion for neck flexion is with the chin nearly touching the chest. The normal range of neck rotation should be left and right from the center with the chin pointed directly toward the shoulder. The normal range of motion for lateral neck flexion is with the ear halfway toward the relaxed shoulder. Any perceived tautness or pain of the muscles with a slight decrease in range of motion in these movements is often caused by trigger points. However, cervical osteoarthritis, ankylosis, and other joint problems may also cause limitation. Passive and active stretching of the neck muscles can be accomplished with the exercise shown in Fig. 4. In this exercise, slow movement with avoidance of crepitation is

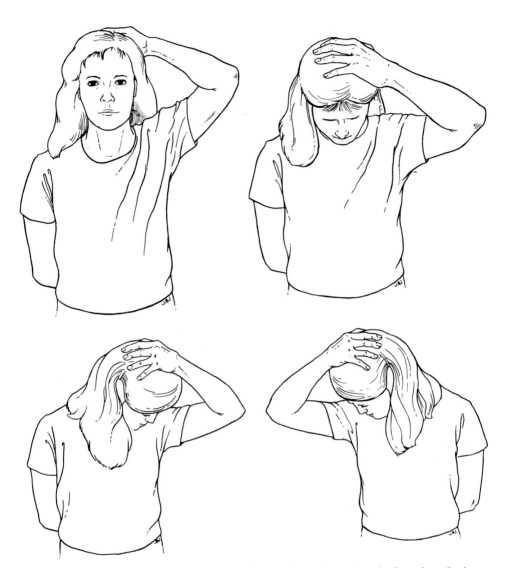

FIG. 4. Neck stretching exercise. This exercise can be performed gradually and gently six times daily for 1 min each time; simultaneous application of heat or ice can be used to reduce pain. Patient should be cautioned to avoid overstretching with an acutely strained neck, severe cervical osteoarthritis with nerve compression, dics disease, or recent surgery in the area. (From Fricton J, Kroening R, Hathaway K. *TMJ and craniofacial pain; Diagnosis and management.* St. Louis: IEA publisher. 1988, with permission.)

eliminating medications, setting a date for resolving litigation or returning to work, or establishing a written mutual agreement to ensure that the patient avoids discussing and pain outside of the clinic and avoids seeing any other health professionals for the pain while being managed within the clinic.

Emotional and behavioral contributing factors play a significant role in indirectly perpetuating muscle disorders through increased anxiety and muscle tension or directly through development of maladaptive habits such as bruxism and clenching. Anxiety and depression can result from chronic pain and make it more difficult to tolerate or manage pain, which may be why a variety of psychological and behavioral approaches are successful in treating MPS. Biofeedback, meditation, hypnosis, stress management, counseling, psychotherapy, antianxiety medications, antidepressants, and even placebos have been reported to be effective in treating myofascial pain (6–8,23–27). Many of these treatments are directed toward reducing muscle tension–producing habits such as bruxism or bracing of muscles. Teaching control of habits is a difficult process because of the relationship that muscle tension may have to psychosocial factors. Simply telling a patient to stop the habits may be helpful with some but with others may result in noncompliance, failure, and frustration. An integrated approach involving education, increased awareness, and other treatments such as behavior modification, biofeedback, hypnosis, or drug therapy may prove to be more successful.

INTERDISCIPLINARY MANAGEMENT

Patients with MPS that becomes chronic may present a frustrating medical situation, which may include persistent aggravation of pain, long-term medications, repeated health care visits, and an ongoing dependency on the health care system. Success is frequently compromised by the chronic nature of the disease and by long-standing maladaptive behaviors, attitudes, and life styles that may result from the illness and actually perpetuate it. Failure to help the patient change these factors often plays a major role in failure to obtain successful long-term management of these disorders.

Our traditional medical system often fails to educate and support the patient in making these changes. Even when these problems in living are recognized by the clinician or the patient, the ability to help deal with factors involved as limited by the nature of dental or medical training, the system in which dentistry or medicine is practiced, and the complex nature of each factor. The past president of the American Congress of Physical Medicine and Rehabilitation, William Fowler, stated, "Schools continue to emphasize diagnostic skills, quick complete cures, and the patient with acute disease as the teaching model for medical students and house staff . . . as a result, clinical management as well as research and teaching regarding chronic disease and rehabilitation tends to take second place and is often done outside the usual academic channels" (28). This may be partially because the practice of health care focuses on evaluation and management of a chronic illness by a single practitioner. It is unrealistic and unwise to expect a single clinician to address the multitude of contributing factors that may be present in a patient with chronic pain. In addition, most treatment of these disorders is singular and varies according to the clinician's favorite theory of etiology. Roydhouse (29) succinctly phrased it (with credit to Lewis Carroll): "Clinicians see what they treat and treat what they see." Clinicians seeing a biochemical etiology treat with medication and clinicians seeing a stress etiology treat with stress management. As a result, success of treatment is often compromised by limited approaches that only address part of the problem.

To improve this situation, evaluation and management systems using a team of clinicians have been developed (11,30–32). Although each clinician may have limited success in managing the "whole" patient alone, the assumption behind a team approach is that it is vital to address different aspects of the problem with different specialists in order to enhance the overall potential for success.

Although these programs provide a broader framework for treating the whole complex patient, they have added another dimension to the skills needed by the clinician: those of working as part of a coordinated team. Failure to adequately integrate care may result in poor communication, fragmented care, distrustful relationships, and eventually confusion and failure in management. However, team coordination can be facilitated by a well-defined evaluation and management system that clearly integrates team members.

A prerequisite to a team approach is an inclusive medical model and conceptual framework that places the physical, behavioral, and psychosocial aspects of illness on an equal and integrated basis (33). With an inclusive theory of human systems and their relationship to illness, a patient can be assessed as a whole person by different clinicians from diverse backgrounds. Although each clinician understands a different part of the patient's problems, s/he can integrate them with other clinicians' perspectives and see how each part is interrelated in the whole patient. For example, a physician or dentist will evaluate the physical diagnosis, a physical therapist will evaluate poor postural habits, and a psychologist will evaluate emotional problems or social stressors. Each factor will become part of the problem list to be addressed in the treatment plan. In the process, the synergism of each factor in the etiology of the disorder can become apparent to clinicians. For example, social stressors can lead to anxiety, anxiety can lead to poor posture and muscle tension, and the poor posture and muscle tension can lead to MPS; the pain then contributes to more anxiety, and a cycle continues. Likewise, a reduction of each factor will work synergistically to improve the whole problem. Treatment of only one factor may improve the problem, but relief may be partial or temporary. Treatment of all factors simultaneously can have a cumulative effect that is greater than the effects of treating each factor individually.

TABLE 4. *Problem list for chronic pain*

Symptoms (chief complaints and associated symptoms)
Physical
Emotional

Diagnosis (physical or psychiatric)
Primary
Secondary

Contributing factors (initiating, perpetuating, resultant)
Biologic
Behavioral
Social
Environmental
Emotional
Cognitive

Source: From Fricton J, Kroening R, Hathaway K. *TMJ and craniofacial pain: diagnosis and management.* St. Louis: IEA Publishers, 1988, with permission.

Applying these concepts requires an interdisciplinary team in an evaluation and management system in which the providers of health care accept responsibility for evaluating and managing the multifaceteds problems that exist. The problem list for a patient with a specific chronic illness includes both a physical diagnosis and a list of contributing factors (Table 4). This broad understanding of the patient is then used in a long-term management program that both treats the physical diagnosis and helps reduce the contributing factors. The purpose of treatment includes four goals: (a) alleviating the symptoms, (b) improving functional capacity, (c) reducing the negative effects of the illness on the patient's life style, and (d) restoring the patient's independence from the health care system. Treatment of the physical problem includes the accepted dental, medical, or physical therapy for that diagnosis. Reduction of contributing factors is accomplished through appropriate behavioral or psychological techniques such as education, behavior modification, biofeedback, family therapy, and exercise. Clinicians must rely on the self-responsibility of the patient for making changes through a home program of self-care (34). This self-care must be facilitated in a supportive environment in which the patient hears the same message from multiple clinicians and gains the sustained insight, support, and care needed to make the changes that both reduce the pain and improve health and independent functioning.

The Team Approach: A Clinical Model

The following discussion describes one example of an outpatient interdisciplinary program that has been implemented in three different settings. The

TABLE 5. *Components of the evaluation and management system*

Team member	Intervention
Physician or dentist	Education, splints, medication adjustment, surgery, team manager
Psychologist or behavioral therapist (Ph.D., M.S., M.S.W.)	Education, stress management, counseling or behavior intervention, family therapy
Physical therapist or other therapists (R.N., P.T., O.T., P.A.)	Education, exercise or diet program, occupational or physical therapy
Patient	Keep appointment, perform home program, follow therapeutic agreement, reduce medication, change habits
Family	Support changes, ignore illness behaviors, follow therapeutic agreement

Source: Ref. 10.

original model was established at the University of Minnesota and subsequently it has been implemented in health maintenance organization (HMO) type and private office health care delivery systems. Despite the differences in the reimbursement mechanism for clinicians and patients in each system, each model has been successful (35). These studies demonstrate that this model is adaptable enough to be successfully implemented in most health care settings with a combination of three clinicians: a physician or dentist, a psychologist, and a physical therapist. Tables 5 and 6 outline the structure and clinical paradigms of the evaluation and management system. Patients in this system undergo three phases: evaluation, management, and follow-up, as diagrammed in the flow chart in Fig. 5.

A patient with a recurring problem presents to the clinic and is examined

TABLE 6. *Shifting doctor or patient paradigms: concepts to follow for patient with chronic TMJ and craniofacial pain*

Concept	Statement
Self-responsibility	You have more influence on your problem than we do.
Self-care	You will need to make daily changes in order to improve your condition.
Education	We can teach you how to make the changes.
Long-term change	It will take at least 6 months for the changes to have an effect.
Strong doctor-patient relationship	We will support you as you make the changes.
Patient motivation	Do you want to make the changes?

Source: From Fricton J. Kroening R, Hathaway K. *TMJ and craniofacial pain: diagnosis and management.* St Louis: IEA Publishers, 1988, with permission.

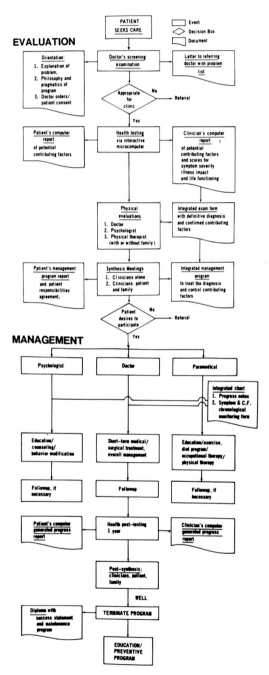

FIG. 5. Patients within this interdisciplinary outpatient pain program undergo three phases: evaluation, management, and follow-up. Evaluation and management include three clinicians, a physical or dentist, a psychologist, and a physical therapist, and take at least 6 months.

by the dentist or physician to determine the physical diagnosis and whether the patient can be helped by the team approach. The clinician explains the diagnosis (if known), what diagnostic tests are necessary, and how the patient can be helped by the team program:

"The symptoms you are experiencing are caused by (*physical diagnosis*). This diagnosis is characterized by (*signs, symptoms, and pathophysiology in lay terms*). As you can see, these characteristics fit your situation closely. However, in addition to the diagnosis, there are other factors such as (*direct contributing factors*) that will lead to (*physical diagnosis*) and need to be considered. These factors will (*put strain on muscles or joints, irritate blood vessels, or nerves*). We need to do (*diagnostic tests or consults*) to confirm the diagnosis and (*IMPATH, Minnesota Multiphasic Personality Inventory, behavioral evaluation*) to evaluate other contributing factors. The treatment program is designed to reduce the (*signs and symptoms*) by treating the (*diagnosis*) and reducing the (*contributing factors*) This is done by teaching you to (*do exercises, change habits*), doing physical therapy to make the muscles and joints more comfortable, and asking you to use a splint or lift to protect and improve the posture of the muscles and joints (*if needed*). In addition, we can help you get back to your normal life style by helping to change (*indirect contributing factors*). Although we can do some things to help you here in the office, most of the work is done by you, at home or work . . . and it does take time. If you do the things necessary, you should expect to feel much better in 6 months. Although you still may have some pain, you usually will notice it less and, if you do, you will learn how to manage it on your own. Does this all make sense to you? What questions do you have? Do you want to participate in such a program?"

If and when the patient desires management, further evaluation can begin with any diagnostic tests or other consultations to confirm the diagnosis, determine health and illness history, establish a contributing factor list, and measure problem severity. This is followed by an evaluation session with each of three clinicians (dentist or physician, psychologist, physical therapist) to assess the characteristics of the problem and establish the patient's unique problem list. The list includes the chief complaints, the corresponding physical diagnoses, and a list of the contributing factors. The evaluation is followed by a synthesis meeting (treatment planning conference), first among the team members and then with the patient and family or significant others to review diagnosis and contributing factors, explain the interrelationships of the factors, assure mutual understanding, and present an integrated management program designed to treat the diagnosis and reduce the contributing factors (Table 7). The purpose of this meeting is to educate the patient and family and to ensure consistent treatment planning and communication among the clinicians, patient, and family. In some situations where compliance and understanding are questionable, a therapeutic agreement should be used to ensure clarity of goals.

The patient then undergoes a long-term individualized management program (with the same team) that integrates long-term patient education and

TABLE 7. *Synthesis meetings (interdisciplinary treatment planning conferences) are designed to enhance communication between the clinicians, patient, and patient's significant others*

Clinician synthesis
1. All clinicians included.
2. Timing: 5 to 20 minutes.
3. Establish problem list and individual patient characteristics.
4. Establish specific goals and priorities of treatment, prognosis, and potential problems.
5. Determine individual clinician responsibilities in management program.

Clinician-patient-family synthesis
1. All clinicians, patient, and significant others, if needed.
2. Timing: 15 to 30 minutes.
3. Dentist or physician reviews diagnoses and their characteristics and how symptoms are caused.
4. Physical therapist reviews related behavioral and postural contributing factors and physical therapy treatment.
5. Psychologist reviews behavioral and psychosocial contributing factors, how they relate to physical diagnoses, and how to change them.
6. Review goals of improving symptoms by treating diagnoses and reducing contributing factors.
7. Each clinician describes his or her role in the overall program.
8. Describe prerequisites to beginning program, guidelines of the program, and pragmatic aspects.
9. Verify patient understanding and desire to proceed.

Source: From Fricton J. Kroening R, Hathaway K. *TMJ and craniofacial pain: diagnosis and management.* St Louis: IEA Publishers, 1988, with permission.

training with short-term traditional medical or dental care. The primary goals of the program include reducing the symptoms and their negative effects while helping the patient return to normal function without need for future health care. The patient first participates in an educational session with each clinician to learn about the diagnoses and contributing factors, why it is necessary to change these factors, and how to do it. The dentist or physician is responsible for establishing the physical diagnosis, providing short-term medical or dental care, and monitoring medication and patient progress. The psychologist or behavioral therapist is responsible for providing instruction about contributing factors; diagnosing, managing, or referring for primary psychological disturbances; and establishing a program to support the patient and family in making changes. The physical therapist is responsible for providing support, instruction, and a management program on specifically assigned and common contributing factors, such as an exercise and posture program. Depending on the therapist's background and the patient's needs, this person may also provide special care such as appliances or occupational therapy. Each clinician is also responsible for establishing a trusting, supporting relationship with the patient while reaffirming the self-care philosophy of the program, reinforcing change, and assuring compliance. The patient is viewed as responsible for making the changes. The team meets weekly to review current patient progress and discuss new patients.

The management program typically involves a sequence of weekly to monthly visits for over 6 months. At the end of the management phase, a brief follow-up synthesis meeting is scheduled with the patient to provide positive reinforcement of progress, terminate the program, and provide goals for maintaining improvement. This is followed by follow-up sessions with one clinician to reinforce the changes every 2 to 3 months. The changes are considered to be temporary unless they are sustained for over a year. If a sustained exacerbation of the problem occurs, the clinician and patient determine why and decide if the team should resume efforts. Reasons for failing to achieve the four goals are many and varied. Assuming the correct physical diagnosis, contributing factors, and treatment plan, two common reasons for lack of symptom reduction are: (*a*) the presence of a diagnosis with pain that is intractable, such as continuous neuralgia, and (*b*) lack of compliance or ability to change a major contributing factor. In these situations, it is important to help prepare the patient for living with the pain, preferably without addictive medications. This can be facilitated by helping the patient achieve the other three goals (reduce effects of pain, improve function, and achieve independence from the health care system) and providing palliative relief with use of a home program of self-care, regular behavioral techniques, home care modalities, or over-the-counter analgesics.

Summary

One of the major factors that leads a patient with a short-term problem into developing a chronic pain syndrome is the lack of adequate recognition and treatment of the whole problem during the first few months of the pain. Thus, in order to prevent development of a chronic pain syndrome, a patient needs to be managed comprehensively from the beginning. Although individual clinicians can do this, the time commitment and training required to provide dental or medical treatment, teach exercises, and address contributing factors by one clinician is often prohibitive, typically less effective, and ultimately frustrating for the solo clinician. However, not all patients with pain require a team approach, since singular treatments such as splints or biofeedback are effective alone. A decision needs to be made at the initial evaluation as to whether there is need for a team or not. Criteria for making this decision include factors such as long duration of pain, overuse of medication, the presence of emotional disturbance, potential for secondary gain, gross confusion, and significant parafunctional habits. The use of a screening instrument such as IMPATH can readily elicit the degree of complexity of a case at initial evaluation (36). The more complex the case the greater the need for a team approach. The decision to use a team must be made at the time of evaluation and not part way through a singular treatment plan that is failing.

REFERENCES

1. Bonica JJ. *JAMA* 1957;164:732–738.
2. Graff-Radford SB, Reeves JL, Jaeger B. *Headache* 1987;27:186–190.
3. Hameroff SR. *Anesth Analg* 1980;60:752–755.
4. Jaeger B, Skootsky SA. *Pain* 1987;4(suppl):560.
5. Melzack R. *Pain* 1975;1:357–373.
6. Travell J. Bonica J, Albe-Fessard D, eds. *Advances in pain research and therapy*, vol 1. New York: Raven Press, 1976;919–926.
7. Travell J, Simons DG. *Myofascial pain and dysfunction: The trigger point manual*. Baltimore: Williams & Wilkins, 1983;63–158.
8. Turner JA, Chapman CR. *Pain* 1982;12:1–12.
9. Fricton J, Kroening R, Haley D. *Oral Surg* 1982;60:615–623.
10. Fricton J, Hathaway K, Bromaghim C. *J Craniomandib Disord Facial, Oral Pain* 1987; 2:00–00.
11. Aronoff G, Evans W, Enders P. *Pain* 1983;16:1–11.
12. Jaeger B, Reeves JL. *Pain* 1986;27:203–210.
13. Cifala JA. *Osteopath Med* 1979;3:31–36.
14. Cooper AL. *Arch Phys Med* 1961;42:704–709.
15. Dorigo B, Bartoli V, Grisillo D, Beconi D. *Pain* 1979;6:183–190.
16. Lewit K. *Pain* 1979;6:83–90.
17. Fine PG, Milano R, Hard BD. *Pain* 1988;32:15–20.
18. Fricton JR. *Neuro Clinics* 1989;7(2):413–427.
19. Glyn JH. *Proc R Soc Med* 1971;64:354–360.
20. Jensen K, Anderson HO, Oleson J, Lindblom U. *Pain* 1986;25:313–323.
21. Travell J, Rinzler SH. *Postgrad Med* 1952;11:425–434.
22. Fricton J. Paper presented at American Congress of Rehabilitation Medicine, October.
23. Bell WH. *J Am Dent Assoc* 1969;79:161–170.
24. Clarke NG, Kardachi BJ. *J Periodontol* 1977;48:643–645.
25. Gessel AH. *J Am Dent Assoc* 1975;91:1048–1052.
26. Moldofsky H, Scarisbrick P, England R, Smythe H. *Psychosom Med* 1975;37:341–351.
27. Rodin J. In: Karoly P, Kanfer FH, eds. *Self management and behavioral change: From theory to practice*. New York: Pergamon Press, 1974.
28. Fowler WM Jr. *Arch Phys Med Rehabil* 1982;62:1–5.
29. Roydhouse RH. In: Sessle BJ, Hannam AG, eds. *Mastication and swallowing, biological and clinical correlates*. Toronto: University of Toronto Press, 1976;83–95.
30. Ng LK, Lorenz K, *New approaches to treatment of chronic pain: A review of multidisciplinary pain clinics and pain centers*. NIDA Research Monograph Series, no 36. Washington, DC: US Government Printing Office, 1981.
31. Rothberg JS. *Arch Phys Med Rehab* 1981;62:407–410.
32. Stieg RL, Williams RC, Gallagher LA. *J Occup Med* 1981;23:94–102.
33. Schneider F, Kraly P. *Clin Psychol Rev* 1983;3:61–86.
34. Bandura A. *Psychol Rev* 1977;84:191–215.
35. Nelson A, Fricton J. *Report to Group Health, Inc., of the implementation of an outpatient pain clinic*. Minneapolis: University of Minnesota.
36. Fricton J, Nelson A, Monsein M. *J Cranio* 1987;5:372–381.

Subject Index